COMMUNICATION DISORDERS in INFANTS and TODDLERS:
Assessment and Intervention

COMMUNICATION DISORDERS in INFANTS and TODDLERS:
Assessment and Intervention

Frances P. Billeaud, MA, CCC-SLP, FASHA

Associate Professor of Communicative Disorders and
Director of Clinical Activities (ret.),
Department of Communicative Disorders
University of Louisiana at Lafayette
Lafayette, Louisiana

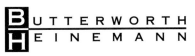

BUTTERWORTH
HEINEMANN

An Imprint of Elsevier Science

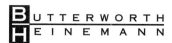

An Imprint of Elsevier Science

11830 Westline Industrial Drive
St. Louis, Missouri 63146

NOTICE

Speech therapy is an ever-changing field. Standard safety precautions must be followed, but as
new research and clinical experience broaden our knowledge, changes in treatment and drug
therapy may become necessary or appropriate. Readers are advised to check the most current
product information provided by the manufacturer of each drug to be administered to verify the
recommended dose, the method and duration of administration, and contraindications. It is the
responsibility of the licensed prescriber, relying on experience and knowledge of the patient, to
determine dosages and the best treatment for each individual patient. Neither the publisher nor
the editor assumes any liability for any injury and/or damage to persons or property arising
from this publication.

Previous editions copyrighted 1993, 1998

International Standard Book Number 0-7506-7421-0

Acquisitions Editor: Kellie White
Developmental Editor: Jennifer Watrous
Publishing Services Manager: Linda McKinley
Project Manager: Rich Barber
Designer: Julia Dummitt

Printed in the United States

Last digit is the print number: 9 8 7 6 5 4 3 2 1

Contributors

Shalini Arehole, PhD, CCC-A
Associate Professor of Audiology
Department of Communicative Disorders
University of Louisiana at Lafayette
Lafayette, Louisiana

Frances P. Billeaud, MA, CCC-SLP, FASHA
Associate Professor of Communicative Disorders and Director of Clinical
Activities (ret.), Department of Communicative Disorders
University of Louisiana at Lafayette
Lafayette, Louisiana

Donna B. Broussard, MEd
Early Interventionist and Family Services Coordinator
University Medical Center
Lafayette, Louisiana
Louisiana State University School of Allied Health
Baton Rouge, Louisiana

Thomas G. Rigo, PhD
Associate Professor of Audiology
Arizona School of Health Sciences
Mesa, Arizona

Suzanne G. Thurmon, MS, CCC-SLP
Former Director
Acadiana Early Intervention Program
Lafayette, Louisiana

Theodore F. Thurmon, MD
Professor of Pediatrics
Louisiana State University School of Medicine
Shreveport, Louisiana

▼

This work is dedicated to all of the children and families who have taught us all so much about communication development and the obstacles many young children and their families have to overcome when developmental problems arise. We also dedicate the book to our own families who have allowed us the time to join together as a team of professionals to produce it. Our hope is that our fellow professionals who use the book will find it a helpful resource as they provide services to their young patients and their concerned families in the future.

▲

Preface

The last month of the year 1999 marked the end of the twentieth century and the not-quite-term delivery of the author's youngest grandchild. His infancy and toddlerhood were marked by a number of complications that contributed to delayed onset of speech. Our family's experiences personalized and deepened appreciation for the concerns and experiences of all families whose tiniest members are at risk for developmental delays and disorders. Although my professional knowledge helped in analyzing the day-to-day issues our family confronted and provided significant guidance in selecting management options, it contributed very little to alleviating the psychological and emotional reactions to the unexpected and repeated crises that arose as the baby battled sleep apnea, hypoxia, and frequent medical treatments. It did nothing to mitigate the worries of the parents as they rotated duty during the baby's hospital stays. Happily, the health issues of our grandson have been resolved; his language system appears to be intact. Although his speech continues to be delayed at this writing, he is acquiring new words on a regular basis, and the prognosis for developing normal communication abilities is good.

In the face of a somewhat complex medical history, why is there concern for acquisition of communication skills? Communication is the most complex of all human endeavors. *Communicative competence is the basic academic skill*—a fact so fundamental that it is seldom stated so bluntly. Similarly, the fact that air is necessary to sustain life is assumed to universal knowledge and, therefore, not necessary to reiterate. The dramatic consequence of depriving an individual of air, however, draws immediate attention to itself and is attended to with heroic measures. In contrast, disorders of communicative development in young children are often overlooked—even by people who know there is (or suspect there may be) a problem. Despite the fact that delayed or disordered communication deprives the child of typical experiences during the period of optimal brain development, the urgency to provide early intervention for atypical preverbal and early symbolic communicative development has only recently become an area of concern. Perhaps it is the very complexity of the processes involved in developing communication competence that mitigates against actions that might be taken early on to address atypical communicative development.

Development of communicative competence begins before birth and is pivotal to cognitive, psychoemotional, behavioral, and social development. The ability to comprehend the communication of others (receptive ability), to process one's own emotions and ideas and code the message one wishes to convey (mapping), and to convey that information to a communicative partner (expressive ability) is communicative competence. Communication is achieved through a variety of means: gestures and body language, symbolic representation (e.g., the language system of the child's family), written symbols, and other symbolic representations (e.g. musical scores and mathematical formulas).

The earliest interactions between mother and infant set the stage for a child's linguistic and communicative development. Most babies begin using words meaningfully by the end of the first year of life, and rapidly build a repertoire of spoken words—and an even larger repertoire of words that they understand. During the first 3 years of life, most children master the essentials of oral language: basic phonology, semantics, morphology, syntax, and pragmatics. By age 3, children are usually quite adept at relating their feelings and experiences and in conversing with others. By the third year of life, we expect the typically developing child to be reasonably intelligible to most listeners.

The development of communicative competence is dependent on a range of basic factors, all of which interact with and have the capacity to influence each of the other factors. Between 6% and 10% of infants born each year fail to follow the typical course of language development as a result of some disturbance in the synergistic relationships among the basic elements that promote developmental processes. At any given time in the United States, there are 630,000 to 1,050,000 infants and toddlers in the birth-to-36-month age group who are experiencing significant problems with communicative development. Those problems in turn affect their social, emotional, behavioral, and pre-academic abilities.

Atypical communicative development may be associated with a wide range of causes and perpetuating factors, the nature, seriousness, and timing of which affect the prognosis for a favorable outcome. Sometimes the communicative problem stands as the sole area of a child's developmental difficulty; sometimes the communicative problem is only one aspect of a complex of problems that affect physical growth, cognitive and motor functions, and other areas of development.

A great deal of research across a range of professional disciplines has been generated in the area of communicative development and disorders in recent years. Since publication of the second edition of this work, extensive information bearing on communicative development has emerged from the Human Genome Project, from medical and social sciences research, and from clinical activities in the area of early intervention. This interdisciplinary knowledge base has improved our ability to predict which risk factors are associated with atypical communicative development and to identify, assess, diagnose, and manage communicative problems in the infant-toddler population. Significant progress has been made in technology and pharmacology for sustaining the lives of smaller and smaller premature babies and infants born with a variety of medical conditions and sensory impairments. Knowledge of management techniques for infants in the preverbal stages of development and those who are experiencing an array of perplexing delays and disorders has mushroomed. Simultaneously, many changes have occurred in the arena of health care delivery systems, with managed care emerging as a "megaforce" that affects all areas of professional activities for communicative disorders specialists and their colleagues in related professions: pediatrics, social work, nursing, occupational therapy, physical therapy, psychology, early childhood education, and medical subspecialties that deal with infant-toddler health and development.

This book is intended for communicative disorders specialists (and colleagues in related professions) who are interested in serving the youngest group within the pediatric population. It is meant to be a clinical reference tool for professionals and a guide to practical resources applicable to working with children who are diagnosed with or at risk for communicative delays or impairments. Because a great deal of the work done in this arena involves interacting effectively with families and peer professionals in related fields, an effort has been made to provide information about the processes of teaming, referral, collaboration, and communicating efficiently and effectively with others in the face of demands placed on the system of care by forces of fluctuating public policy and of managed care. It may also serve as a resource for preservice training programs in their endeavor to address the needs of the communicatively impaired across the life span. It is also appropriate for consideration as a text for a graduate course in serving the needs of infants and toddlers with disabilities and their families.

This edition of *Communication Disorders in Infants and Toddlers: Assessment and Intervention* supplements the content of previous editions with new information throughout. Two new sections have been added—a chapter of autistic spectrum disorder (ASD) in infants and toddlers and an appendix focusing on Internet resources, which both professionals and families will find helpful. An effort has been made to distill and synthesize findings and information reported in the research literature from a variety of professional disciplines. Although a volume of this scope can only sample such studies, references are provided for further study. A handy reference section for contacting pertinent organizations and suppliers of materials and equipment is also included.

A special note of appreciation goes to the contributing authors: pediatrician and medical geneticist Theodore F. Thurmon, MD; Suzanne G. Thurmon, MS, CCC-SLP, former director of one of the first early intervention centers in the country; Donna B. Broussard, MEd, infant-toddler coordinator servicing three private and public hospitals and a member of the staff of the LSU School of Allied Health Professions; and audiologists Thomas G. Rigo, PhD of the Arizona School of Health Sciences, and Shalini Arehole, PhD of the University of Louisiana at Lafayette. My thanks are also extended to all of the individuals and groups that have contributed so generously of their time and have shared their expertise to make this new edition a reality. It is our sincere collective hope that readers will find this work to be a useful tool in their dedication to the families and babies in need of special care and understanding. Their welfare is our common bond.

Frances P. Billeaud
Lafayette, Louisiana
2002

Contents

1   Communication Impairment in Infants and Toddlers: A Frame of Reference, 1
Frances P. Billeaud

2   Causes of Developmental Delays and Disorders in Infants and Toddlers: Implications for Communication Competence, 31
Frances P. Billeaud

3   Selected Medical Aspects of Communication Disorders, 49
Theodore F. Thurmon and Suzanne G. Thurmon

4   The Early Intervention Team: Giving and Getting the Right Kind of Help, 69
Frances P. Billeaud

5   The Role of the Speech-Language Pathologist in the Neonatal Intensive Care Unit: Preemies, Micropreemies, and Medically Fragile Infants, 83
Frances P. Billeaud and Donna B. Broussard

6   Identification and Assessment of Hearing-Impaired Infants and Toddlers, 101
Thomas G. Rigo and Shalini Arehole

7   Autistic Spectrum Disorder: Special Considerations in Assessment and Intervention with Infants and Toddlers, 121
Frances P. Billeaud

8   Assessment: Examination, Interpretation, and Reporting, 141
Frances P. Billeaud

9   Optimizing Communication Development: Treatment, Management, Intervention, 173
Frances P. Billeaud

10   Habilitation and Communication Development in Hearing-Impaired Infants and Toddlers, 201
Thomas G. Rigo

11   Marketing What We Have to Offer: Why? How?, 221
Frances P. Billeaud

Appendix A   Normal Development and Infant Assessment Tools,   229

Appendix B   Assessment and Intervention Tools and Procedures,   249

Appendix C   Administrative References,   267

Appendix D   Internet Resources for Professionals and Families,   275

Glossary,   285

COMMUNICATION DISORDERS in INFANTS and TODDLERS:
Assessment and Intervention

CHAPTER 1

COMMUNICATION IMPAIRMENT IN INFANTS AND TODDLERS

A Frame of Reference

Frances P. Billeaud

This book is about people and their relationships. It is about parents and families whose babies are different. It is also about men and women who come into the lives of these families because of their children's atypical development.

This book is packed with data about conditions that result in communication disorders and about the system of care available to affected children and their families. There is information about treatment and intervention strategies, research, and technology. Mere possession of knowledge and technical expertise, however, is not enough. Ultimately, the professional's knowledge, skills, and competencies are only effective to the extent they are applied for the benefit of individual children and their families in specific circumstances.

This book is about challenges and hopes. It is also about facts that are hard to hear and hard to deliver. It is about interactions with professional peers, babies, and families. It is about real people like those whose stories follow.

CASE STUDY 1-1

Ellen

"There's something wrong with my child," Ellen's mother told the pediatrician. She was assured that her fear was unfounded. As the mother of 3-month-old Ellen, Ann was told that she was expecting too much too soon of her beautiful little daughter. Ellen's constant crying and infrequent periods of sleep were ascribed to "just a little colic," possibly complicated by transmission of her mother's anxieties during caregiving activities. The pediatrician assured Ann that once Ann herself could get a little more sleep and relax and enjoy the baby, Ellen would settle down too. Over the next several months, the doctor reassured Ann that everything was normal, despite Ann's repeated assertions that something was wrong. The doctor pointed to the child's continued weight gain, her normal head circumference, blood-test results, and other physical evidence that Ellen met expectations for development.

By the time Ellen was 15 months old, she was still not sleeping well. She had frequent bouts with ear infections. She frequently cried for hours at a time. Although she was sitting up, she tended to wobble. She was not walking, and she did not talk. She drooled constantly. Ann was exhausted. She was also frustrated; it seemed that no one would take her fears about Ellen's development seriously. Ann's husband Roger was concerned too, but his business had not been going well, and he was spending all of his time trying to avoid losing it. In desperation, Ann begged the doctor to refer Ellen to a pediatric neurologist in a nearby town. He agreed that it was time to look into Ellen's problems with walking and talking. Six weeks later (the earliest appointment that could be arranged) Ann drove the 80 miles to keep Ellen's 10:00 AM appointment with the neurologist. By noon, Ann had the diagnosis: Ellen had cerebral palsy.

CASE STUDY 1-2

David

David, at 36 months of age, was an active little fellow who loved playing with his collection of toy trucks. He was a bit of a picky eater, but his mother found it easy to please him with the few foods he enjoyed eating—pizza, French fries, and fish sticks. He was not impressed when his baby sister arrived. The family was pleased that the new baby did not have the feeding problems David had in the early months: David was hospitalized once because he became so dehydrated. After the mother's difficult delivery with David, it seemed ages before he was finally healthy. However, once he was able to keep food down, he grew and developed. David's father, Henry, was in his final year of medical school. It was fortunate that David's early medical problems received prompt attention thanks to Henry's connections at the teaching hospital. It was also fortunate that the family's finances allowed Victoria, David's mother, to be at home with the children on a full-time basis.

Victoria quizzed Henry about why David's speech was so slow in developing. He was saying three or four words, but he did not use them often. When he used them, they were very hard to understand; sometimes his few words were not even pronounced the same way from one utterance to the next. Henry arranged to have David's hearing tested at the hospital. The results indicated no problem, ruling out the most likely cause of the scant speech development. Victoria knew there was some logical explanation and urged Henry to check the resources in the medical library. He did not find any leads there, but he promised to keep trying, even though he knew his schedule did not allow much time for personal research.

It was obvious to everyone in the family that David was intelligent. He was adept at constructing elaborate structures with his blocks. He seemed to understand everything that was said to him. He was intrigued with his grandfather's farm equipment and had learned to identify many different types of trucks and farm implements, easily choosing the right one from the array of pictures in his favorite book when asked to do so.

It was true that David's attention span was brief, but he seemed interested in so many different things, and he *was* able to sit down with his dad to look at books for 15 to

20 minutes when Henry had time to play with his son. David especially liked sitting in Henry's lap, supported snugly against his dad's warm chest and surrounded by his big arms as they looked at pictures of combines, reapers, dump trucks, and highway tankers. Henry was especially proud that David liked this particular activity, because David usually rebuffed his parents' and grandparents' attempts to offer affectionate little pats and strokes.

Victoria finally convinced Henry that a speech-language pathologist (SLP) might be able to tell them something they could do to help David talk more. An SLP from the nearby university, a friend of the SLP at the hospital, agreed to go to the house to see David in surroundings that were familiar to him, where he had access to his toys. The SLP found David to be quite active, just as his mother had described when the appointment had been set up by phone. He was cooperative, bringing requested items to the SLP for inspection, opening his mouth willingly to allow a view of the oral mechanism, and offering the visitor a cookie before drinking apple juice from his covered cup. The SLP noticed that the sipping flange of the plastic cup had obviously been chewed. Victoria explained that David seemed to need to "bite down on the cup" to swallow liquids. She guessed it was the result of taking his bottle away before the baby came. When Victoria tried to give him juice from an open-top cup or tumbler, he "always got too much at one time" and choked. Victoria added that he also liked to "suck on his food," often discarding portions of it, such as toppings other than cheese on the pizza.

After observing David in several activities, the SLP asked Victoria to take David to the university's speech and hearing clinic for further evaluation. The SLP disclosed that she suspected the child had oral-motor coordination problems that could be directly related to his difficulty in producing speech. That diagnosis was subsequently confirmed. David now continues to receive speech therapy from a private practitioner in the city where his father is the newest member of the medical community.

CASE STUDY 1-3

Kent

Kent's mother and father describe him as "all boy." He is the younger of two children born to Courtney and Michael. Kent's sister is 3 years older and is in first grade. Michael is an engineer. Courtney quit her job when Kent was born to become a full-time mom. She would like to return to work, at least part time, now that Kent is 3 years old, but she has been unable to locate a daycare center willing to take him. He is unusually handsome and loves playing outdoors. He is not yet fully toilet trained and does not talk much. Courtney worries about his speech, because the times he has spoken have been few and far between. Words she has heard him use seem to have disappeared, almost as if "he said them once and then lost interest in doing it again." His sister's friends have begun asking questions about why Kent doesn't talk and why he "acts funny." She just laughs and responds, "That's just how boys are." But she knows there must be something else and wonders why Kent doesn't play with her or use his toys "the right way."

Courtney describes Kent as affectionate "when he wants to be," checking frequently to be sure she is nearby, but not responsive to her cuddling, which his sister loved when she was his age. Kent seems unable to concentrate on most things but is "able to totally immerse himself in a cartoon or action show on TV." His mother and father agree that he is "the most stubborn child" they know when he does not want to do something, even when it is something as simple as getting dressed in the morning or turning off the TV set.

Michael and Courtney know that they have to watch carefully what Kent eats because he has allergies to many cereal grains. Foods that contain even small amounts of corn sweetener or many other cereal products cause him to have stomachaches and set off extreme hyperactivity, sometimes lasting far into the night and requiring one parent or the other to remain awake to prevent the child from going outside "to run off his energy."

Because Kent does not always respond to requests or comply with directions, Michael and Courtney fear that the child will be viewed as "retarded." They point out that he is quite intelligent "in his own way." They are aware that his lack of social interaction and speech will cause problems in school when the time comes, and they would like to enroll him in a program for children with delayed onset of speech. However, when they visited the program, they were alarmed to see that some of the children had strange behaviors. The other children did not seem to pay much attention to each other or their surroundings, and Kent's parents were afraid Kent might pick up "some bad habits" by watching them. The teacher told them that Kent would have to be tested to be sure that he was eligible for enrollment in the program. They were sure that Kent "could not cooperate" well enough to be tested and feared that he might be "labeled" if they gave their permission to try. They were emotionally torn and frustrated by the seemingly limited avenues open to them.

CASE STUDY 1-4

Cedric

Ruby's teenage daughter ran away from home only 2 weeks after giving birth to Cedric, a full-term, healthy, beautiful little boy. Cedric is 4 years old, and Ruby is the only mother he has ever known. She is proud of Cedric. On the days Ruby works, he stays with a neighbor who cares for two other children in her home. The sitter brags that Cedric is the best child she has ever looked after. He is polite and bright, helping his grandmother with household chores, keeping his room neat, and even helping the sitter care for the two younger children when he is there. Although Cedric is eligible to attend Head Start, Ruby feels that he will have plenty of time to "be in school" and prefers having him in a child care setting with which she is familiar. Ruby's one concern is that Cedric has never talked. He does communicate, however, in a very lively way. His eyes dance when he is excited, his facial expressions are captivating, and he has an extensive repertoire of gestures that help him get his points across. It is almost as if he does not really need to talk.

When Ruby took Cedric to the university speech and hearing clinic, she did so only because the babysitter suggested that it would be a good idea to "have him checked out before school starts." As a standard part of the communication evaluation, a hearing test was administered. The audiologist, who suspected that the child probably had a hearing loss, was startled to find that Cedric had a profound bilateral sensorineural hearing loss. When Ruby was told of this, she vehemently denied that it could be true. She insisted on "showing" the staff how well Cedric could hear. Because she was so agitated, the staff agreed to let her demonstrate her point and watched through a one-way mirror as she gave Cedric directions (which he followed with ease), made requests of him (with which he readily complied), and responded to his spontaneous and elaborate nonverbal communication efforts.

Satisfied that she had proven to the staff that Cedric could, indeed, hear despite what the "machines" said, Ruby emerged from the observation room all smiles. When she was asked to allow an examiner to go into the room with Cedric while she watched and listened from the other side of the one-way mirror, she readily agreed. Once again, Cedric responded to the adult's bids for communicative interaction. However, when the examiner turned her back on Cedric and made requests, he continued playing with the toys without responding. Ruby was embarrassed that Cedric was being uncharacteristically "rude" to the examiner. When it was pointed out that Cedric could not see her face when she spoke, Ruby insisted that it ought not to make a difference. The staff member sitting with Ruby offered to let her use the intercom microphone to communicate with Cedric. She accepted the offer and began giving specific directions to the child: Cedric did not respond at all. She attempted several times to get his attention but could not. When the examiner in the room with him stated that she thought Cedric was an exceptional speechreader but did not hear what she was saying, Ruby dissolved in tears, acknowledging Cedric's hearing impairment for the first time.

CASE STUDY 1-5

Bitsy

She was nicknamed Bitsy because her real name—Elizabeth—seemed far too big for the tiny premature child lying in the neonatal intensive care unit (NICU). She would be going home in a few days if everything continued to go well. The NICU was the only home she had known since her birth 2 months ago. Although she weighed less than 4 lb at birth, the main worry was her cleft palate and cleft lip, which interfered with her ability to get sufficient nutrition when she was strong enough to be taken off nasogastric feedings. The nurses said she had to be watched carefully because she sometimes forgot to breathe. Bitsy's mom, Karen, had learned a lot from the nurses about caring for her, and she felt fairly comfortable feeding her with them nearby to help in case anything went wrong. Bitsy's head had to be supported while she was positioned upright during feedings so that she would not choke. A special bottle and nipple had to be used because her sucking was not normal. After the surgeries to close Bitsy's lip and palate, the nurses said she would do much better with her feedings. Karen was excited about taking Bitsy home to her new room with the ruffled curtains and freshly painted bassinet, but she was also scared. There was so much to do just to take care of Bitsy. Karen caught herself daydreaming about Bitsy's future: How would she sound when she started to talk? Would other people be able to understand her? Would she have a scar on her face that would cause her embarrassment, especially when she reached her teenage years? Karen had only known one other person who was born with a cleft lip and palate, her mother's older cousin, and her speech was very nasal. Who could help her teach Bitsy how to talk so that she didn't have that kind of speech? Karen was stirred from her daydreaming when Bitsy coughed.

CASE STUDY 1-6

Brendan

Brendan was born into an upper middle class family within a year of his older sister's arrival. Both parents are college-educated, and both are employed in fast-paced, demanding jobs. Fortunately Brendan's mother was able to take a 6-week maternity leave after his birth. Brendan's sister Ann was already enrolled in a day care center, where she seemed well-adjusted to the routines and personnel. From the beginning, Ann loved her baby brother.

Brendan had had a series of problems from the outset. His mother was able to add another 3 weeks to her maternity leave in order to be with him through the most difficult period. His problems included hypoxia at delivery (which had been induced), sleep apnea that lasted throughout his first year of life, repeated ear infections, and environmental allergies. Although he had excellent medical care, his growth pattern placed him somewhat below the norms for height and weight at age 24 months, and his speech and expressive language skills were significantly delayed. Brendan's receptive language seemed age-appropriate, but his play skills were below expectations for his age. He pointed at objects and engaged adults and other children in looking at objects of interest to him. However, if an object was given to him, he simply carried it around until he lost interest in doing so.

In contrast to Ann's rapidly developing communication skills, Brendan did not seem interested in experimenting with the sounds or intonation patterns he heard at home or at the child care center. Because he was clever in making his needs known by pointing, grunting, or getting what he wanted by himself if it were within reach, his parents were not concerned with his delays in saying words. As yet, he had not combined any words in phrases or sentences and was actually using only about 10 words consistently. Except for three or four of those, they were not clearly understood by anyone outside of the family. Most of the words he said began with [b]; vowels were inconsistent, and no final consonants were present.

Brendan was considered the opposite of his vivacious and precocious sister, who talked and sang and asked questions most of her waking hours. The little boy, on the other hand, was quiet, compliant, observant, and "laid-back." He did, however, protest loudly when his sister or a little friend took a toy he was holding. He seemed to prefer the company of familiar adults to that of his peers.

He loved being outside, climbing, sliding, and being in the water. Because he was so quiet, he had to be watched carefully lest he jump into the swimming pool or climb too high on play equipment designed for much older children. His parents regarded him proudly as "all boy." They often commented that because he *was* a boy, they accepted his communication delays as being characteristic of (a) boys, (b) being the younger of two children close in age, (c) his sister's tendency to speak for him, and (d) the family's busy and noisy lifestyle, which didn't allow him much time to do any talking. They made it a habit to read to him daily. He loved this activity and would bring book after book to them. He delighted in pointing to the pictures as the stories progressed.

When an evaluation was suggested by a close friend of the family, Brendan's parents were not enthusiastic. Although he had had repeated ear infections—and probable temporary conductive hearing losses as a result—his parents pointed out that he had always had prompt medical care when his ears bothered him and that he seemed to hear "just fine." They obviously loved and cared for their beautiful and affectionate little boy and were confident that he would soon "catch up" in developing his communication skills. After all, they'd been reassured by his pediatrician that he was in good health, well-coordinated, and had no apparent hearing or cognitive problems. *"Let's wait until he's 3—if he's still behind in talking, we'll do something about it then,"* is what Brendan's parents had decided to do.

▼ FAMILIES AS STATISTICS IN THE EPIDEMIOLOGICAL DATABASE

Ellen, David, Kent, Cedric, Bitsy, and Brendan are parts of an epidemiological database; however, first and foremost they are children with caring families whose concern for their welfare is obvious. Some of these families learned of their child's communication problems early, and others learned later. Some had to deal with other, sometimes life-threatening, issues before turning their attention to the communication difficulties. In each case, the impact of the child's communication disorder is far reaching and affects the entire family unit. The hopes, dreams, and expectations of the families of these children have been altered in significant ways by the existence of the child's communicative difficulties.

Statistical Overview

Accurate statistical data on the number of children affected by communicative disorders in this country are difficult to obtain for many reasons. The primary reason is the variability in categories of reporting used by different governmental agencies and by different professional groups that view the population from different perspectives. As the Assistant Secretary for Planning and Evaluation of the U.S. Department of Health and Human Services pointed out,[1] "Few data sources exist on children with disabilities, and estimates vary by how disability is defined. In December 1992, 548,700 children under 18 received SSI (Supplementary Social Security Income), which provides cash assistance to certain low-income children with disabilities" (p. 1). By way of contrast, the U.S. Department of Education[2] reported that a total of 3,507,488 children in the 6- to 21-year age group received special education services in categories of disability usually served by communicative disorders specialists (i.e., hearing impairment, speech-language impairment, multiple disabilities, and specific learning disabilities). On the other hand, agencies that track prevalence and incidence figures relevant to public health often use categories related to childhood chronic illness and use different criteria to define disability or impairment of function resulting from those categories. Newacheck and Taylor[3] (p. 364) summarized methodological problems in identifying affected populations, which are spawned by the definitional variations and frustrate the effort to arrive at reliable figures:

> *Partly because common definitional criteria are lacking, the research community has generated widely differing estimates of the prevalence of childhood chronic conditions. Additional variation results from the different methods used in collecting prevalence data [studies based on population, clinical studies, parental reports, medical records review, types of conditions reported]. As a result of these different methods, published estimates of the proportion of children with one or more chronic illnesses range from less than 5% to more than 30%.*

To complicate the issue, the term *disability* is defined differently by policy makers in dealing with issues of education and those dealing in issues of health. The 1992 National Health Interview Survey, conducted by the Census Bureau for the National Center for Health Statistics, used a household survey to survey the noninstitutionalized U.S. population. In that study, *disability* was broadly defined to include "any limitation in activity due to a chronic health condition or impairment."[4] For children under 5 years of age, whose ability to engage in play was used as the gauge of disability, 2% were reported to have been so affected. The criterion for disability in this study changed (from ability to engage in play to ability to attend school) for children between 5 and 17 years of age, making comparisons among age groups difficult at best. Some social service and health tracking systems define disability in terms of a condition or set of conditions that interfere with activities of daily living.

The 1991-1992 Survey of Income and Program Participation collected information about chronic conditions, including functional limitations related to those conditions, using the extended International Classification of Impairments, Disabilities, and Handicaps that encompasses the personal and social consequences of diseases. "For children aged 0 to 5 years, disability was defined as (1) limitation in the usual kind of activities done by most children the same age or (2) receipt of therapy or diagnostic services by the child for developmental needs. For children over 6 years, disability was any limitation in the ability to do regular school work"[5] (p. 1).

According to Wenger and colleagues,[4] 5 million conditions cause disabilities among 4 million children, an average of 1.2 conditions per child. The fifth most common group of disabling conditions among children in the National Health Interview Survey was "speech impairments," which affect 335,000 or 6.7% of children under 18 years of age. Statistics cited in this survey for other groups often served by communicative disorders specialists included an additional 190,000 (3.8%) children under 18 years of age with hearing impairments, 167,000 (3.4%) with learning disabilities, 108,000 (2.2%) with congenital anomalies, and 99,000 (2%) with cerebral palsy.

Diagnostic Classifications

To further confound the difficulty of obtaining accurate epidemiological data, diagnostic classifications count some children more than once and others not at all. Consider the difficulty of comparing children who have some or many labels that cross the boundaries among specific medical diagnostic categories as listed in the following sources: *Current Procedural Terminology (CPT)*[6] and *International Classification of Diseases-CM (ICD)*[7] used by physicians, its new companion publication—(for the forthcoming ICD-10-CM—), the World Health Organization's *International Classification of Functioning, Disability, and Health (ICF)*[8] adopted by ASHA as the framework for assessment and intervention in the "2001 Revised Scope of Practice in Speech-Language Pathology,"[9] the American Academy of Pediatrics' *Classification of Child and Adolescent Mental Diagnoses in Primary Care*,[10] the codes for psychological and psychiatric diagnoses outlined in the *Diagnostic and Statistical Manual* of the American Psychiatric Association,[11] the *Diagnostic Classification of Mental Health and Developmental Disorders of Infancy and Early Childhood*,[12] Individuals with Disabilities Education Act (IDEA) educational eligibility guidelines (which vary from state to state for infant, toddler, and family services covered under Part C),[13] and various state guidelines for services under Section 504 of the Rehabilitation Act of 1973.[14]

Whatever the actual figures may be, the U.S. Department of Education recognizes that the number of infants and toddlers receiving services under Part C of IDEA is below expectations in terms of reaching children who are eligible because of diagnosed medical conditions, documented developmental delays, or both. The federal government is urging states to find and provide services to all eligible children.[15] At the same time, professionals in early intervention are pleading with their colleagues to help children with "less severe disabilities" who often go untreated (and whose disabilities sometimes go unrecognized by parents and professionals) until they are 5 to 8 years of age.[16]

▼ PRACTICAL APPROACHES TO FRAMING THE ISSUES

In the short time between birth and the third birthday, most children progress from being 100% reliant on others to recognize and respond to their needs to being individuals capable of moving about in familiar surroundings, thinking about their experiences, comprehending what is being said to them, and using speech with a reasonable level of intelligibility to share their feelings and intentions. These important milestones are the outcomes of typical or "normal" child development and evolve from a broad range of interdependent variables, each of which is capable of affecting the others. Table 1-1 is a condensed display of elements contributing to communicative development.

TABLE 1-1
Elements Affecting Early Language Development*

Physical and Neurophysiological Factors	Developmental Domains
Integrity of body structures: oral, auditory, respiratory mechanisms	Sensory integration
Regulatory capacity	Physical growth
Sensory integrity	Gross- and fine-motor control
Myelination process	Emotional adjustment
Cortical integrity	Cognitive skills
Physical health	Communication skills
	Social skills
Early Language Sequences	**Emotional and Environmental Factors**
Perception of stimuli	Attachment and emotional security
Memory for experiences	Experiential exposure
Presymbolic (R) (e.g., sound discrimination)	Need and motivation to communicate
Presymbolic (E) (e.g., babbling, vocal play)	Opportunity to communicate
	Impact of communicative intent (i.e., choices, rewards, power to affect others or the environment)
Synergistic Activities	
Sensory integration	
Phonatory dynamics	**Communication Skills**
Resonatory dynamics	Symbolic, vocal/nonverbal (E,R)
Articulatory dynamics	Symbolic, nonvocal (E,R) (e.g., gestures, "baby signs")
Gross- and fine-motor control functions	Symbolic: first words and holophrasis (E)
Cognitive processing	Symbolic complexity (E,R) (e.g., semantics, syntax, and morphology)
Executive function (e.g., intonation, stress)	
Integration of social and cultural conventions	

E, Expressive modality; R, Receptive modality.
*Language development, both typical and atypical, occurs in conjunction with simultaneous maturation and development across many parameters. Anything that disturbs development in one area has the potential to affect development in other areas (transactional theory of development).

Transactional Factors in Development

Hallett and Proctor[17] pointed out the interdependency of biological structures, maturation of the central nervous system, and environmental processes on the developing child:

"By the second or third year of ... life, the cerebral cortex begins to approach the metabolic rate and dendritic complexity of the adult brain. Thus, at least five-sixths of dendritic branching occurs postnatally during the period of language development."

They report further that the "neural architecture" of the brain itself (i.e., proliferation or location of synapses) may be affected by experiential stimuli during the first 3 years of the child's life—the primary language development period (pp. 12–13). Thus an ongoing, delayed, or disordered function or element shown in Table 1-1 must be considered in the context of the effects on the child's total developmental framework.

Typical and Atypical Language Development

For a myriad of reasons—some well understood and others as yet unclear—some infants and toddlers fail to move along a developmental course toward attainment of the expected level of communicative competence by their third birthday. Most, if not all, readers of this work have a thorough understanding of typical sequences of language development, probably having completed a specific course in that subject. Several relevant references are provided in Appendix A for readers who would like a quick review of expected sequences of language acquisition during the first 3 years of life.

When children fail to follow the typical course of communicative development, even during the presymbolic period, it is a cause of concern. Approximately 6% to 10% of infants born each year do not follow the expected developmental course as a result of some disturbance in the synergistic relationships among the basic elements that promote communicative competency. It is estimated that the number of individual infants and toddlers so affected ranges between 630,000 and 1,050,000.[4] For those children and their families, the impact is manifested in social, emotional, behavioral, and preacademic abilities.

Development of communicative competence begins before birth and is pivotal to cognitive, psychoemotional, behavioral, and social development. The ability to comprehend the communication of others (receptive language ability), to process one's emotions and ideas and code the message one wishes to convey (linguistic mapping), and to convey that information to a communicative partner (expressive language ability) is communicative competence. The earliest interactions between mother and infant set the stage for a child's linguistic communicative development. By the end of the first year of life, most babies begin using words meaningfully and rapidly build a repertoire of spoken words and an even larger repertoire of words they understand. During the first years of life, most children master the essentials of oral language: basic phonology, semantics, morphology, syntax, and pragmatics. By 3 years of age, children are usually adept at relating their feelings and experiences in conversing with others.[18]

It is obvious that atypical communicative development can be associated with an array of causal and perpetuating factors, the nature, seriousness, and timing of which affect the prognosis for a favorable outcome. Sometimes the communicative problem is one aspect of a complex of problems that affect the child's health, physical growth, cognitive ability, motor functions, and other areas of development. Sometimes the communicative delay or disorder is the only identified developmental problem.

▼ HISTORICAL PERSPECTIVE OF EARLY INTERVENTION

An understanding of today's approach to early intervention must take into account the parallel efforts of a number of professions and of families of infants, toddlers, and preschool children with special needs. Over the past decade, major advances in knowledge have resulted from contributions of clinicians and researchers in child development and education, medicine and allied health, social services, and other professions. Recent research across a number of professional disciplines, including medicine, nursing, physical therapy, occupational therapy, speech-language pathology, audiology, the biological sciences, social work, and early childhood education, along with clinical experiences of pediatric practitioners, have provided a rich mix of data establishing the value of early intervention for children with developmental delays and disabilities.[19-26]

Education Legislation and Its Role in Development of Early Intervention

Precursors to recent advances in knowledge about working with young children were generated by projects completed in the 1970s and 1980s that generally focused on children in the 3- to 5-year age group, which was then considered the appropriate target for early-intervention efforts. A great deal of what is known about infant-toddler development and effective intervention practices emerged from studies and pilot demonstration programs that followed in the late 1980s and early 1990s. School systems established preschool programs in many states in response to federally funded incentives to serve young children with identified "handicaps." The number of preschool children (ages 3 to 5 years) served under Part B of IDEA (formerly known as Public Law 94-142) increased from 260,931 in 1986 (under the Education for the Handicapped Act) to 478,617 in 1993 (by which time the reauthorized law was known as *IDEA*).[27] Although results of the early model programs and the subsequent proliferation of preschool programs for children with special needs were giant steps forward, groundwork laid during that time period clearly indicated that habilitation for young children with developmental delays and disabilities needed to be undertaken much earlier than the preschool years to be optimally effective.

From the beginning, states were given the option under Public Law 94-142 (Education for the Handicapped Act) to establish programs for children from birth to 21 years of age. States were mandated to serve children from 6 to 21 years of age and encouraged to serve preschool children in the 3- to 5-year age group. In 1990, the Education for the Handicapped Act was reauthorized by Congress under a different title (IDEA).[28] In 1986, an amendment to the act was added in the form of Public Law 99-457,[29] which was later amended as Public Law 102-119 and became known as *Part H*.[30]

Part H mandated that participating states that had not already done so establish programs for 3- to 5-year-old children with special needs. Further, it encouraged states, using self-determined guidelines, to establish a multidisciplinary, community-based, family-focused, interagency system of services for infants and toddlers with special needs and their families. The unique features of Part H included (1) a 5-year planning period during which funding was provided to participating states to get their system up and running; (2) the authority of each state to name its own "lead agency" to oversee establishment and administration of the system; (3) the authority of each state to establish its own eligibility requirements for participation in the system, so long as children with medical diagnoses indicative of developmental delays or disabilities and those with established delays or disparities were included; (4) a requirement that the needs of *families* of eligible children be addressed to assist them in enhancing their child's optimal development; (5) the authority of each state to develop its own procedures and guidelines to see that an Individual Family Service Plan (IFSP) is in place for each family with an eligible child; (6) unprecedented short timelines to comply with required assessment and evaluation processes to establish eligibility for services following referral of a child; (7) a mandate of family service coordination (previously referred to as *case management*); and (8) the provision of services, to the extent possible, in naturalistic environments. *Naturalistic environments* were defined as those in which children of the same age who do not have developmental disabilities would normally be found; this is generally interpreted as homes and child care facilities.

The intent of Part H legislation was clearly to promote optimal development of infants and toddlers with special needs. In many states, especially in those whose "lead agency" is the state department of education, the focus on preparing children for school experiences has become a primary focus of Part H efforts. In fact, many children who transition out of the Part H system are transitioned at 3 years of age to Part B (special education) programs for preschool children with special needs.

Reauthorization of IDEA in 1997 changed the infant-toddler statutory reference from Part H to Part C, strengthened the role of families, and expanded the requirements for transition planning.[31]

From the perspective of policy makers and legislators who allocate and administer taxpayer dollars, it is important to see that children are prepared to enter school ready to learn (a theme articulated in those very words in the Goals 2000 education initiative). Interestingly, that effort to date has not taken particular notice of that preparation's dependence on communicative competence, despite the fact that most children in "noncategorical preschool" programs (which succeeded "preschool programs for the handicapped") have significant delays in communication skills.

Communicative Competence and Education

From the perspective of performance in the classroom, communicative competence is *the basic academic skill*—a fact that is so fundamental that it is often overlooked. Wetherby[32] reviewed statistical data on special education services provided nationally and concluded, "Problems in communication and language are the most common symptoms across categories of developmental disabilities." Young children with communicative disorders have no capacity for personal comparison of their language systems with those of their peers. There is generally no physical pain or discomfort associated with communicative delays or impairments; they do not portend physical degeneration or other "scientifically measurable" deficiencies; they are not fatal; they are usually not accompanied by traits that distinguish affected children from their age peers. Children with communicative difficulties are often judged by parents, teachers, or other adults to be "immature" or "slow." It is usually not until the child is expected to be able to transfer oral-communication skills to deriving meaning from new sets of symbols (i.e., letters and numerals) in literacy tasks that the language difficulty becomes evident to educators. The very complexity of the processes involved in communicative development—and their interdependency—seem too often to mitigate against actions that can be taken early on to address difficulties, especially in the absence of accompanying physical impairments.[33] Since the passage of Part C, all states have elected to establish early intervention programs, and many families and children from birth to 36 months of age are being served.

Preparation for literacy, however important, cannot be the total focus of the impact of delays and disorders of communicative development; the entirety of a child's life is affected when significant communication difficulties are present.

Health Care and Early Intervention

Advances in providing prenatal care in typical and high-risk pregnancies, dramatic improvements in neonatology, gene therapy, prenatal surgery for some conditions, and the availability of increasingly effective pharmacological management for a variety of diseases have contributed to the medical community's ability to preserve the lives of infants who in earlier times would not have survived. It is not uncommon today for babies born at 6 months' gestation to survive. Only a few years ago, children born with birth weights under 1500 g were not considered viable; now infants born at 1000 g (and sometimes less) are surviving, thanks to advances in knowledge and technology.

Advances in neonatal care extend beyond the availability of specialized equipment, pharmacological products, and highly trained medical practitioners. Developmental specialists in nursing, occupational therapy, physical therapy, and medical social work contribute to improved outcomes for compromised babies and their families. The work of Heidelese Als and her colleagues has changed the concept of the nurturing environment of the NICU.[34–39] When the best practices are used, lights are dimmed and noise levels are lowered to reduce the sensory stimulation with which the fragile newborns have to contend. In some units, family members and volunteer staff offer skin-to-skin contact ("kangaroo care") for babies who were born too soon. The emotional needs of the infants and their families are being given high priority in implementing treatment that previously focused only on the medical requirements called for simply to preserve life. Procedures to enhance the infant's quality of life, attachment, and emotional adjustment are considered important parts of the treatment plans for at-risk babies.

It has become relatively commonplace for SLPs in large hospitals to be included as members of the NICU team. In such cases, SLPs participate in developmental assessment; counsel families and professional colleagues in early communicative interactions between infants and their caregivers; and assist physicians, nursing staff, and occupational therapists in determining whether a given infant is ready for oral feedings and how that process can be optimized by use of specialized feeding equipment and appropriate positioning. These roles for the SLP are relatively new and obviously require specialized training and skills. More detailed information about the role of the SLP in the NICU is covered in Chapter 5.

Audiologists also play an important role in newborn care. Electrophysiological measurements of integrity of the auditory system, along with traditional audiometric assessment, have become commonplace in dealing with the needs of infants and toddlers. Early detection of hearing impairment and early application of appropriate habilitation strategies—including early fitting of amplification or provision of cochlear implants when indicated—have contributed to improved developmental outcomes for hearing-impaired children. Additional information about assessment and management for hearing impairment in infants and toddlers is provided in Chapters 6 and 9.

The results of advances in prenatal and neonatal care are mixed. On one hand, ever increasing numbers of infants are surviving preterm delivery; many medically compromised infants are being treated successfully; and early management of some congenital anomalies is making it possible for larger numbers of children to look forward to brighter futures. On the other hand, it is impossible to establish conditions that guarantee a "normal" developmental course for all of these infants. Many survivors continue to have problems that compromise their development in one or more areas. Some of the residual impairments are highly visible (as in cerebral palsy, severe craniofacial anomalies, and some syndromes), whereas others are not superficially apparent (as in certain chronic diseases, some neurological conditions, most receptive communicative disorders, and some expressive communicative disorders). The bottom line is that there are larger numbers of children surviving with conditions that are likely to be predictive of significant developmental delays or disorders, which require management by knowledgeable practitioners from many professional disciplines.

Physicians who care for infants and toddlers have children other than NICU "graduates" among their patients. The majority of newborn infants are not admitted to NICUs; most children born in U.S. hospitals are admitted for a day or two to regular newborn nurseries or are allowed to room-in with their mothers during a brief hospital confinement. Additionally, home births attended by midwives or nurse practitioners are prevalent in some parts of the country. Infants and toddlers who appear to be physically healthy sometimes exhibit significant developmental delays or disorders that may or may not be detected by their physicians. Wajda and Brorson[40] reported only 48% of children with global developmental delay, 38% of children with autism, 38% of children with language delay, and 24% of children with voice disorders were correctly selected for referral for SLP assessment by a panel of 21 physicians in their 2001 survey. Time pressures imposed by busy medical practices combined with scant training in medical schools pertinent to identification and management of nondisease-related delays and disorders of early childhood often result in lack of attention to those problems and help to explain why so many children are reaching the age of school entry before the seriousness of the problems is detected.

The American Academy of Pediatrics (AAP) and various public health agencies, including the National Institutes of Health, have made significant efforts to address these issues. Reduction of infant mortality rates has been a common goal of all groups, as has improving child (and maternal) health. Public awareness campaigns promoting early and continuous prenatal care; the federally funded nutrition program for women, infants, and children (WIC); the establishment of Kid-Med centers to provide community-based well-child health care; and the Medical Home initiative of the AAP are all examples of nationwide efforts to improve health care for children from conception on.

Unfortunately, the country is battling other societal problems that mitigate against the efforts of those promoting child health and welfare. The explosion of drug use among those in their child-bearing years, the spread of autoimmune deficiency diseases (e.g., acquired immunodeficiency syndrome), the high incidence of sexually transmitted diseases (including syphilis), the increased numbers of smokers among teens and young adults, and the widespread abuse of alcohol in that age group are of concern because of potential increases in developmental disabilities among infants and toddlers born to affected mothers. The combination of low socioeconomic status and low educational attainment of mothers is a further problem that places infants and toddlers at risk for developmental delays and disabilities.[41] Neither the medical community alone nor in conjunction with members of the educational community can hope to deal with problems of this magnitude. Solutions—if they are to be found—must involve political, legal, medical, educational, religious, family, and individual efforts.

▼ Families, Babies, and Early Intervention

Through the years, families of children with atypical developmental patterns have struggled to find ways to help their children. In this country, attitudes toward families of children with special needs have undergone significant changes. Child protection laws, education legislation that mandates services to families of infants and toddlers with special needs, development of standards of practices among medical and allied health professions dealing with the youngest pediatric populations, public health legislation, and other developments of recent times are all reflective of society's attempts to address the issues with which every family with a special-needs child deals.

From an individual family's perspective, however knowledgeable they are about the availability or scarcity of public policies to cover their particular situation, issues related to their child's development, including communication development, are more personal. The issues involve relationships between the child and other members of the family. Parents face any problem involving their child's development with a set of issues unique to their own experiences. Their emotions, expectations, perceptions, levels of information and abilities to process it, present concerns, priorities, and coping mechanisms are factors that affect their decision making.

These factors also affect the family's ongoing relationships with professionals who are in the picture *because* of the child's atypical development and perhaps only for that reason. All families balance a plethora of day-to-day demands on their time, energy, attention, and resources. A family with a child whose developmental problems require the attention of a number of professionals, which is typical of many families who are referred to communicative disorders specialists, may experience a significant amount of stress as they parcel out their time, energy, and other resources to meet the needs of their young child. Figure 1-1 illustrates the demands that face many such families. Each of the elements depicted has positive and negative aspects, as the family attempts to balance daily activities and simultaneously attend to the needs of their atypically developing child.

Any consideration of the perspectives of families must take into account that very few families *expect* to be dealing with anything but a healthy, typically developing child. Consider the implications and functional impact on emotional, financial, marital, and social aspects of family functioning when their new baby has disabilities. The child's problems may require immediate and difficult decisions on the part of the parents with respect to medical or surgical treatment options, impose unexpected and huge financial hardships related to extended stays in NICUs, or may result in the need for long-term management of congenital or acquired conditions or diseases. It takes time for families to adjust to what life is suddenly like, as compared with what the parents *expected* life to be like as they anticipated the birth of a healthy child. Alternatively, if the child appeared to be healthy at birth and experienced no major medical problems, consider the impact of a gradual discovery that the child's development is not proceeding along a typical path.

The growing anxieties—or dealing with the unanticipated pronouncement by a professional whose assessment has revealed a "deficit" or "significant delay"—of whether the child will be able to deal with social situations, adjust to a child care setting, and succeed in school when the time comes are difficult for the family. Some families are better able than others to cope, to identify and use available resources to promote their child's development, and to advocate for their child. It is part of the professional's role to assist those families who need support in those endeavors and to promote their innate abilities to make choices that meet their own and their child's needs. Early interventionists refer to that goal as "empowering" the family. Families often comment that they are *already* empowered to make such decisions; what they *need* is access to the information that enables them to make informed decisions that assist them in optimizing their child's development.

Communication Disorders Specialists and Early Intervention

The frame of reference for understanding the impact of atypical communicative development must include knowledge that the majority of children receiving special education services in the schools, regardless of their primary diagnosis or eligibility label, receive speech-language therapy services. Obviously, these children did not suddenly develop communication delays or disorders at the time of school entry. The fact that they have a communication delay or disorder at the time they enter school places them at risk for academic difficulties in reading and other literacy-based subjects, *because literacy skills are built on the foundation of oral-language competencies*.[30,42] Research indicates that a substantial number of children with many special-education service eligibility labels have coexisting communication delays, disorders, or both. The most heavily documented problems

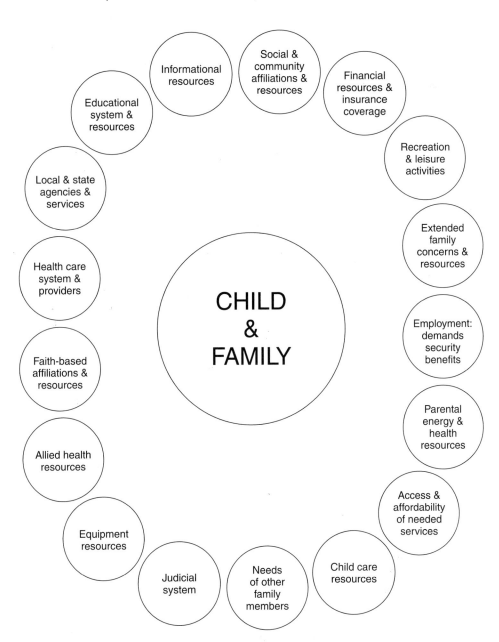

▼ Figure 1-1   Child and family.

in which communication development is also affected are autism, attention-deficit hyperactivity disorder, cerebral palsy, and certain genetic syndromes. In fact, the presence of a communication disorder or significant delay is a hallmark for the diagnosis itself in many instances. This issue is addressed more specifically in Chapters 2 and 7.

Until recently, early communication delays were generally not thought of as being especially noteworthy by the medical community. Parents who exhibited concern about their child's late talking were frequently told by their pediatricians that a referral would be made only if the problem persisted past the age of 3. Information emerging from infant research on cognitive, social, emotional, sensory, and physical factors that contribute to the development of speech and language long before the emergence of the spoken word has become more readily available with advances in, and widespread use of, information technology. Access to the research knowledge base combined with recognition of the advantages of early intervention and efforts of the AAP to encourage physician referrals to early intervention services are changing the way in which the medical community deals with high-incidence, low-visibility problems in the pediatric population. The availability of a legitimate medical diagnostic code for "developmental delay" has also contributed to the emergence of attention to developmental problems earlier in the child's life.[7,9]

Years before the age of school entry (and introduction to literacy), children with communicative difficulties are at risk for a variety of other problems. Children who have problems communicating are at risk for atypical social development. Early interactions with significant others are adversely affected when the child is not appropriately responsive to the efforts of caregivers. Research indicates that children with impaired early interactive and preintentional communicative abilities are responded to differently by their parents and other caregivers.[43–45] Specific preintentional communication intervention strategies are indicated when this is the case. SLPs can be called on to train caregivers to look for small changes in the child's responses to their bids for interaction, rather than simply noting the absence of the expected behaviors of typically developing infants.

Behaviors of toddlers who are frustrated by an inadequate ability to convey their feelings through language are often problematic, compounding the frustrations of their families and other caregivers who wish they could interpret what the child is trying to convey but often cannot. The problematic behavior (e.g., withdrawal, excessive dependence, frequent tantrums) in turn often generates a set of issues that sometimes become the primary focus of the family or child care provider, who often do not consider the communicative difficulty as a precipitator of the behavioral problem.[19] Speech-language specialists can serve as consultants to families and childcare providers to help deal with such situations, helping the adults deal effectively with behavior modification when communicative impairment is the underlying factor triggering undesirable behaviors.

Some conditions associated with communicative delays and disorders have an adverse effect on the child's physical development. Feeding and swallowing difficulties can be present in the child with tongue mobility difficulties or palatal anomalies; the child's nutritional needs may be compromised as a result. The infant with a persistent odd quality of cry may be referred by the SLP to an otorhinolaryngologist (i.e., ear, nose, and throat specialist) for evaluation of specific physical problems (e.g., choanal atresia, laryngeal polypoid growths, vocal fold paresis or unilateral paralysis, submucous or overt palatal cleft). Over time, these specific physical problems could underlie compensatory motor adjustments that impact growth patterns of bony- or soft-tissue structures or interfere with adequate nutrition. Toddlers with extremely poor articulation abilities may have ankylosis of the

lingual frenum with resultant physical growth deformities of dental or mandibu-
lar structures. These issues are dealt with in more detail in Chapters 2 and 8.

High-Incidence, Low-Visibility Disorders

Children with delays and disorders affecting communication development comprise a large portion of the high-incidence, low-visibility population. Although
there is a segment of the pediatric population with high-visibility, low-incidence
developmental disabilities associated with atypical communicative development
(e.g., craniofacial anomalies, syndromes with characteristic physical features such
as Down syndrome), the majority of children with delayed or disordered communicative development look like other children in their age groups. It is often
because they "look normal" that their difficulties with communicative development are downplayed or overlooked entirely. It takes continuing efforts on the
part of those who understand the impact of communicative impairments to
educate the public and the professional community to the pervasiveness of
the problem and its potential to adversely affect other areas of development.
Demonstration through clinical programs that early intervention for communication problems can be effective must be coupled with ongoing communication with
other professionals who work with the population and with families. As Stark[46]
asserts, part of the professional role of the communicative-disorders specialist
serving this population must be to undertake these responsibilities.

▼ MANAGED CARE AND EARLY INTERVENTION

The health care environment, including that segment relating to early intervention,
is demanding adjustment to the rapid proliferation of managed care plans that have
arisen in response to mushrooming health care costs. Under managed care plans,
primary care providers (PCPs) (i.e., licensed obstetricians, pediatricians, and family
practitioners) control access to other services. In effect, they are the gatekeepers for
all health services. Members of a managed care plan are required to access services
through the PCP. A feature of many, if not most, managed care plans is capitation.
Capitation is a basic fee paid to participating PCPs for each member of the plan, based
on a formula devised by the managed care plan administrators or negotiated
between the contracted PCPs and plan administrators. The PCP is awarded a fixed
dollar amount under the contractual arrangement. That dollar amount is designed
to cover charges for all care provided to plan members during a specified term. If the
PCP manages to "save" costs by reducing referrals to specialists and subspecialists
and limiting expensive testing procedures, hospital admissions, or both, any dollars
remaining in the fund at the end of a fixed time period specified in the contract are
awarded to the PCP as a reward for conserving resources. Capitation practices are
a subject of great debate with respect to ethical decision making, the care that is in
the best interests of patient-health outcomes, and the roles of specialists and subspecialists in medicine and allied health fields (e.g., speech-language pathology,
occupational therapy, physical therapy, audiology).[47]

Obviously the PCP's role as gatekeeper, or referring agent, has taken on overtones
of personal economics that are different from the issues involved before the advent

of managed care. Will the hard-won knowledge that a child with developmental delays or disabilities can profit from intervention before the age of 3 years be ignored by persons with authority to make referrals in the interest of protecting the capitation limit? The full impact of managed care plans has yet to be realized, and, in time, there will undoubtedly be changes in the operations of some plans. Practitioners who rely on the PCP for referrals must monitor this situation carefully, if they hope to survive in this environment. An example of the issue for communicative disorders specialists is found in the denial of payment for language-therapy services rendered to a child of a managed care plan participant because the PCP did not make the referral for that service. Precertification for services is a common requirement of managed care plans. Precertification requires PCP referral. It is awarded normally for a specified number of visits, with authority to extend the treatment for additional visits dependent on documentation satisfactory to the managed care certification officer (who may or may not be knowledgeable about communication-therapy regimens) that the extension is warranted.

This is a critical issue for practitioners who are required by Public Law 102-119 and recent amendments to IDEA (Public Law 205-17, Part C, which pertains to the population from birth to 3 years of age) to serve infants and toddlers in naturalistic environments to the extent possible. This is problematic because homes and child care centers do not qualify as health care centers, and many early-intervention programs are operated through community organizations (e.g., the Association for Retarded Citizens) or as a service of local schools. One bright spot is that at least one health maintenance organization has carved out a special division to handle infants and toddlers with special needs.[48]

Maintaining ongoing lines of communication with PCPs is a crucial issue.[49,50] Assisting them in understanding why early referrals are critical is essential. Dealing with the certification officer at the administrative offices of managed care plans is a new area in which professional skills are needed. Understanding what a particular plan requires by way of authorization for services is a particular challenge, because plans differ in their requirements.

▼ FRAMEWORK OF THE FAMILY AND PROFESSIONAL TEAM

An immediate realization of professionals who work with the infant-toddler population is that their families are the true decision makers with respect to the care the children receive. Professionals can and do make recommendations about appropriate management options, suggest intervention or treatment strategies, and provide pertinent information; ultimately, however, the family chooses the paths to take or whether to select any path at all. Whether the family is forced to deal with difficult decisions at the time their child is born (e.g., authorizing surgery or special treatment, selecting one medical specialist over another, finding a way to pay for expensive care for their child with a congenital condition) or faces a set of different decisions later, either as a result of a traumatic event that leaves the child with a disability or through realization that the child's developmental course is impaired, a great deal of emotional energy and personal tension can be expected.

Families move through adjustments at varying rates and with varying degrees of comfort and success. Adjustment is not the same for all members of the family, nor are the issues involved given equal weight by all members of the family. Coping mechanisms vary within the family. Coping and adjustment to a child's developmental delays or disorders is not linear. There are sometimes slow steps forward, and occasionally there are leaps forward only to be followed by a return to an earlier level of dealing with the situation. There can be short or long periods of "plateau," when the family chooses not to deal with the issues or cannot do so for some reason.

The concerns, priorities, and resources of the family may be different from those of the professionals. When there is intersection of family and professional goals to promote the best outcome for the child, opportunities for effective teaming between families and professionals are created.

The author's experiences with families mirrors what is found in the research literature with respect to coping and adjustment. Some families (or members of families) are open and responsive, seek information, and quickly follow through on suggestions and management strategies, whereas others appear to be resistant to any suggestion that something should or could be done, even to the point of denying (overtly or covertly) that a problem exists. Still others wax and wane in their involvement with intervention or treatment plans, even if they helped to create them. Such responses can be attributed to human nature and are not necessarily a comment on either the character traits of family members or the skills of the professionals involved. Additionally, families sometimes report that they cannot work with certain professionals because of their inflexibility or insistence on following a particular course of treatment or management that is unacceptable to the family. The family's choices may be based on religious beliefs, child-rearing practices, social or cultural values, or simply intuition. With the exceptions of parental choices that result in criminal or medical neglect or child abuse, parents are free to make those choices that make the most sense for their families.

As professionals, we must keep reminding ourselves that families are dealing with a myriad of difficult decisions, including but not limited to those we have placed before them. Their lives are more complex than the slices of it with which we are involved because of a particular child. They move at their own pace. Our responsibility is to provide them with enough information to make those decisions that make the most sense to them. We must be open to listening to what their concerns and priorities are. We must also find out what their supports and resources are.

Although the timing of communication intervention is critical and sometimes crucial to a desired outcome, families may not see the situation through the same lens that we use. The family is dealing with balancing the costs of some services against other financial priorities in their lives. Families who are engaged with multiple members of the early-intervention professional team (who can but probably do not practice in the same setting) also have to balance appointment schedules, transportation arrangements, and other matters, in addition to caring for the child and the needs of other family members. Demands of the managed care system, program-eligibility requirements, lifetime insurance caps, availability of and accessibility to services, medications, and needed equipment can take precedence over a professional's desire for an immediate decision by the family about a management recommendation.

Another matter requiring the attention of the family and practitioners with whom they work is the extent to which family members, particularly the mother or primary caregiver, desire to function as members of the early-intervention team. For many people, this concept is not readily acceptable. Their cultural background, values, prior life experiences, educational background, socioeconomic status, belief system, and expectations (especially about disabilities and relationships with professionals) all bear on their concept of what it means to be a team member. Although many professionals have adopted the stance that team membership is the ideal way of addressing early-intervention activities, we must keep in mind that in most cases the whole experience of early intervention is new to every family with whom we come in contact.

Establishing a satisfactory working relationship with any family takes time and patience on the part of both the professional and family members as they adjust to each other and define both their commitment to the process and their expectations of one another. The professional must be able to provide the information and tools with which the family can operate as true partners, if they choose to do so.

▼ SERVICE-DELIVERY MODELS IN EARLY INTERVENTION

Infants and toddlers who have or are at risk for communicative disorders may come to the attention of the SLP through referrals to developmental programs or through clinical programs. Developmental programs are often conducted under the auspices of community-based agencies and operate in keeping with the mandates of Part C of IDEA. Clinical programs more traditionally operate in health care settings and private practices. They tend to be "center based," that is, families take their children to the professional. Conversely, Part C mandates that services be delivered, to the extent possible, in naturalistic environments, which often means that professionals travel to the child's home or child care center.[51] Center-based programs are not prohibited by Part C legislation, but very young children do not typically attend habilitative programs. The very young child's normal environment is the home, and many regularly attend child care during their parents' working hours. Increasingly, the philosophies of both developmental programs and clinical programs are being applied in meeting the needs of atypically developing young children and their families when communicative problems are the primary issue. Developmentally appropriate practices are the hallmark against which every management program should be measured.

Under IDEA *families* are also eligible for services if their children qualify.[52] Many children who could profit from early intervention do not qualify for Part C services, however, either because their developmental delays are "not serious enough" to meet their state's eligibility criteria or because the nature of the risk is excluded from defined eligibility guidelines. For example, environmentally at-risk children (especially those whose low family socioeconomic status is combined with the mother's low educational achievement level) constitute a group who could profit from early intervention.[53] Although states are encouraged to include at-risk groups in their eligibility criteria, financial considerations are substantial, and children in environmentally at-risk groups are omitted from eligibility definitions in most states.

Eligibility for services under clinical service delivery models varies considerably across agencies and practices. As with the Part C model, it is most likely that children who are referred early in life for SLP services under the clinical model are infants or toddlers with physical anomalies (especially craniofacial anomalies), hearing impairment, and those who are multiply handicapped. Eligibility, especially in the private sector, is often dictated by family income level or insurance coverage or other factors unrelated to the child's developmental needs. It should be noted that some families take longer than others to adjust to the many facets of the child's condition and to changes in their own lives that can ensue. Developmental habilitation awaits their readiness to seek it. When they do seek such services, they may choose to start with only one service, adding others as they feel or recognize the need to do so. It is particularly important that all professionals on the child's habilitative team appreciate the advantages of approaching development from the perspective of parallel developmental maturation, of taking advantage of synaptogenesis during the early years of life, and of involving a collaborative team effort to achieve optimal outcomes for affected children and their families.

▼ WHAT ABOUT THE FAMILY: ARE THE CHOICES ONLY EITHER-OR?

As SLPs attempt to forge effective parent-professional partnerships, they must acknowledge that just as individuals differ, families are different. The definition of family has changed from the idea of being exclusively comprised of two parents, one or more children, and extended family (i.e., grandparents, aunts, uncles, and cousins). In most families, blood-related extended family members no longer live with the children and parents under the same roof, as was once commonly practiced, although this practice varies considerably across cultural groups. Large numbers of children now grow up in single-parent households, often headed by women. Close friends or intimates not related by blood are sometimes considered members of the family and function as such, regardless of whether they live under the same roof. Adoptive or foster families may be the people responsible for the child. Even in homes where there are two parents, both of whom may work outside the home, the child may be left during most waking hours in the hands of child care providers in home-based or center-based programs. The staff members of such centers can change often, thereby introducing the child to new faces on a fairly frequent basis. Identification with a "primary caregiver" can be tenuous for some children. These issues are addressed in more detail in Chapter 9, because they can affect child development and planning and implementing management of communicative difficulties.

Ultimately, decisions regarding the child still rest in the hands of the parent(s), of course, but factors influencing the decision-making process must be considered by professionals who work with the child and family. Open-minded professionals recognize that it is possible to combine the service delivery models discussed above to the advantage of all concerned. Children and their families may qualify for Part C services at some points in time and not at others. Families may prefer to use the services of a private practitioner or of a particular clinical program at certain points in the child's life or may choose to address specific needs they feel may be more appropriately handled by a particular practitioner who is not part of the IDEA system. At other times, families may wish to take advantage of the multidisciplinary approach offered through the Part C service model or some specialized pediatric clinical practices. Thus the professional finds that the family's choice of options can vary over time, according to their perception of the child's needs, their priorities, and their resources.

Challenges that may be new to professionals are understanding the scope of available options, sharing information with the family so that they can understand the bases of professional recommendations, communicating openly with the family about advantages and disadvantages of various service-delivery systems, and supporting the family in their choice of services for their child and themselves. Table 1-2 provides an overview of the basic service-delivery models that provide the framework for services to infants and toddlers with or at high risk for disabilities and their families.

▼ PROFESSIONAL COMPETENCIES

Under whatever service-delivery model is employed (the parents may or may not know what model is being applied by a given practice or agency), it is imperative that practitioners who work with infants and toddlers with or at risk for developmental disabilities possess the essential competencies, knowledge base, and experiential background. Table 1-2 compares features of various service delivery models with which every professional should be familiar.

The American Speech-Language-Hearing Association published guidelines for professionals who work with infants and toddlers.[52] Additionally, certain competencies are outlined in Part C implementation rules and regulations. Multidisciplinary guidelines have been developed by the Division of Early Childhood of the Council for Exceptional Children.[54] Suggested guidelines for physicians dealing with developmentally disabled children have been published by the AAP.[55] The *Practice Parameter: Screening and Diagnosis of Autism* guide has been adopted by several professional organizations, including the American Academy of Audiology, the American Occupational Therapy Association, ASHA, the Autism National Committee, and the Society for Developmental Pediatrics.[56]

Families who entrust their children to professionals, often at times of emotional and financial stress, anticipate that they will deal with practitioners who can guide them appropriately as they face making decisions that have the potential to alter their children's lives. Regardless of socioeconomic status, level of intelligence, educational background, or family composition, parents are anxious to secure the best available treatment for their children's needs. Some may have an unrealistic expectation about a possible *cure* for serious disabilities with no known remedy; over time, the family's expectations will become more realistic as a result of their interactions with professionals and through their own life experiences. Professionals must strike a critical balance between the family's hopes for the future of each child and appropriate management leading to optimal developmental outcomes for each child.

The following chapters of this work focus on specific issues of diagnosis, assessment, and management for communication disorders.

TABLE 1-2
Comparative Features of Various Service Delivery Models

Model	Likely Service Setting	Population Served and Approaches Used	Focus
Clinical	Hospital or other medical setting (e.g., NICU) Out-patient services Health care centers, practices, or programs Specialized multidisciplinary teams (e.g., craniofacial anomalies teams, cleft lip or cleft palate teams, feeding teams)	Newborns, infants, and toddlers The service is child-centered The service relies heavily on professional expertise for guidance and selection of treatment and care options The service includes a well-established chain of command (lines of authority) Parents rely heavily on professionals' knowledge and expertise Parents are given options regarding choices, receive training in specialized procedures, and are provided information regarding community resources	Prevention Diagnosis Assessment Treatment/management Discharge planning Team collaboration Parent training and education Health, wellness, and promotion of development
Clinical	Solo or group SLP practice, such as traditional center-based private practice with or without off-site consultants	The population can be limited to or only certain portions of the birth to 3-year-old population, depending on structure of the clinical practice The SLP or audiologist may contract with various agencies to provide services at other sites (e.g., homes, child care centers)	Unidisciplinary, child-centered therapy Family participation directed by practitioner in keeping with clinical goals
Group or multi-disciplinary	Professional practice, often office group practice with or without off-site consultants	Population served varies from inclusion of birth to 3-year-old children and their families to inclusion of selected subgroups (e.g., autism, cerebral palsy language disorders) Services are often specific to needs of children with developmental or physical health needs or those with designated conditions or diagnoses	Child-centered Dependent to a large extent on combination of disciplines comprising the team (e.g., physical therapy, occupational therapy, and SLP; psychology, SLP and social work; SLP and psychology)

Continued

TABLE 1-2
Comparative Features of Various Service Delivery Models—Cont'd

Model	Likely Service Setting	Population Served and Approaches Used	Focus
Developmental	Multidisciplinary early intervention teams (which can be center-based or combination home-based and center-based)	Ages served vary from comprehensive inclusion of birth to 3-year-old children and their families to selected groups (e.g., mental retardation, cerebral palsy, autism) Services are usually family-focused and governed by federal and state early intervention statutes Management by IFSP is commonly used, whether or not it is required by law Services are based on family priorities and objectives are related to enhancing the child's development	Services fall between clinical and educational models Historic origins often traced to developmental disability programs, parent-funded centers for specific problems, or to university training or research programs
Developmental	Multidisciplinary developmental assessment teams that can operate in conjunction with: Health care centers Hospital units Developmental disability centers Local education agencies Centers sponsored by civic organizations (e.g., SERTOMA, Scottish Rite, Easter Seal Society)	The population served can include all of the 3-year-old population and their families or be limited by policy or statutory regulation to a segment thereof Programs offer specialized assessment leading to referral elsewhere for treatment, therapy, or intervention	Diagnosis and assessment for designated purposes conducted in highly specialized settings Generally child-centered but can be more family focused
Transdisciplinary	Same as above	Same as above except team members may also provide family services and direct or indirect intervention services to infants and toddlers	Collaborative, family-focused assessment; role sharing among team's professionals

NICU, Neonatal intensive care unit; *SLP,* Speech-language pathology/pathologist; *IFSP,* Individual Family Service Plan.

▼ REFERENCES

1. U.S. Department of Health and Human Services: Research notes, January 1995.
2. U.S. Department of Education: *Seventeenth report to congress on the implementation of Individuals with Disabilities Education Act,* Washington, DC, 1995.
3. Newacheck PW, Taylor WR: Childhood chronic illness: prevalence, severity, and impact, *Am J Public Health* 82:364–371, 1992.
4. Wenger BL, Kaye HS, LaPlante MP: Disabilities among children. Disability Statistics Abstract, No. 15, Washington, DC, 1996, U.S. Department of Education, National Institute on NIDRR Outcome.
5. U.S. Department of Health and Human Services/Public Health Service: Disabilities among children age 0–17 years—United States, 1991-1992, *MMWR Morb Mortal Wkly Rep* 44:33, 1995.
6. American Medical Association: *Physicians' current procedural terminology,* Chicago, 1996, CPT Intellectual Property Services, AMA.
7. American Medical Association: *International classification of diseases: clinical modification,* ed 9, Dover, Del, 1996, AMA.
8. American Speech-Language-Hearing Association: *2001 Scope of practice in speech-language pathology,* Rockville, Md, 2001, Author.
9. Threats TT: New classification will aid assessment and intervention, *The ASHA Leader* 6(18):12, 2001.
10. American Academy of Pediatrics: *The classification of child and adolescent mental diagnoses in primary care: diagnostic and statistical manual for primary care (DSM-PC) child and adolescent version,* Elk Grove Village, Ill, 1997, AAP Division of Publications.
11. American Psychiatric Association: *Diagnostic and statistical manual of mental disorders,* ed 4, Washington, DC, 1996, American Psychiatric Association.
12. Zero to Three/National Center for Clinical Infant Programs: *Diagnostic classification: 0–3-diagnostic classification of mental health and developmental disorders of infancy and early childhood,* Arlington, Va, 1994, Author.
13. U.S. Department of Education: Assistance to states for the education of children with disabilities and early intervention program for infants and toddlers with disabilities, 34CFR, Part 303: early intervention program for infants and toddlers with disabilities, *The Federal Register* 64(48):12505–12554, 1999. (Full text of final regulations for IDEA available at http://www.icase.org/idea/regulations/12416.htm)
14. Rehabilitation Act of 1973, Sec. 504 (34 CFR 104.3 [j]).
15. OSEP's Hehir voices concern about need for more child-find in Part H, *Early Child Rep* 7:7, 1996.
16. Fewell R: Educator says research points to need for more aid for children with less severe disabilities (excerpts from keynote address of Rebecca Fewell at the 1996 Conference of the Division of Early Childhood), *Early Child Rep* 8:3, 1997.
17. Hallett T, Proctor A: Maturation of the central nervous system as related to communication and cognitive development, *Infant Young Child* 8(4):1–15, 1986.
18. Roeper T, deVilliers P: *What every three-year-old needs to know.* Seminar presented at the ASHA Convention, New Orleans, La, Nov 17, 2001.
19. Prizant BM, Meyer EC: Socioemotional aspects of language and social-communication disorders in young children, *Am J Speech-Lang Pathol* 2:56, 1996.
20. Catts HW: The relationship between speech-language impairments and reading disabilities, *J Speech Hear Res* 36:948, 1993.
21. Lockwood SL: Early speech and language indicators for later learning problems: recognizing a language organization disorder, *Infant Young Child* 7:43–52, 1994.
22. Menyuk P: Syntactic and reading disabilities. In Stark J, Menyuk P, Wurtzel S, eds: *Language learning and reading disabilities: a new decade,* New York, 1980, Queens College Press.
23. Ramey CT, et al: Infant health and development program for low birth weight premature infants: program elements, family participation, and child intelligence, *Pediatrics* 89:454, 1992.

24. Bryant DM, Ramey CT: An analysis of the effectiveness of early intervention programs for environmentally at-risk children. In Guralnick M, Bennett FC, eds: *Effectiveness of early intervention*, Orlando, Fl, 1987, Academic Press, p 33.
25. Campbell RA, Ramey CT: Effects of early intervention on intellectual and academic achievement: a follow-up study of children from low-income families, *Child Dev* 65:684, 1994.
26. Shonkoff JP, Hauser-Cram P: Early intervention for disabled infants and their families: a quantitative analysis, *Pediatrics* 80:650, 1987.
27. Preschool program data, *Early Child Rep* 5:7, 1994.
28. Education for the Handicapped Act of 1975, Pub L No. 94-142.
29. Amendments to the Education for the Handicapped Act of 1986, Pub L No. 99-457.
30. Individuals with Disabilities Education Act of 1990, Pub L No. 101-476.
31. Wetherby AM, Prizant BM: Toward earlier identification of communication and language problems in young children. In Meisels SJ, Fenichel E, eds: *New visions for the developmental assessment of infants and young children*, Washington, DC, 1996, Zero to Three/National Center for Clinical Infant Programs, p 289.
32. Wetherby AM: *First words project: improving identification of communication disorders.* Seminar presented at the Louisiana Speech-Language-Hearing Association 2000 Convention, Baton Rouge, La, Nov 6, 2000.
33. Alfonso DD, Wahlberg V, Persson B: Exploration of mothers' reactions to the kangaroo method of prematurity care, *Neonatal Network* 7:43, 1989.
34. Als H: Individualized, family-focused developmental care for the very low birthweight preterm infant in the NICU. In Friedman SL, Sigman MD, eds: *Advances in applied developmental psychology*, vol 6, Norwood, NJ, 1992, Ablex.
35. Becker PT, et al: Outcomes of developmentally supportive nursing care for very low birthweight infants, *Nurs Res* 40:150, 1991.
36. Lawhon G, Melzar A: Developmentally supportive interventions. In Cloherty JP, Stark AR, eds: *Manual of neonatal care*, ed 3, Boston, 1991, Little, Brown, p 581.
37. McCormick MC: Advances in neonatal intensive care technology and their possible impact on the development of low birthweight infants. In Friedman SL, Sigman MD, eds: *The psychological development of low-birthweight children: advances in applied developmental psychology*, Norwood, NJ, 1992, Ablex, p 37.
38. Parker SJ, et al: Outcome after developmental intervention in the neonatal intensive care unit for mothers of preterm infants with low socioeconomic status, *J Pediatr* 120:780, 1992.
39. Schmidt E, Wittreich G: *Care of the abnormal newborn: a random controlled clinical trial study of the "kangaroo method of care for the low birth-weight newborns."* Paper presented at the 1996 World Health Organization Interregional Conference on Appropriate Technology Following Birth, Rome, Italy, October 1986.
40. Wajda V, Brorson K: *Referrals for speech and language services: are medical students/residents prepared?* Poster session presented at the ASHA Conference, New Orleans, La, Nov 15, 2001.
41. Bendersky M, Lewis M: Environmental risk, biological risk, and developmental outcome, *Dev Psychol* 30:484, 1994.
42. Scarborough HS: Very early language deficits in dyslexic children, *Child Dev* 61:1728, 1990.
43. Barnard KE, Kelly JF: Assessment of parent-child interaction. In Meisels SJ, Shonkoff JP, eds: *Handbook of early childhood intervention*, Cambridge, Mass, 1990, Cambridge University Press, p 278.
44. Barnard KE: Influencing parent-child interactions for children at risk. In Guralnick M, editor: *The effectiveness of early intervention.* Baltimore, Md, 1997, Paul H. Brookes, p 249.
45. Hudson KM, Giardino AP: Child abuse and neglect. In Meisels SJ, Shonkoff JP, eds: *Handbook of early childhood intervention*, Cambridge, Mass, 1997, Cambridge University Press, p 278.
46. Stark RE: Early language intervention: when, why, how? *Infant Young Child* 1:44, 1989.
47. Shapland C: Be aware that managed care can affect children with disabilities, *Pacesetter* 20:12, 1997.

48. HMO makes an important connection to early intervention, *Early Child Rep* 7:1, 1996.
49. Droter D: But where are the data? Planning services for infants and families in an era of managed care, *Infant Young Child* 9:vi, 1996.
50. Barnett WS, Escobar CM: Economic costs and benefits of early intervention. In Meisels S, Shonkoff JP, eds: *Handbook of early childhood intervention*, Cambridge, Mass, 1990, Cambridge University Press, p 560.
51. U.S. Department of Education: Early intervention program for infants and toddlers with disabilities, *Federal Register* Sec. 303.361; 40968, July 30, 1993.
52. Ramey CT, Yeates KO, MacPhee D: Risk for retarded development among disadvantaged families: a systems theory approach to preventive intervention, *Adv Special Educ* 4:249, 1984.
53. American Speech-Language-Hearing Association: The roles of speech-language pathologists in service delivery to infants, toddlers, and their families, *ASHA* 32:4, 1990.
54. DEC Task Force on Recommended Practices: *DEC recommended practices: indicators of quality programs for infants and young children with special needs and their families*, Reston, Va, 1993, Council for Exceptional Children pp 47, 69.
55. Liptak GS: The role of the pediatrician in caring for children with developmental disabilities, *Pediatr Ann* 24:232, 1995.
56. Filipek PA, et al: Practice parameter: screening and diagnosis of autism. Report of the Quality Standards Subcommittee of the American Academy of Neurology and the Child Neurology Society, *Neurology* 2:468–479, 2000.

CHAPTER 2

CAUSES OF DEVELOPMENTAL DELAYS AND DISORDERS IN INFANTS AND TODDLERS

Implications for Communication Competence

Frances P. Billeaud

A s a preface to the materials included in this chapter, a brief discussion of terminology is in order. Terminology used by professionals who work with very young children who have or are at high risk for developmental delays and disorders can be somewhat confusing in that descriptors applied to conditions and behaviors have somewhat different meanings for different groups of professionals. It is important that practitioners not assume the definitions they are accustomed to using are understood or applied universally by other professionals working with the same child. Issues of terminology have been complicated further by the current societal trend to be "politically correct." Thus the term *mental retardation* is customarily used by psychologists in defining limited mental capabilities and in applying diagnostic labels, whereas the same individual who is so diagnosed or described by the psychologist may be labeled as *developmentally delayed* by teachers and other professionals who work in agencies serving persons with physical and mental disabilities. Persons who work in special education programs may refer to the same individual as *cognitively challenged* or *mentally handicapped* and may add a further qualification implying the degree to which the individual is affected (e.g., *mild-moderate* or *severe-profound*). Such labels are usually dictated by rules and regulations of governmental agencies, professional practice criteria, or by organizations devoted to serving selected groups of individuals with exceptionalities. Statutory language included in federal and state laws sometimes provides definitions that apply to eligibility for services, thus making use of particular terms imperative in qualifying individuals for the services to which only certain groups are entitled.

With those cautions in mind, this chapter provides information about infants and toddlers who exhibit a range of conditions or behaviors of concern to professionals. It is essential that practitioners recognize the status of a child who has been referred.

▼ RECEIVING REFERRALS AND DETERMINING WHICH CHILDREN ARE AT RISK

Decisions about whether a given child is in need of treatment or management hinge on the child's condition or status in the eyes of the professional(s) to whom the referral has been made. Physicians look for specific physical conditions, disease processes, and anomalies that affect health or development. Psychologists and others look for identifiable behaviors, cognitive abilities, and indicators of mental and emotional status and development. Educators and early childhood development specialists look at child development across a number of "domains" (e.g., physical, social, self-help, cognitive) to make judgments about the child's readiness for instruction. Physical and occupational therapists evaluate the child's neuromotor maturation, physical capabilities, balance, use of concurrent sensory stimuli, and movement patterns. Speech-language pathologists (SLPs) assess certain sensory characteristics—oral, neuromotor, qualitative, and quantitative characteristics of the child's receptive and expressive communication. Strengths, capabilities, and potential for development are also evaluated. Practitioners from other professional disciplines are trained to look at other aspects of the child's present levels of functioning and discern the probable potential for further development.

All professionals, each approaching his or her task from different perspectives based on training and experience, make decisions about a given child's status. They also make decisions as to whether interpretation of the data they have at their disposal suggests that the child's condition and behaviors represent one, or a combination, of the following possibilities:

- *Difference:* a condition or behavior that is somewhat unusual in certain circumstances but represents a variation of normal within the child's family, culture, or society (e.g., regional linguistic dialect patterns, short stature).
- *Delay:* a physical condition, state, or behavior having the potential to develop that is currently judged to be below expectations for the child's age, sex, or physical condition when measured against accepted norms or performance criteria. When no specific etiological cause for late onset of language has been identified, such children are often said to be *language delayed*. Readers should note that the term *developmental delay* is also used by some groups of professionals to mean that the child has and will continue to have, perhaps for a lifetime, the identified condition (e.g., "pervasive developmental delay," "cognitive delay" when used as a synonym for mental retardation).
- *Disorder:* a condition or behavior that impairs functional abilities in one or more areas of development (e.g., language disorder, autistic spectrum disorder). Some disorders can be remediated, whereas others require development of

compensatory skills, and still others can continue to exist despite all habilitative or rehabilitative efforts.

- *Deficit:* an identified absence or significant limitation in a specified physical attribute, function, or skill. Readers should note that the term *deficit* is used by some professionals in the same way *developmental delay* or *cognitive delay* are used by colleagues in other professional disciplines. Both terms may imply that there is a lifelong deficit in cognitive ability. Optimized functioning of the individual with that condition can occur with early intervention and continued specialized training, but there will always be a deficit. Proponents of using the alternate term *developmental delay* recognize the presence of cognitive limitations but assert that it is unkind and unwise to use terminology that implies there is little prospect for improved functional abilities among affected individuals. They note that ongoing development does occur in most cases, although it is likely to be limited in scope.
- *Disability:* a limitation in the ability to perform certain tasks in a typical manner (e.g., learning disability, language disability). The implication is that with proper assistance, alternative or adaptive methods can be employed to compensate for the condition that underlies the disability, allowing the affected individual to achieve a level of functional competence. CAUTION: Readers should note that *disability* is sometimes used, especially among nonprofessionals, interchangeably with the term *handicap*.
- *Handicap:* the degree to which an impaired condition or behavior prevents the affected person from engaging in life activities appropriate to others of the same age. What comprises a handicap for one person or situation may not do so for another. For example, unilateral vocal cord paralysis or developmental verbal dyspraxia would be a handicap for the respective purposes of singing or developing a "normal" speaking voice or articulation, but would not necessarily affect successful communication by alternative communication strategies or competent use of augmentative communication devices. Profound deafness, on the other hand, constitutes a continuing handicap across a variety of life situations for affected individuals.

The Goal: Promoting Functional Abilities of Infants and Toddlers

Functional abilities of the developing child are affected by many factors, including congenital (present at birth) and acquired conditions and disorders. Among the common problems encountered by the SLP in work with the infant-toddler population are those related to (1) disease processes, (2) conditions (e.g., cerebral palsy), (3) structural anomalies (e.g., craniofacial clefting), (4) syndromes (collections of symptoms that are identifiable with specific genetic, chromosomal, physical, or psychoneurological disorders), (5) sequences (a connected series of *conditions,* such as CHARGE sequence), (6) spectrum disorders (an array of *symptoms* related to a specifically diagnosed condition that can be predictive of a favorable prognosis or one that is less favorable, such as autistic spectrum disorder), and (7) physical or psychological trauma.

Some conditions with which infants are born or that develop in very early infancy can be identified by SLPs who are members of developmental care teams in neonatal nurseries. Many such conditions are complex and have serious consequences for the health and well-being of the infants who possess them, yet some of the very early symptoms or characteristics of the conditions appear simply as unusual vocal cry features, feeding difficulties, asymmetrical oral structures, or asymmetrical movements of the facial complex. Special training in assisting in the diagnosis and management of such conditions is imperative for practitioners in hospital and other health care settings that serve infants and young toddlers. However, general information about the conditions and knowledge of when referrals to specialists are indicated are essential for all SLPs who serve the pediatric population.

As was pointed out in Chapter 1, early intervention has the advantage of being applied at a time when the child's biological development is characterized by rapid proliferation of synaptic connections in the brain. Although that process does not overcome severe physical impairments (e.g., cerebral palsy) or correct anatomical anomalies (e.g., palatal clefts), it does optimize the neurophysiological ecological environment in which habilitation can occur.

In terms of language development, "[t]he differential growth of the cortex of the cerebral hemispheres is of vital importance for speech and language function because the majority of neural structures for communication are integrated there. The cortical association areas lag behind the development of the cortical receptor areas that are present and active at birth" (p. 257).[1] Further, as Love and Webb[1] point out,

> [A]t 1 year the normal child has a vocabulary of one or more word approximations, usually names for objects that have been seen and sometimes touched. This stage of language development requires the ability to mix neural information from the auditory, somesthetic, and visual association areas. The rapid growth of vocabulary in the second and third years of life may well be a correlate of the maturation of [the] significant posterior association area in the parietal lobe, which combines information from surrounding association areas (p. 258).

Because of the "plasticity" of the brain in the early years of life, when the very young child's brain is known to have been damaged, undamaged areas sometimes are capable of assuming the respective function(s) of the damaged area(s).[1,2] Hence, early maturation and growth of the brain itself work in favor of early-intervention efforts.

Appropriate early-intervention practices take into account environmental influences that support and are likely to promote positive developmental outcomes. Ideally, those practices are family focused, culturally sensitive, and specific to the child's needs.

The Concept of Prevention

As Wetherby and Prizant[3] pointed out,

> [E]arly identification of communication and language problems and appropriate intervention can prevent a number of difficulties that may be closely related to, and may possibly result from, early language and communication disorders. Although many questions remain regarding causal relationships, most investigators agree that infants and toddlers with communication delays or disorders are at high risk for the development of emotional and behavioral disorders (p. 290).

Prevention is a term that is often used in medical practices and other health care settings in a slightly different context than is usually applied by the general public. In the arena of health care, separate forms of prevention are recognized.

- *Primary prevention* is comprised of measures taken to prevent the occurrence of an undesirable outcome (e.g., genetic counseling that results in a couple's decision not to bear a child because the risk of a particular problem is considered too high).
- *Secondary prevention* consists of curing or ameliorating a problem that has occurred (e.g., surgical procedures employed to close a palatal cleft, install a cochlear implant, or clip a short lingual frenum; conducting speech-language therapy when full habilitation or rehabilitation is the goal).
- *Tertiary prevention* is reducing the negative effects of a given condition through treatment if amelioration of the condition is not possible (e.g., prescribing pharmacological products to reduce or eliminate seizures, conducting speech-language therapy when compensatory skills are the goal, fitting appropriate amplification devices to optimize hearing in the presence of a known hearing loss).

Screening, Evaluation, Diagnosis, and Assessment

The causes of problems in communicative development are sometimes identifiable but often are not. It is highly desirable that the causes, if they can be identified, be understood, because the treatment or management plans for a given condition can differ from appropriate plans for other conditions. For example, the management approach for a child with a profound hearing loss is different from the one used for a child whose hearing is known to be within normal limits. Likewise, a child diagnosed with a particular syndrome or spectrum disorder is likely to benefit from a treatment-management plan designed to address the functional components affected by the cluster of characteristics associated with the syndrome or sequence. For example, management options for a child diagnosed with autism are quite different from those designed to optimize communication function in a child diagnosed with Down syndrome or Usher syndrome. Targeted goals for treatment of children with certain rare syndromes (e.g., Beckwith-Wiedemann syndrome, Smith-Magenis syndrome, Smith-Lemli-Opitz syndrome) may best be attained by attending to specific aspects of oral language production in a planned sequence.[4]

Rubin[5] emphasized the importance of an accurate etiologic diagnosis:

... An accurate etiological diagnosis aids the understanding of pathological mechanisms and hence the prevention of specific conditions (e.g., congenital infections, perinatal asphyxia, lead toxicity) (p. 25).

Rubin supports the concept that an accurate diagnosis is also important to identifying and planning for implementation of appropriate medical, therapeutic, and educational management. He noted, however, that the process of obtaining an accurate diagnosis is not always easy, may take time, and may in fact be elusive.[5]

As pointed out above, terminology used in identifying children in need of further assessment varies across professional disciplines. Almost all practitioners agree that screening is the first level of identification. Screening can be formalized (i.e., specific protocols and criteria are applied to select a subgroup that meets the criteria for further assessment). Screening can also be informal (e.g., a family member or caregiver may sense that a child's behaviors or abilities are "different" from those of peers). Hearing screenings, cholesterol screenings, and lead-exposure screenings are common types of formal screenings with which almost everyone is familiar. Once a subgroup or individual of concern has been identified, the next level of investigation can involve assessment or evaluation of functional abilities or can move directly to the level of diagnosis.

A possible complication in arriving at a common understanding of the term *diagnosis* has to do with the level of confidence with which a particular diagnosis is invested. Technically, a diagnosis can be any one of the following: confirmed, differential, or definitive diagnosis (most reliable); presumptive diagnosis (highly probable on the basis of symptoms and testing conducted); and descriptive diagnosis (implies the presence of a specific condition or set of behaviors with a commonly used label without actually confirming its presence by scientific means). Each of the diagnostic levels has practical applications, but each also has certain limitations. For example, a confirmed or differential diagnosis meets criteria for a specific label (e.g., acquired immunodeficiency syndrome, recurrent respiratory papillomatosis, fragile X syndrome, cephaloceles, sensorineural hearing loss) but fails to delineate expectations for functional abilities of the individual child diagnosed with the condition or disease. Such a diagnosis, however, is associated with general expectations with respect to probable response levels, behaviors, and prognosis.

Generally speaking, it is worth the effort to get as refined a diagnosis as possible, so that the implications of the condition or disease are well understood and treatment and management plans can be appropriately designed. Additionally, early diagnosis is a strong protective factor for prevention of secondary disabilities that often ensue. Superneau's statement[6] in this regard could be applied to any disorder and not exclusively to fetal alcohol syndrome (FAS) and fetal alcohol effects (FAE): "The early and appropriate diagnosis of FAS and FAE should be made to enhance the long-term outcome and reduce the disabilities experienced by affected individuals and their families."[6,7]

It is possible that a definitive or differential diagnosis requires documentation of characteristics that emerge over a period of several months or years, because many conditions derive from a failure of development or a disruption in developmental processes that typically proceed in an orderly and predictable manner. Cerebral palsy and autism are two examples of conditions that become evident with the passage of time.

Assessment of conditions and functions, however, is an ongoing process. The process of ongoing assessment is crucial to the concepts of prevention and the benefits of early intervention. In fact, early intervention legislation requires frequent assessment of each child throughout the first 3 years of life. The recognition of atypical characteristics and functions as they emerge in the child's development can signal the need for specific management strategies to optimize development before a definitive diagnosis of a specific condition can be made. Assessment procedures and tools are discussed in Chapters 7 and 8.

There is a certain level of tension between proponents of the so-called *medical model* of viewing atypical development and proponents of the so-called *developmental model*. On the one hand, it is argued that the medical model is based on identifying "deficits" and labeling children with terms that have negative implications, thus increasing the difficulties with which such children and their families must contend. The developmental model, on the other hand, identifies strengths and needs at given points of development and hence provides a more positive approach that is "family friendly." In truth, both models are useful and need not be mutually exclusive. Parents can choose to disclose a diagnostic "label" or keep it confidential; some individuals with whom the family comes in contact have a negative reaction to a child who is "different," no matter how unfair that attitude may be. Insensitivity is impossible to avoid, but it is not universal. Practitioners should know both the array of causes of atypical development *and* be competent in assessing current and potential skills and methods of facilitating optimal outcomes. Such competencies require working in collaboration with families and members of the professional community. Tracking developmental outcomes across individuals and diagnostic groups is an important responsibility of professionals who work with the infant and toddler population.

Because the lives of increasing numbers of very small, very sick infants are being saved in neonatal care facilities, and because those children are being seen increasingly in early intervention practices and preschool settings, it is also important that their progress be monitored and documented carefully so that improved prognoses for children with like problems can be formulated for the future. The following sections of this chapter are devoted to exploring specific factors that can cause a child to have a delay or disorder in development of communication and how those factors are identified. Chapter 8 provides more detailed information about assessing common effects of those factors on early communicative development.

▼ CAUSES OF COMMUNICATIVE DISORDERS

Genetic and Chromosomal Aberrations

One method of discovering causes of disorders of human development is the application of knowledge in human genetics. Genetic and chromosomal problems associated with communicative disorders have become the focus of many professionals who specialize in the practice of medical speech pathology. Many, but not all, genetic and chromosomal problems are evident at or before birth and are often associated with a set of specific biological characteristics (phenotypes). Medical geneticists and SLPs have a natural alliance in following the course of infants and toddlers diagnosed with such disorders.

Willner[8] put it this way: "Recent advances in the molecular biology of embryogenesis and development have led to the identification of genes and mechanisms that when disrupted result in human malformation syndromes. Identification of these genes and their mutations permits accurate DNA diagnosis, genetic counseling, and prevention of recurrence, which are now integral to the up-to-date management of patients with craniofacial disorders." This writer suggests that the same is true of up-to-date management of patients with other forms of genetic disorders.

Because many children with chromosomal or genetic anomalies were doomed to early death until recent advances in medical technology improved the outlook, the literature on long-term outcomes for such children is limited and may, in fact, be unreliable in many instances. Now that more of these children are surviving and receiving early-intervention management from teams of professionals, it is becoming evident that the quality of life they can access, along with a more favorable outlook for developing functional abilities, can result in improved prognoses for many of them. Careful documentation of developmental outcomes among affected children is crucial to establishing more appropriate predictions of what other children diagnosed with the same disorders can achieve. Such information is critical to parental decision making and to the process of genetic counseling.

Congenital Anomalies, Syndromes, Sequences, and Spectrum Disorders

Chapter 3 provides detailed information about congenital syndromes and conditions associated with communicative disorders. It also includes a table showing common communicative disorders associated with recognized syndromes (see Table 3-5). Although the relative frequency of occurrence of all syndromes is quite small, a significant number of affected children are referred to communicative-disorders specialists. Bearing in mind that children with syndromes are first and foremost children who have the same needs of all children, those who are born with identified syndromes comprise a group whose treatment plans must address additional, and usually very specific, elements related to the characteristics of the specific syndrome(s) involved.

Recent discoveries have verified that chromosomal problems seen in affected individuals are somewhat variable even when the same chromosome is affected. This is so because the aberration on a given chromosome can occur at differing locations and can have different configurations (e.g., breaks, extra material, deletions, distortions), producing different effects. The important thing to remember is that not all persons with an identified chromosomal aberration have the same traits. Ongoing scientific research seeks to reveal specific sites with which particular traits are associated. Certain syndromes have already been "mapped." Clinical descriptions of characteristics and behaviors of individuals with such problems are urgently needed and are beginning to appear in the professional literature with increasing frequency.[9]

Other Diseases and Conditions Associated with Communicative Disorders

Acquired Diseases

Any disease that has the potential to affect cognition or central nervous system functioning has the potential to have an adverse effect on communicative development and function. Table 2-1 lists some of the more commonly encountered acquired diseases that can have a negative impact on communicative development.

Trauma

Infants and toddlers are subject to physical trauma from the prenatal period through all stages of development during childhood. Damage to the respiratory system, the central nervous system, and to anatomical structures of the speech mechanism can occur as a result of mechanical pressures experienced by the fetus

TABLE 2-1
Etiologies Associated With Communicative Delays and Disorders

Delays and Disorders	Etiologies
Allergies (especially those that are chronic and affect the respiratory system or mucosal tissues of the mouth, nose and throat)	Cytomegalovirus
	Encephalitis, meningitis
	Fetal alcohol effects
	Herpes
Asphyxia and extended or repeated episodes of hypoxia	Human immunodeficiency virus and acquired immunodeficiency syndrome
Chronic illnesses resulting in persistent depressed energy and attentional levels	Rh incompatibility (untreated)
	Rubella (German measles)
	Syphilis
Congenital or acquired infections, diseases, or conditions	Toxoplasmosis
Other diseases and anomalies of the speech mechanism	Choanal atresia
	Gastroesophageal reflux disease
	Laryngeal clefts (posterior or laryngotracheosophageal)
	Laryngeal papillomas
	Laryngeal stenosis or atresia
	Laryngeal stridor
	Laryngeal web (glottic or subglottic)
	Polyps
	Space-occupying oropharyngeal lesions (cephaloceles, macroglossia)
	Vocal fold nodules
	Vocal fold cysts
Physical anomalies (related to disorders of language)	Brain anomalies
	Agenesis of the corpus callosum
	Anencephaly
	Encephalocele
	Holoprosencephaly
	Hydrocephaly
	Intraventricular hemorrhage (especially Grades II–IV)
	Seizure disorders
	Stroke
	Other central nervous system anomalies and conditions (i.e., cerebral palsy, hypotonia [floppiness])
Physical injury and trauma	Accidents resulting in damage to physical mechanisms involved in understanding and producing language and speech
	Birth injuries resulting in damage to the recurrent laryngeal nerve (usually resolves with time)
	Congenital, perinatal, in later infancy, and early childhood
	Extended periods of intubation
	Injuries resulting from repeated intubation
	Radical surgical interventions required to treat injuries, diseases, and anomalies resulting in damage to mechanisms involved in understanding and producing speech and language
	Tracheostomy

Continued

TABLE 2-1
Etiologies Associated With Communicative Delays and Disorders —Cont'd

Delays and Disorders	Etiologies
Psychoemotional disorders (see Box 2-1)	Attentional disorders* • Attention deficit disorder (ADD) • Attention deficit hyperactivity disorder (ADHD) Autism spectrum disorder (ASD) Pervasive developmental disorder (PDD)
Sensory impairment	Hearing (congenital, acquired; conductive, sensorineural) Other sensory impairments (vision, balance, hyper- or hyposensitivity to sensory stimuli)
Side effects or reactions to drugs or sera	Allergies to components of the drug, suspension, or coating agents used in its delivery Ototoxic drugs Reactions to components of serum injections resulting in catastrophic effects
Syndromes	See Table 3-5 for comprehensive details

*Although these disorders are classified as psychogenic in the *Diagnostic and Statistical Manual* (4th ed.) and other standard references, evidence exists that these conditions are actually neurogenic.

in the womb, adverse effects of treatment designed to preserve life (e.g., use of ototoxic drugs), or unanticipated problems at the time of delivery (e.g., damage caused by surgical instruments). Other factors that can occur at any time include surgical trauma (e.g., removal of malignancies requiring resections of adjacent structures involved in speech production or language development, inadvertent severing of a branch of the vagus nerve during surgical procedures unrelated to the speech mechanism), mechanical trauma (e.g., gunshot wounds to crucial organs, shaken baby syndrome[10]), and other injuries incurred as a result of events such as near drowning, automobile accidents, and falls.

Infants and toddlers who require tracheostomies are of particular interest for a number of reasons. Simon and McGowen[11] stated that tracheostomies in infants can be indicated for babies who are ventilator dependent and who have subglottic stenosis (narrowing of the airway below the glottis), tracheomalacia (softening of the tracheal cartilage), neuromuscular disorders, congenital anomalies (e.g., craniofacial anomalies, laryngeal neoplasms, cardiac anomalies, croup), and epiglottitis (inflammation of the epiglottis). They observed that, "[t]he development of speech and language in the tracheostomized child has been found to be related to the time of cannulation. If the child receives a tracheostomy during the prelinguistic stage of development, speech and language therapy may be needed for both the establishment of a communication system and for early vocal production" (p. 1).[11]

Other types of trauma can lead to residual effects that impair speech or language development. This category includes such things as extensive scar tissue resulting from electrical burns to the oral structures (e.g., incurred when a child bites into a connected electrical cord), scar tissue residual to chemical burns (e.g., seen in children who swallow drain cleaners), and deleterious effects on the nervous system from exposure to heavy metals such as lead (which may be contained in paint chips ingested by children).

Regulatory, Emotional, and Mental Health Problems

Regulatory disorders in neonates are discussed in some detail in Chapter 5, but such problems are not limited to newborns. Children who are difficult to please and who seem "out of sorts" most of the time are exhibiting hypersensitivity to the requirements of adjusting to the demands of daily living and exhibiting that difficulty as behaviors that are described as "fussy" or "irritable." Such children may experience unsatisfactory interactions with their caregivers. DeGangi and colleagues[12] state that "children who are fussy, irritable, and demanding are extremely challenging for parents" (p. 115). They observed that responses to such a child's behaviors may take the form of understimulation by parents who fear risking new episodes of difficult interactions if their child seems to be content for a time. At the other end of the spectrum, parents of children who are extremely distractible may react by overstimulating (presenting too many toys or activities) under the assumption that the child can only be kept happy by catering to the child's apparent need for constant change.

Diagnosis of specific psychosocial or psychoemotional disorders is rare in children under the age of 3 years. However, a number of such problems have as part of their diagnostic criteria specified onset before age 3 years (e.g., autism). Clinical practitioners are encouraged to document persistent atypical behaviors in infants and toddlers that can lead to a subsequent diagnosis of attentional disorders, conduct disorders, and temperament and personality disorders, many of which have symptoms that appear in early childhood.

Post-traumatic stress disorder has been documented in children under the age of 3 years.[13–15] Such problems can manifest themselves as elective mutism and other types of speech problems that have a low rate of occurrence but are familiar to clinical practitioners (e.g., atypical stress, rate, fluency).

Landy and Peters[16] commented about young children who exhibit excessively aggressive behavior:

> Delays of development in these children may be due primarily to neurologic or physiologic problems or to attachment disorders resulting from previous interactional difficulties. These problems may lead to difficulties in interacting with others, delays in symbolization (such as language and pretend play), and failures in impulse control (p. 28).

The Hinks-Dellcrest Center, at which Landy serves as head of the Infant and Preschool Program, reported in 2002 that about half the children attending mental health clinics at their site have language impairments.[17]

Box 2-1 lists an array of psychoemotional disorders that can be associated with difficulties in communicative development.

▼ SINGLE AND MULTIPLE RISK FACTORS: THEIR ROLE IN DIAGNOSIS AND ASSESSMENT

Communicative disorders specialists must be aware of a variety of factors that place a child at risk for problems in developing speech and language. As Russell

Box 2-1
Psychoemotional Disorders Having Known or Potential Association With Communicative Development

Attachment disorders
Childhood disintegrative disorder
Emotional disorders resulting from maltreatment, abuse, or neglect
Oppositional defiant disorder
Post-traumatic stress disorder
Separation defiant disorder
Pervasive developmental disorder
Autism
Asperger syndrome
Landau-Kleffner syndrome
Pervasive developmental disorder, not otherwise specified

and Free[18] observed, for example, "[c]hildren exposed to potentially harmful substances ... during the vulnerable developmental period before birth often grow up in a childhood environment where the mother continues to abuse drugs and where there are limited mother-child interactions and learning experiences, placing the infant at both biological and environmental risk" (p. 181).

Preterm delivery *per se* is not a reliable predictor of developmental delays or disorders. However, preterm infants as a group, especially the subgroup in which neonatal complications are known to have occurred, are at risk for developmental difficulties. Hack and colleagues[19] observed that "neonatologists are saving 34% of infants of less than 751 g birth weight, 66% of those between 751 and 1000 g, 87% of those weighing 1001 to 1250 g, and 93% at 1251 to 1500 g. By obstetric measures of gestation, survival was 23% at 23 weeks, 34% at 24 weeks, and 54% at 25 weeks" (p. 587). Because many of these children develop severe intracranial abnormalities, it is estimated that 60% of those who do will have handicaps. Severe handicaps are found among 50% of infants born at 23 weeks, 38% of those born at 24 weeks, and 8% for those born at 25 weeks.[20] Ruff and Lawson[21] observed that preterm babies with low birth weight observed at play at 9 months and 24 months exhibited less focused attention, lower levels of response to novel objects, and less reactivity than their full-term peers. They concluded that:

> [t]hese data suggest that measures of attention may be important indicators of a child's present and future functioning. A child who engages in relatively little focused attention and exploration of objects in the latter half of the first year may learn less about objects and their properties and at the same time develop fewer strategies for gathering more information. The consequences could be serious for developing knowledge of the world and for emerging language (p. 122).[21]

Although some research (see Chapter 5 for full discussion) suggests that infants born preterm who suffer from bronchopulmonary dysplasia (BPD) are likely to have delayed or disordered language development, others question that conclusion. Lewis and colleagues[22] conclude that although children with BPD are at risk for poor language outcome, it is the condition in combination with other factors (gestional age, birth weight, neurological risk, and septicemia) that magnifies the risk for language disorders present at age 8 years.

Hack and colleagues[23] compared a group of 242 very low birth weight (VLBW) survivors with a control group who had normal birth weights and found that only 74% of the VLBW group had graduated from high school (vs. 83% of controls); VLBW survivors had lower mean I.Q. scores (87 vs. 92). Neurosensory impairments were 10% (vs. less than 1% for controls). They concluded that "(e)ducational disadvantage associated with VLBW persists into early adulthood" (p. 149).

In another study, Hack and colleagues[24] studied a group of 221 extremely low birth weight (ELBW) survivors at age 20 months. All had a history of admission to a tertiary level neonatal intensive care unit at a university hospital. The researchers found that 24% of the children had major neurosensory abnormalities, including cerebral palsy, deafness, and blindness. Neurodevelopmental impairment was present in 48% of the group (p. 725).

In their 1994 study, Hack and colleagues[25] compared 68 school-age children with VLBW (<750 g) to 65 low birth weight (LBW = 750–1499 g) and 61 children born at term (normal birth weight). The VLBW group "were inferior to both comparison groups in cognitive ability, psychomotor skills and academic achievement." They also had more behavioral problems and problems with attention. Of particular note were the higher rates of mental retardation: 21% (vs. 8% and 2% for the respective control groups) and cerebral palsy: 9% (vs. 8% and 2%). Their conclusion: "Children with birthweights under 750 g who survive represent a subgroup of very-low-birth-weight children who are at high risk for neurobehavioral dysfunction and poor school performance" (p. 753).

Neonatal predictors of school-based services used by neonatal intensive care unit (NICU) graduates at school age were studied by Lindeke and colleagues.[26] They noted that their study was prompted in part by the Lindeke study published in 1998 in which a "two-fold increase in special services use at school entry compared to preschool services use" was documented. The 2001 study, which excluded children with chromosomal or congenital anomalies, metabolic disorders, or who had been in the NICU for less than 5 days, concluded that the neurobehavioral risk score (NBRS), a sum of illness factors related to brain damage, and length of stay in the NICU were positively related to later need for school-based services among their subjects.

The presence of one or more risk factors is not in and of itself predictive of atypical communicative development but indicates to the practitioner that the child may have a greater likelihood than other children of experiencing such difficulties. Even the indirect effects of some conditions, in areas seemingly unrelated to communication skills, can contribute to the confounding of atypical language and speech development. For example, lack of normal childhood experiences, which can be related to unusual child-rearing practices, can affect vocabulary acquisition or the child's level of curiosity, thus discouraging attempts to communicate. A family's overprotectiveness at one extreme or neglect at the other can discourage the child's desire to communicate. Impaired development of fine-motor skills, which are usually thought of as the province of occupational therapy, can have a counterpart in developmental dyspraxia of speech, a condition related to delayed and disordered speech in young children.

The SLP must be sensitive to all possible implications of information provided by the family or other knowledgeable informants when the case history is provided.

TABLE 2-2
Overview of Causes of Communicative Disorders in Infants and Toddlers

Category and Onset	Examples of Diagnoses	Comment
Inherited disorders and syndromes *Time of onset:* conception	Down syndrome Goldenhar syndrome Usher syndrome	See Chapter 3 for detailed discussion.
Acquired diseases and disorders *Time of onset:* can occur pre-, peri-, or postnatally	Fetal alcohol syndrome Encephalitis Toxoplasmosis Papillomatosis Hearing loss resulting from ototoxic drugs	This category covers a broad range of viral, bacterial, and teratogenic etiologies.
Disruptions of growth in utero producing anomalies of structures or systems crucial to language and speech development *Time of onset:* prenatal	Certain forms of facial clefting Branchial arch deformities Anencephaly Laryngeal stridor Laryngeal web	Effects can range from conditions not clinically significant regarding communication (e.g., amniotic band syndrome affecting an extremity) to those that are crucial to communication development.
Sensory impairments *Time of onset:* usually prenatal but can occur in peri- or postnatal periods	Congenital or acquired hearing loss Multiple sensory impairments Extreme hyper- or hypo-sensitivity	Sensory impairments can result from congenital conditions or be acquired as a result of trauma, illness, or drug reactions.
Physical injury and trauma associated with conditions related to communicative development *Time of onset:* can occur pre-, peri-, or postnatally	Cerebral palsy Shaken baby syndrome Prolonged intubation Chemical burns affecting the speech mechanism Paresis or paralysis of one or both vocal cords	Physical injury and trauma can occur accidentally or result from surgical procedures or intentional physical abuse.
Severe or prolonged emotional trauma *Time of onset:* postnatal	Post-traumatic stress disorder Child abuse and neglect	The prevalence of child neglect and abuse is reportedly higher among children with developmental delays.
Disorders associated with global developmental delays and disorders *Time of onset:* prenatal or postnatal	Lead poisoning Certain metabolic disorders Failure to thrive	This category encompasses a wide range of possible problems.
Psychogenic disorders *Time of onset:* can be present but undetected at birth or appear in early childhood	Autism Pervasive developmental disorder not otherwise specified Childhood disintegrative disorder	Differential diagnosis is essential to selection of appropriate treatment options.

TABLE 2-2
Overview of Causes of Communicative Disorders in Infants and Toddlers—Cont'd

Category and Onset	Example of Diagnoses	Comment
Delays and disorders arising from socioenvironmental factors *Time of onset:* variable	Extreme poverty coupled with low maternal educational level Extreme isolation and lack of stimulation	The factors noted have multiple effects that can involve poor nutrition and housing, immediate surroundings in which toxic particles are plentiful, lack of access to basic health care with consequent complications from common childhood diseases, lack of availability of appropriate speech-language models, and atypical child-rearing practices.
Other neurophysiologic factors known to have a high co-occurrence of language development disorders *Time of onset:* variable	Attention deficit hyperactivity disorder Central auditory processing disorder Sensory integration disorder Learning disability	Many of the neurophysiologic mechanisms underlying these disorders are thought to be common to those underlying communicative functions. The effects of variable attention or atypical learning styles are likely to be disruptive of normal acquisition of selected language functions.

It is sometimes the case that a combination of factors, rather than a single element, is the cause of a communication delay or disorder. Risk factors may reflect circumstances that were once operative in the child's life but no longer exist or, conversely, may be ongoing influences that may or may not be amenable to modification as part of the therapy program. An overview of causes of communicative disorders in infants and toddlers is provided in Table 2-2.

Potential etiologies associated with specific conditions are shown in Table 2-3. Obviously the process of differential diagnosis dictates the direction of appropriate management, including referral and treatment options.

If atypical development is displayed, professionals are expected to untangle the "mysteries" with which they are presented when a family entrusts their child to the professionals' care. In addition to comparing the child's development to normative expectations, the SLP considers at least two other sources of information: (1) reports from others who have cared for the child and family, and (2) completion of a thorough case history that explores an array of information the SLP finds indispensable to understanding a given child's situation. Examples of formats for

TABLE 2-3
Communicative Disorders and Related Conditions

Condition	Occurrence	Variable Effects
Speech or language impairments	20.8% of disabled school-age children have speech or language impairments. 3%-10% of the general population have speech or language impairments.	Misarticulation Disorders of phonation Fluency disorders Receptive and expressive language disorders Occurences shown are for primary speech or language disorders; such disorders often occur as part of other conditions and syndromes.
Hearing impairments	1:1000 children is born with congenital deafness. Up to 5% of children from 0-18 years of age have hearing impairments. 1.3% of disabled 6-21 year olds have hearing loss. 1% of the general population are affected; 0.2% have severe losses.	Conductive hearing loss Sensorineural hearing loss Mixed hearing loss Deafness Condition can be acquired or congenital. Delayed or disordered speech and language commonly occur.
Developmental delay	2%-5% of children under the age of 5 years have developmental delay.	Delays are frequently observed in the area of communication development in isolation or in combination with generalized delays across modalities.
Autism	15:10,000 children are affected. 0.5% of disabled 6-21 year olds are affected. Autism affects 0.5% of the population when combined with figures for pervasive developmental disorder.	Severely impaired language Idiosyncratic behaviors Disorders of social interaction
Multiple disabilities	1.8% of disabled 6-21 year olds have multiple disabilities.	Many multiple disabilities involve communicative disorders as a feature.
Traumatic brain injury	0.1% of disabled 6-21 year olds have traumatic brain injury.	Many children with traumatic brain injury experience communication problems.
Specific learning disabilities	51.1% of disabled 6-21 year olds have specific learning disabilities. 70%-80% of learning-disabled children have language disorders.	Note that the federal definition of dyslexia includes any problem with reading, writing, listening, or speaking.

▼
▼
TABLE 2-3
Communicative Disorders and Related Conditions—Cont'd

Condition	Occurrence	Variable Effects
Attention deficit disorder	2.2% of disabled 6-21 year olds have attention deficit disorder.	A large number of children with attentional disorders also have language delays and disorders. Attention deficit hyperactivity disorder can be diagnosed in some children before the age 3 years.
Cerebral palsy	3%-7% of all live births have cerebral palsy. 0.5% of the general population are affected.	Cerebral palsy is diagnosed before the age of 3 years. Up to 50% of children with cerebral palsy have communicative disorders.

documenting more detailed or supplementary case-history information specific to identifying risk factors and family histories that are useful in determining when to refer families for genetic consultations are provided in Appendix A.

The potential for delayed or disordered communicative development inferred from the presence of single or multiple risk factors must be ascertained. Practitioners take into account prenatal, perinatal, and postnatal events and conditions; family history; environmental risks and adverse societal conditions; infant temperament and capacity for self-regulation regarding formation of attachments; and the emotional stability of the child. Reliable conclusions can be drawn only after balancing the known risks with known protective factors such as family stability, a secure and nurturing environment, physical health, cognitive ability, and emotional health.[27]

It is not always possible to obtain a confirmed diagnosis, especially in very young children. In such cases, it is the presence or absence of one or more risk factors that may lead the practitioner in the direction of a presumptive diagnosis, on which the selection of management or intervention strategies is based. In many situations, it is essential that a team of professionals work alongside the parents in identifying the parameters of the problem(s) at hand and in devising optimal care and management plans. Chapter 4 addresses the concept of teams and processes of effective team operations.

▼ REFERENCES

1. Love RJ, Webb WG: *Neurology for the speech-language pathologist*, ed 3, Boston, 1996, Butterworth-Heinemann.
2. Fox N, Leavitt L, Warhol J: *The role of early experience in infant development*, St. Louis, 2000, Johnson & Johnson Pediatric Institute.
3. Wetherby AM, Prizant BM: Toward earlier identification of communication and language problems in infants and young children. In Meisels SJ, Fenichel E, editors: *New visions for the developmental assessment for infants, toddlers, and young children*, Washington, DC, 1993, Zero to Three/National Center for Infants, Toddlers, and Families, p 289.

4. Solomon BI, Sonies BC: *Oral-motor, speech and swallowing functions in three rare genetic syndromes.* Seminar presentation at the 2001 ASHA Conference, New Orleans, Nov 16, 2001.
5. Rubin IL: Etiology of developmental disabilities, *Infant Young Child* 3:25–32, 1990.
6. Superneau D: *Fetal alcohol syndrome and fetal alcohol effects: clues to detection and behavioral implications.* Presentation at the Contemporary Forums Conference on The Child with Special Needs, New Orleans, April 1997.
7. Hymbaugh K: Data analysis: fetal alcohol syndrome surveillance network, *MMWR* 51:433–435, 2002.
8. Willner JP: Genetic evaluation and counseling in head and neck syndromes. In Rothschild MA, editor: Syndromic and other congenital anomalies of the head and neck, *Otolaryngol Clin North Am* 33(6):1159–1170, 2001.
9. Weistuch L, Schiff-Myers NB: Research note: chromosomal translocation in a child with SLI and apraxia, *J Speech Hear Res* 39:668, 1996.
10. Committee on Child Abuse and Neglect, American Academy of Pediatrics: Shaken baby syndrome: rotational cranial injuries—technical report, *Pediatrics* 108(1):206–210, 2001.
11. Simon BM, McGowan JS: Tracheostomy in young children: implications for assessment and treatment of communication and feeding disorders, *Infant Young Child* 1:1–9, 1989.
12. DeGangi GA, Craft P, Castellan J: Treatment of sensory, emotional, and attentional problems in regulatory disordered infants: parts 1 and 2, *Infant Young Child* 3(3):1–8, 9–19, 1991.
13. Zeanah CH: The assessment and treatment of infants and toddlers exposed to violence. In Osofsky JD, Fenichel E, editors: *Caring for infants and toddlers in violent environments: hurt, healing, and hope,* Arlington, Va, 1994, Zero to Three/National Center for Clinical Infant Programs, p 29.
14. Zeanah CH, Boris N, Scheeringa M: Psychopathology in infancy, *J Child Psychol Psychiatry* 38:81, 1997.
15. Zeanah CH: *Disorders of attachment.* Paper presented at the Contemporary Forums Conference on The Child with Special Needs, New Orleans, April 1997.
16. Landy S, Peters RD: Identifying and treating aggressive preschoolers, *Infant Young Child* 3:24–38, 1990.
17. Hinks-Dellcrest Center of Toronto: Research agenda statement of the clinical programs of the Hinks-Dellcrest Center of Toronto. Available at: http://www.hincksdellcrest.org.
18. Russell FF, Free TA: Early intervention for infants and toddlers with prenatal drug exposure, *Infant Young Child* 3(4):78–85, 1992.
19. Hack M et al: Very low birth weight outcomes of the National Institute of Child Health and Human Development Neonatal Network, *Pediatrics* 87:587, 1991.
20. Allen M, Donohue P, Dusman A: The limit of viability: neonatal outcome of infants born at 22–25 weeks gestation, *N Engl J Med* 329:1597, 1993.
21. Ruff HA, Lawson KR: Assessment of infants' attention during play with objects. In Schaefer CE, Gitlin K, Sandgrund A, editors: *Play diagnosis and assessment*, New York, 1991, Wiley, p 115.
22. Lewis BA et al: *Predictors of speech-language outcomes in VLBW and BPD children.* Presentation at the 2001 ASHA Conference, New Orleans, La, Nov 16, 2001.
23. Hack M et al: Outcomes in young adulthood for very-low-birth-weight infants, *N Engl J Med* 346(3):249-157, 2002.
24. Hack M et al: Neurodevelopment and predictors of outcomes of children with birth weights of less than 1000 g: 1992-1995, *Arch Pediatr Adolesc Med* 154(7):725–731, 2000.
25. Hack M et al: School-age outcomes in children with birth weights under 750 g, *N Engl J Med* 22;331(12):753–759, 1994.
26. Lindeke L et al: Neonatal predictors of school-based services used by NICU graduates at school age, *Matern Child Nurs* 27(1):41–46, 2002.
27. Landy S, Tan KK: *Understanding the contribution of multiple risk factors on child development at various ages.* Working Paper of the Applied Research Branch Strategic Policy, Human Resources Development Canada, Quebec, Oct 1998.

CHAPTER 3

SELECTED MEDICAL ASPECTS OF COMMUNICATION DISORDERS

Theodore F. Thurmon
Suzanne G. Thurmon

The medical aspects of communication disorders can be either acquired or congenital in nature. In both categories, it is necessary to use testing to establish the presence of speech and language deficits and to assess capabilities. Deficits and capabilities can vary widely within diagnostic categories. Acquired disorders usually result from injury (e.g., trauma, infection, toxins). Their mechanisms can be better understood when it is possible to confer with the physician who evaluated or treated the injury.

Focal lesions of the central nervous system, peripheral nerves, and the organs of articulation can produce specific speech and language disorders (Figure 3-1). It is easy to see how trauma or infection can destroy any of these structures, but some toxins have focal effects also. Aminoglycoside antibiotics (e.g., gentamicin, kanamycin, neomycin, streptomycin, tobramycin) have a specific eighth nerve toxicity in persons who are genetically predisposed to this effect. The cochlea and retina are exquisitely sensitive to anoxia and noxious agents. Heritable aberrant development of the perisylvian speech and language areas is seen in persistent developmental stuttering.[1]

Asphyxia, such as that which complicates some births, also produces a cognitive defect because of general brain injury. Many noxious agents also result in generalized brain injury. Equivalent degrees of brain malfunction can also result from poor brain formation or microcephaly, which is typical of Down syndrome and a number of other congenital disorders. Congenital microcephaly in progeny is the most frequently identified result of consanguineous matings in population isolates. Consanguineous mating means reproduction by a man and a woman who are relatives. Varying degrees of unusual brain development is seen in most persons who have cleft lip/palate.[2] When severe, it may affect cognition.

Locations	Levels: Structures. Symptomatology.

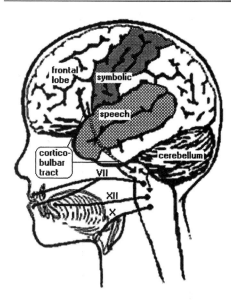

Level 5: Frontal lobes. Stuttering.

Level 4: Temporoparietal cortex.
Expressive and receptive
aphasia.

Level 3: Cerebellum. Broken,
monotone speech.

Level 2: Corticobulbar tract. Poorly
coordinated speech.

Level 1: Cranial nerves VII, X, XII.
Dysarthria, distortion.

▼ **Figure 3-1**   Locations of neurological lesions and resulting speech and language disorders. (Modified from Bakes FP: Chapter 14, Speech, language, and hearing. In Falkner F, editor: *Human development*, Philadelphia, 1996, WB Saunders.)

Congenital means that a disorder is present at birth but not due to events complicating the birth. Congenital disorders are the focus of this section. Although present, such disorders may not be noticed at birth but may become evident as the child grows older. These various disorders have little in common and can be understood only through study of the individual disorders.

▼ EFFECTS OF TERATOGENS

Congenital disorders are usually heritable, though, in rare cases, an injury to the developing fetus can result in a congenital disorder. Fetal injury, caused by teratogens, is much less frequent than is commonly thought. Few pregnancies pass uneventfully, but the events rarely harm the fetus. That fact, combined with the difficulties of diagnosing heritable causes, leads to the frequent erroneous assumption of acquired disease or injury. There is also a time-honored tendency at all levels of society to turn to fables to explain our undesirable features.[3] The very word *teratogen* derives from a Greek term for importunate actions of the gods.

Table 3-1 is a list of known teratogens and their effects. Most of them must be delivered directly to the fetus in large doses in the first 10 weeks of gestation if ill effects are to be realized. When this occurs, the degree of affectation of the fetus can vary because of heritable differences in defense mechanisms of the fetus (i.e., the same dose can produce severe defects in some fetuses and little or no effect in others). *There is a potential for speech and language disorders in all patients who have visible effects of teratogens.*

TABLE 3-1
Currently Characterized Human Teratogens

Medications

Direct Effects (same as postnatal)	Teratogenic Effects (continued)
Dependency-inducing drugs • Withdrawal	**Cocaine** • Limb, heart and neural tube defects
Hormones and antihormones • Endocrine effects: developmental in fetus also	**Fluconazole** • Craniofacial and skeletal anomalies
Streptomycin, daraprim, quinine • Deafness	**Hydantoins** • Wide face, nail hypoplasia, fingertip hypoplasia
Tetracyclines • Dental malformation	**Lithium** • Ebstein anomaly of heart
Obstetric drugs • Fetus more sensitive	**Methyl mercury** • Deafness, blindness, paralysis
Delayed Effects	**Penicillamine** • Skin hyperelastosis
Diethylstilbestrol • Genital metaplasia	**Smoking** • Low birth weight
Teratogenic Effects	**Trimethadione** • V-shaped eyebrows, dental and palatal anomalies
Poor fetal growth and development are common to all	**Thalidomide** • Phocomelia, heart malformation, deafness
Alcohol • Blepharophimosis, faint philtrum	**Valproic acid** • Brachycephaly, microstomia, spina bifida
Aminopterin • Dwarfism, hypoplastic cranium	**Vitamin A cogeners (retinoic acid)** • Microtia, clefts, brain anomalies
Anticoagulants • Stippled epiphyses, hypoplastic nose	
Carbamazepine • Up-slanting eyes, short nose, nail hypoplasia	

Infections

Maternal Infections	Fetal Infections
Defects result from focal thrombotic vascular occlusions in the fetus. Purulent infections Viral infections Amnionitis	Low birth weight, vision and hearing defects, mental retardation are common to all. Cytomegalovirus Rubella Syphilis Toxoplasmosis Varicella

Continued

TABLE 3-1
Currently Characterized Human Teratogens—Cont'd

Maternal Disorders	
Diabetes mellitus • Conotruncal defects, caudal regression	Myasthenia gravis • Newborn myasthenia
Hypertension • Low birth weight, microcephaly, PDA	Myotonic dystrophy • Arthrogryposis, mental retardation

Hyperthermia
• Arthrogryposis, low birth weight,
  neural tube defect
	Phenylketonuria
	• Microcephaly, dwarfism, prominent
	  mid-face

Malnutrition • Low birth weight	Twinning • Disruption, sirenomelia, exstrophy of cloaca

Hazardous Procedures and Trauma	
Maternal Trauma and Surgical *Complications*	*Direct Fetal Trauma*

Fetal cerebral blood flow cessation causes
  defects.
Maternal hypotension
Maternal hypoxia
	Hypertonic intravenous contrast material
	• Focal thrombotic vascular occlusions
	
	X-ray (therapeutic or catastrophic, not
	  diagnostic)
	• Microcephaly, eye and genital
	  malformation

From Thurmon TF: *A comprehensive primer on medical genetics,* New York, 1999, Parthenon Publishing Group.

    The impact of a teratogenic disorder on speech and language results either from damage to anatomic structures that are important to speech production and language development or from neurologic damage. Teratogens usually damage multiple areas at once, producing syndromes (*syn* = together, *drome* = run), in which anomalies of multiple structures are observed together. Single genes may also cause syndromes if they affect the development or function of multiple organs or body structures. Important remarks about syndromes follow the Common Heritable Anomalies section below.

    Fetal injury should not be accepted as the cause of a congenital disorder, except when there is forthright documentation of the actual injury. For example, the inherited disorder chorioretinal cerebral dysplasia[4] so closely mimics congenital toxoplasmosis that these disorders cannot be differentiated without accurate serologic testing. *Nearly every other teratogenic disorder also has a genetic equivalent.* This may seem to be of little consequence to the speech and language therapist, but greater comprehension of a problem comes from the understanding of its etiology. Assumptions about causation can be sharpened also. Hearing impairment arising from congenital toxoplasmosis infection is often said to be common; however, studies based on serologic diagnosis disclose that only about 2 of 1000 newborns with serologic evidence of congenital toxoplasmosis infection have congenital hearing impairment.[5] In contrast, careful evaluation of families of cases of newborns with congenital hearing impairment discloses a heritable cause in at least 50%.[6]

▼ CHROMOSOME ABNORMALITIES

Chromosome 21 trisomy is associated with maternal age. Some other chromosome abnormalities are also, but the causes of most of them are not known. Mechanisms that cause them experimentally do not appear to cause actual cases. Some result from segregation of a chromosome aberration in a parent (carrier), and subsequent conceptuses of that parent have a high risk of related chromosome abnormalities.

Large numbers of genes of various types are duplicated or deleted in chromosome abnormalities, but the exact manner of production of the phenotypes is not known. Certain features are common: Poor growth and development, communicative disorders, and multiple dysmorphic features. The evaluation of a patient with these features should always include a chromosome analysis.

Typical syndromes are associated with many chromosome abnormalities. The better known ones include autosomal trisomies (chromosomes 13, 18, and 21), Turner syndrome (monosomy of the X chromosome), and the cri-du-chat syndrome (deletion of the short arm of chromosome 5). Trisomies of the sex chromosomes (XXX, XXY, and XYY) are among the more common chromosome abnormalities but are difficult to recognize because their features are subtler. They are often discovered during evaluation of behavioral disorders in older children and adults.

▼ COMMON HERITABLE ANOMALIES

A number of heritable anomalies that affect speech and language development are much more common than teratogenic disorders. They are most frequently found as isolated defects in an otherwise normal person (nonsyndromic). These common heritable anomalies occur even more frequently among relatives of affected persons than in the general population; in fact, the frequency of such an anomaly among immediate family members is the square root of the population frequency.[7] Extensions of that mathematical relationship have developed the theory of polygenic inheritance. This theory holds that some traits are caused by the total effects of all genes and all environmental factors. The effects must be strong enough to produce a degree of the trait that can be perceived. There are gradations in the strengths of the effects above that level, so the trait has gradations from mild to severe. Though polygenic inheritance remains a theory, it allows differentiation from other etiologies and prediction of frequency with which a given disorder may occur in relatives. Figure 3-2 and Table 3-2 illustrate that concept.

Common heritable anomalies can affect speech and language functions through either anatomic or neurologic aberrations. Clefts of the lip or palate interfere with articulation and resonance. The same primordial structures of the embryo contribute to formation of both the heart and the organs of articulation. Hence, cleft palate and high-arched palate are often associated with heart malformation, as are middle- and inner-ear anomalies, retrognathia, glossoptosis, and laryngeal hypoplasia, any occurrence of which can adversely affect speech. Members of the immediate family may have similar disorders that are clinically evident. However, a more insidious problem is that parents may instead have milder forms such as velopharyngeal incompetence and may thus prove to be poor role models for speech development (i.e., an affected child's speech defect may be in part a learned pattern).

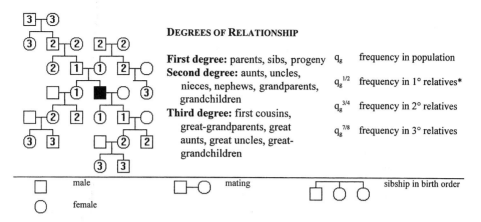

DEGREES OF RELATIONSHIP

First degree: parents, sibs, progeny q_g frequency in population

Second degree: aunts, uncles, nieces, nephews, grandparents, grandchildren $q_g^{1/2}$ frequency in 1° relatives*

 $q_g^{3/4}$ frequency in 2° relatives

Third degree: first cousins, great-grandparents, great aunts, great uncles, great-grandchildren $q_g^{7/8}$ frequency in 3° relatives

□ male   □—○ mating   sibship in birth order

○ female

▼ **Figure 3-2**   Calculation of frequencies of a polygenic disorder among relatives of a patient. The patient is represented by the darkened symbol. Numbers in the symbols represent degrees of relationships.* The notation is in fractional exponents, for example, $q_g^{1/2} = \sqrt[2]{q_g}$. A frequency is a fraction; a fractional exponent of a fraction has a larger numerical value: If frequency is 1 in 10, or 0.1, the square root is 0.32, or 1 in 3. (Modified from Thurmon TF: *A comprehensive primer on medical genetics*, New York, 1999, Parthenon Publishing Group.)

Webs, clefts, atresia and stenosis of the larynx occur as features of syndromes. The first three also occur as isolated heritable traits. These are important problems as the severe cases can threaten the life of the newborn and the mild cases can lead to permanent lung damage as well as significant speech problems ranging from hoarseness through weak voice to aphonia. Diagnosis is by visualization and usually requires the services of an otolaryngologist.

TABLE 3-2
Observed Frequencies of Polygenic Disorders Among Relatives

	NORMAL PARENTS		AFFECTED PARENT	
Disorder	**Population Frequency**	**Risk of Second Affected Child**	**Risk of an Affected Child**	**Risk of Second Affected Child**
Cleft of lip or palate	0.1%	2%	NA	NA
Bilateral	NA	6%	NA	NA
Heart malformations	0.5%	2% (same type)	14% (if mother)	NA
Additional risk	NA	4% (other type)	NA	NA
Neutral tube defects				
U.S.	0.1%	3.2%	4%	8%
U.K.	0.3%	5%	NA	NA

Modified from Carter CO: Multifactorial genetic disease. In McKusick VA, Claiborne R, editors: *Medical genetics,* New York, 1973, Hospital Practice Publishers.
NA, Statistically significant data are not available.

The neural tube is an embryonic structure that, when projected onto the completely formed human, extends from the glabella at the nasal root to the coccyx at the base of the spine. The central nervous system and associated bony structures derive from the neural tube. Well-known anomalies of the neural tube include anencephaly, encephalocele, and myelomeningocele (spina bifida). Although these may appear to be localized, there is, in truth, aberrant development throughout the nervous system, and speech production and language development are often affected.

The tangible nature of these common heritable anomalies has facilitated the confirmation of their heritability. However, development of speech and language appears to also be heritable in the same manner (i.e., polygenic).[8] Well-known congenital disorders of speech and language, when occurring in an otherwise normal person, also affect family members in frequencies similar to those of the common heritable anomalies.[9] As with the common heritable anomalies, occurrence of a speech and language disorder in a parent complicates therapy. The spectrum of pervasive developmental disorder-autism-Asperger syndrome occurs in families at the frequencies expected of polygenic disorders. Members of the immediate family who do not fall into the spectrum do tend toward similar speech and psychologic disorders.

Approximately 5 of 1,000 children have isolated, nonsyndromic, congenital mental deficiency (simple familial mental retardation) that is also polygenic.[4] Language deficit is the most significant communication problem among those children, and those with very poor mental functions may exhibit poor articulation skills as well. As with the common heritable anomalies, parents may have either the same or milder degrees of affectation that can contribute to learned speech aberrations and can lead to compliance problems in continuing therapy. Cultural language differences, also familial but not heritable, can coexist with these developmental disorders and confuse the diagnosis. Careful neurologic and developmental assessment may be required for differentiation.

▼ IS IT AN ISOLATED PROBLEM OR IS IT PART OF A SYNDROME?

A major pitfall to the understanding of congenital disorders is the fact that, although they usually occur as isolated problems in otherwise normal persons, they are also found as a feature of various syndromes in other persons. For example, about half of cases of heritable hearing impairment have a syndrome instead of an isolated deficit.[6] Syndromes can have diverse causes, as well as many features other than those associated with speech and language impairment, so that all patients cannot be approached in the same way. Table 3-3 compares frequencies of isolated versus syndromic anomalies.

In general, persons with syndromes have more limited potentials than do persons with isolated defects. Some features of the syndromes can limit their ability to respond to speech and language therapy. Management requires a multidisciplinary approach. The practical difficulty of securing and coordinating multidisciplinary management is another limiting factor. Although some of the syndromes can be recognized on sight, diagnosis usually requires the services of an experienced physician such as a medical geneticist or a dysmorphologist. Table 3-4 illustrates the breadth of issues to be considered.

TABLE 3-3
Isolated Versus Syndromic Forms of Common Anomalies

Disorder	Isolated	Syndromic
Cleft lip	88%	12%
Cleft palate	60%	40%
Heart malformation	75%	25% (half are chromosomal)
Neural tube defects	90%	10%

Modified from Thurmon TF: *A comprehensive primer on medical genetics*, New York, 1999, Parthenon Publishing Group.

TABLE 3-4
Examples of Syndromes Associated With Neural Tube Defects

Syndrome	Findings	Etiology
Goldenhar syndrome	Hemifacial microsomia, preauricular tags, epibulbar dermoid, microtia, hemivertebrae	Polygenic
Chromosome 18 trisomy	Gestational dwarfism, microcephaly, prominent occiput, small ears, small face, short sternum, overlap of index finger onto middle finger and little finger onto ring finger, contractures of hips and fingers, septal heart malformations	Chromosomal
Fetal valproate syndrome	Fetal flow heart malformations, neural tube defects, telecanthus, short nose, small mouth, long fingers	Teratogenic

Modified from Jones KL: *Smith's recognizable patterns of human malformation*, ed 4, Philadelphia, 1988, Saunders.

▼ MENDELIAN DISORDERS

Mendelian disorders are those heritable disorders that have discrete inheritance (i.e., dominant, recessive, X-linked). The term *discrete* has a mathematical basis. It means that a person either has the gene or does not have the gene, and there are no gradations. Figures 3-3 through 3-6 illustrate Mendelian inheritance patterns.[6]

A number of Mendelian disorders (about 150 are known) produce speech and language deficits, and all are rare. They range from anatomic abnormalities through neurologic aberrations to specific disorders of speech and language. Some are isolated abnormalities, but most are syndromes. The best guide to Mendelian disorders is the encyclopedic publication by McKusick[4] (Internet address: http://www3.ncbi.nlm.nih.gov/Omim/). The isolated disorders provide insight

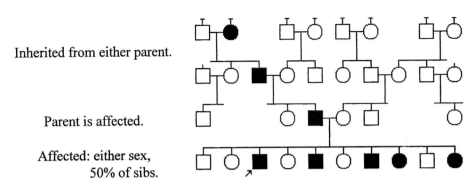

Inherited from either parent.

Parent is affected.

Affected: either sex,
50% of sibs.

▼ **Figure 3-3** Autosomal dominant inheritance.

into the genetic basis of speech and hearing, since a normal congener must exist for each abnormal gene identified.

A large family study of children with specific language impairment, not accompanied by any disorder, associated the problem with a locus on chromosome 13q21. Data were most consistent with autosomal recessive inheritance but could not rule out dominant inheritance with variable penetrance. The causative gene has not yet been identified within the locus. A single nucleotide G-to-A transition in exon 14 of the FOXP2 gene on chromosome 7q31 causes an autosomal dominant disorder known as speech and language disorder with orofacial dyspraxia, characterized by an inability to generate syntactic rules for tense, number, and gender. Older studies indicated that a gene for orofacial dyspraxia was on the X chromosome. A locus for a syndrome with a similar speech-language disorder (Wieacker-Wolff syndrome) has recently been found at chromosome Xq13-q21. A more subtle syndrome, autosomal dominant rolandic epilepsy and speech dyspraxia, involves oromotor apraxia with difficulty organizing and coordinating movements necessary to produce fluent speech [but without dysarthria], and mild impairment of perceptive language. The gene has not been found for it or for familial developmental dysphasia, an isolated autosomal dominant trait in which the development of spoken language is severely delayed. Language-based learning impairment characterizes three autosomal dominant forms of dyslexia, which

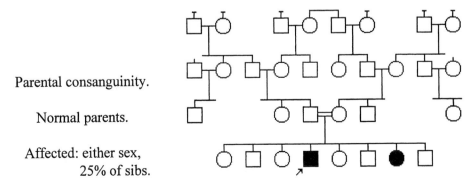

Parental consanguinity.

Normal parents.

Affected: either sex,
25% of sibs.

▼ **Figure 3-4** Autosomal recessive inheritance.

Female carriers are heterozygotes.

No male to male transmission.
More frequent in males.
Affected female: heterozygous
    mother, hemizygous father.
Progeny of heterozygote:
    50% of sons affected,
    50% of daughters are carriers.

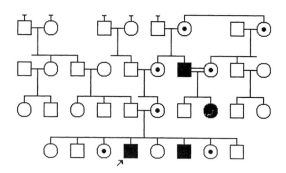

▼ **Figure 3-5** X-linked recessive inheritance.

have been mapped to chromosomes 2p16-p15, 6p21.3, and 15q21. Specific mutations have not yet been identified. Dyslexia is also a feature of several syndromes.

Congenital dysphagia probably occurs only as a feature of syndromes (about 50 in number). The only other regularly occurring feature of the Opitz G/BBB syndrome is wide-spaced eyes so, in it, dysphagia may appear to be an isolated autosomal dominant disorder (chromosome 22q11.2) or X-linked disorder (chromosome Xp22). Other features occurring less uniformly are anteverted nares, clefts (pharynx, larynx, or esophagus); hypertelorism; hypospadias; and developmental delay. Various forms of heritable pharyngeal muscular dystrophy cause later onset dysphagia, which may initially appear to be an isolated trait.

Nonsyndromic hearing loss is one of the better-defined isolated Mendelian traits.[10] Tests for some of the genes are emerging; however, even a very careful evaluation may provide little guidance as to which gene to test for. Really practical laboratory diagnosis in the form of a battery of gene tests is yet to come. Connexin 26 mutations cause one of the more frequent autosomal recessive forms and a less common autosomal dominant form. Complete sequencing of the connexin 26 gene is available. Generally, there is a different mutation in each family so this is the ideal approach for a new case.

Loci for 22 autosomal recessive forms of nonsyndromic deafness have been mapped. Most are prelingual (onset before language development) and stable. Twenty-five autosomal dominant forms have been mapped. Most are postlingual

More frequent in females.

Milder in heterozygous female.
Hemizygosity may be lethal.

Homozygosity may be lethal.
No male to male transmission.
Progeny of heterozygote:
    50% affected, either sex.

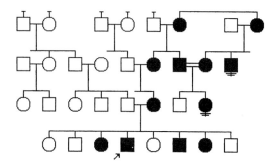

▼ **Figure 3-6** X-linked dominant inheritance.

(onset after language development) and progressive. Of great interest, in some genes, different mutations can cause either dominant or recessive forms, as well as syndromic forms. Over the last few years the number of X-linked nonsyndromic forms has diminished with the recognition that some of them were syndromic. Two of the X-linked forms are postlingual progressive; one has been mapped. Three prelingual stable forms have been mapped. Three other X-linked forms have not yet been fully defined.

Diagnosis of Mendelian disorders often requires the services of an experienced physician. However, these disorders may be present among relatives, and this can be discerned through genealogy evaluation. Even without a precise diagnosis, clinical expectations can be formulated for a new case by cataloguing the characteristics of other cases in the family. Public records of marriages, births, deaths, and successions are the most accurate sources of genealogic data, but recollections of family members are the most commonly used. The Catholic Church and the Mormon Church are also good sources of data and are frequently consulted by health professionals who specialize in diagnosing genetic disorders.

The most informative data are found among the descendants of the patient's great-grandparents and are often limited to a small section of the family's genealogy. There is a standardized manner of recording genealogic information that allows one to recognize inheritance patterns, providing sufficient family data exist. A genealogy chart is also a very compact representation of large amounts of family data. Charting conventions are variable, so a legend should be included with a given patient's chart. Figure 3-7 shows the standard charting method.

Parents of young children with heritable disorders may seek, or be advised to seek, information about the possibility that they may have other children with the same disorder, or they may be interested to know whether their affected child or siblings are likely to bear children with the same disorder. Such counseling should be provided by qualified health care professionals, such as medical geneticists and genetic counselors, to whom other practitioners can refer the family. Due to experience in handling the wide breadth of genetic disorders, the medical geneticist is also in a unique position to assist the speech and language practitioner in coordination of the management of the more complex congenital disorders of speech and hearing.

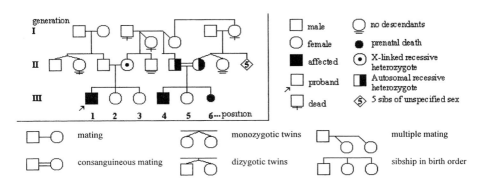

▼ **Figure 3-7**   Guide to genealogy charting. (From Thurmon TF: *A comprehensive primer on medical genetics*, New York, 1999, Parthenon Publishing Group.)

▼ THE HUMAN GENOME

The genome project identified all of the human genes, but the functions of many of the genes are not known, and an unexpected complexity has been found: Parts of genes may combine with each other or with parts of other genes to produce different functions. There also remains a large number of heritable disorders for which no causative genes have been discovered. Many of the disorders with discrete inheritance have been assigned to at least one gene. Here, too, there is complexity. Ostensibly identical cases of a disorder may be caused by different genes with different inheritance patterns.

Linkage studies have been valuable in these pursuits. Linkage is physical closeness of genes on the same strand of DNA. It is analyzed by counting the frequency that sibs who have a specific allele at a gene locus also have a specific allele (DNA *marker*) at a nearby gene locus on the same chromosome. If the gene loci are widely separated, crossovers will occur and *recombine* the alleles with those on the other chromosome. The frequency of that is the recombination fraction. The lower the fraction, the tighter the linkage between the two genes.

Linkage methodology has been extended into polygenic disorders. DNA markers at regular intervals throughout the genome are typed in a large group of sibs in families with a genetic disorder. For each sib pair, a computation is done to assess the difference in disease severity (both affected, one affected, or neither affected). It is plotted on the Y-axis of a graph. Sibs must share either 0, 1, or 2 marker alleles by descent. For each locus, this status is graphed on the X-axis. If the slope of the resulting line for both affected is negative, the marker is near a gene that influences occurrence of the disease. The meaning of the results is probably that, given an individual's polygenic propensity to a disease, there are modifying genes scattered in the genome whose functions may influence actual occurrence of the disorder and its severity. Given the great numbers of genes required to produce polygenic frequencies, it is unlikely that any of these *oligogenes* or any combination thereof could directly cause a polygenic disease.

Association studies extend these concepts. While linkage is studied within families, association studies compare the prevalence of a particular DNA marker, or set of markers, in affected and unaffected individuals in a population. Single nucleotide polymorphisms (SNPs) are the most popular markers. These are ubiquitous sites throughout the genome where individuals may differ by one nucleotide, e.g., one person may have an adenine at that site while another may have a thymine. Within each interval that can be analyzed by the sib pair method, there are very many SNPs. Hence, it is a much higher resolution methodology. It promises to reveal the remaining undiscovered genes for disorders with discrete inheritance and to define all of the modifying genes for polygenic disorders.

▼ FREQUENCIES OF DISORDERS

Among all of the categories and individual disorders discussed here, which are the common ones? There are at least two levels of answers to that question: (1) the perspective of the individual speech and language practitioners and (2) the population frequency.

Many factors govern the actual frequencies at which individual disorders occur in a particular speech and language practice. For example, some speech and language practitioners are associated with a special interest group, such as a craniofacial surgery team. Disorders that are extremely rare, such as Apert syndrome, can be seen frequently in such situations. Other categories of disorders may be treated by other special interest groups that do not ordinarily include a speech and language practitioner. Although those disorders may, in truth, be quite frequent and may frequently entail speech and language aberrations, they may not often come to the attention of the speech and language practitioner. Heart malformations are a good example of this type of disorder.

Many population frequency data have already been mentioned in the discussions of the individual disorders. Perhaps the most frequent individual disorder is Down syndrome, which occurs in 0.16% of newborns per year. Actual population prevalence is higher because modern medical care enables prolonged longevity of individuals with this syndrome. Heart malformations as a group are a bit more common than Down syndrome at birth, but individual types of heart malformations are less common. Cleft lip and palate, neural tube defects, deafness, nonsyndromic speech and language disorders, and nonsyndromic mental deficiency are a bit less common. Most other congenital disorders occur at low frequencies in the general population.

The basal (lowest) frequency of an autosomal dominant Mendelian disorder is the mutation rate, approximately 0.001%. For an autosomal recessive disorder, the basal figure can be smaller or larger, as it is a function of both mutation and the mating structure of the population. Various types of selection mechanisms result in polymorphisms of many Mendelian disorders. A *polymorphism* is a situation in which a disorder occurs at a frequency that is higher than the basal rate. Some Mendelian disorders can also attain high frequencies in specific population isolates due to either genetic drift or selection.

Most teratogenic disorders are also quite rare. Only a few (i.e., fetal effects of alcohol, cytomegalovirus, tobacco) occur at frequencies above basal levels of autosomal dominant Mendelian disorders. This is due, in part, to dose dependency, but surveillance and control have also played important parts in keeping these problems at bay. Surveillance and control mechanisms for teratogens will become increasingly important as our society develops more technological complexity.

Considering teratogenic and Mendelian syndromes, those that affect communication number in the hundreds. All are rare, and relatively few have received any specific study of the communicative component,[11] which points out the importance of diagnostic evaluation of each patient by the speech and language practitioner. Table 3-5 summarizes available data about the clinically recognizable syndromes that have had some study of the communicative component.

A number of other syndromes have had some study of the communicative component but are not as recognizable. In some cases, the affected body systems may not be evident. The King-Kopetzky syndrome is an example.[12] It is characterized by normal pure tone audiometry but difficulties in understanding speech. Other syndromes may be recognizable only by the neurologist on the basis of a set of neurologic abnormalities. The communicative component is usually nonspecific and ranges from absent speech in the worst cases to delayed speech and language in

TABLE 3-5
Clinically Recognizable Syndromes That Have Had Some Study of the Communicative Component

Syndrome	CLP	NE	LI	A	C	R	V	CHL	SNL
Aarskog hypertelorism, brachydactyly, shawl scrotum				P	O				
Ablepharon-macrostomia				F	F			F	P
Achondroplasia				O		F	F	F	
Acrodysostosis				F	F			O	
Acroosteolysis				P	P			O	
ADAM fetal mutilation, constricting bands	F			F	F	F		F	
Albers-Schonberg osteopetrosis				F	F			F	F
Alport nephropathy and deafness									F
Alstrom deafness, retinitis pigmentosa, obesity, diabetes									F
Angelman jerky gait, large mouth, mental deficiency			F		F				
Aniridia, cerebellar ataxia, mental deficiency		F	F						
Apert acrocephaly, mitten syndactyly				F	F	F		F	
Beckwith-Wiedemann exomphalos, macroglossia, gigantism				F	F				
Bilateral femoral dysgenesis-unusual facies	F			F		F		F	
Binder maxillonasal dysplasia				O					
Bloom dwarfism, actinic dermatitis					O		F		
Branchiooculofacial syndrome				F					
Carpenter acrocephalopolysyndactyly				F	F	F		F	
Cerebrocostomandibular syndrome			F	F					
CHARGE association			F	F	F	F	F	F	F
Chondrodysplasia punctata (Conradi-Hunermann)				F				F	
Chromosome 10q+				F		F			
Chromosome 11p+				F		F	F		
Chromosome 18p–				F	F	F			
Chromosome 18q–	F			F	F	F	F	F	
Chromosome 1q+	F			F	F	F	F	F	
Chromosome 21 trisomy (Down)				F	F	F	O	F	I
Chromosome 3p+	F			F	F	F	F	F	
Chromosome 4p–	F			F		F	F	F	
Chromosome 4p+				F		F			
Chromosome 5p– (Cri-du-chat)				F		F		F	
Chromosome 6q–	F			F	F	F	F	F	
Chromosome 7q+	F			F	F	F	F	F	

TABLE 3-5
Clinically Recognizable Syndromes That Have Had Some Study of the Communicative Component—Cont'd

Syndrome	CLP	NE	LI	A	C	R	V	CHL	SNL
Chromosome 8 trisomy			F	F	F				
Chromosome 9p–			F		F				
Chromosome 9p+	F		F		F	F		F	
Chromosome X– (Turner), short stature, sexual infantilism	O			O	I	O		F	F
Chromosome X (Fragile) large ears, long face, cluttering speech			F		F				
Chromosome XXY (Klinefelter)			F	F	F				
Clasped thumb, mental retardation		F	F						
Clefting and oral teratoma	F			F	I	F		F	
Cockayne precocious senility			F	F	F	I	F	F	F
Coffin-Siris coarse face, hypoplastic fifth digits			F						
Cohen hypotonia, obesity, prominent incisors			F	P	F				
Costello faciocutaneoskeletal syndrome		F	F						
Crouzon craniofacial dysostosis				F	O	F		F	
Cryptophthalmia	O			O	O	O	O	F	F
De Lange synophrys, dwarfism, limb reduction	F		F	F	F	F	F	F	
Diastrophic dwarfism				O		F	F	F	
DiGeorge syndrome (CATCH-22)	F							F	
Dominant craniometaphyseal dysplasia				F		F		F	O
Dubowitz short asymmetric eye slits, eczema, short stature	O		F	P	F	O	F	O	
Dysautonomia		F		F	F	F	P		
Ectrodactyly, ectodermal dysplasia, cleft palate (EEC)	F			F	O	F		F	
Ehlers-Danlos hyperelasticity, fragile tissues				O				O	
Extrapyramidal disorder, hypogonadism, alopecia		F	F						
Facio-auriculo-vertebral sequence				F	O	F		F	
Fetal alcohol growth deficiency, microcephaly, blepharophimosis	F		F	F	F	F		F	
Floating-Harbor short stature, triangular face, language delay						F			
Foix-Chavany-Marie suprabulbar paresis			F	F	F	F	F		
Freeman-Sheldon whistling face, ulnar deviation of hands					F		F		P

Continued

TABLE 3-5
Clinically Recognizable Syndromes That Have Had Some Study of the Communicative Component—Cont'd

Syndrome	CLP	NE	LI	A	C	R	V	CHL	SNL
Frontometaphyseal dysplasia								F	O
Frontonasal dysplasia	O			O	O	O		O	
Gilles de la Tourette vocal and motor tics, self-mutilation						F			F
Growth retardation, small puffy hands and feet, eczema		F	F						
Hall-Riggs mental retardation, depressed face, bone dysplasia			F						
Hallerman-Streiff microcephaly, small nose, hypotrichosis				P	F	O			
Hallervorden-Spatz late infantile neuroaxonal dystrophy		F	F						
Homocystinuria ectopia lentis, malar flush, osteoporosis		F	F	P	F	P			
Hydrocephalus, agyria, retinal dysplasia		F	F						
Hypochondroplasia				O	F	F		O	
Hypoglossia-hypodactyly	O			F		O		O	
Immune deficiency, centromeric instability, tongue protrusion				F	F				
Johanson-Blizzard hypoplastic alae nasi, hypothyroidism		F	F		F				F
Kabuki make-up syndrome			F	F					
Kniest flat face, thick joints, plastyspondyly, short stature	F			F		F		F	
Langer-Geidion trichorhinophalangeal syndrome			F		O			F	
Larsen flat face, joint luxations, short fingernails	F			F		F		F	
Leopard lentigines, hypertelorism, deafness, pulmonic stenosis					F				F
Macrocephaly, lipomas, hemangiomas			F		F				
Male pseudohermaphroditism, mental retardation-Verloes type			F		F				F
Maxillofacial dysostosis		F		F					
Mental retardation, X-linked-6, gynecomastia, obesity*			F		F				
Mental retardation-Buenos Aires type†			F		F				
Mesomelia-synostoses	F			F					
Moebius sequence of facial diplegia				F	F	F			
Mohr cleft tongue, deafness, bifid hallux (OFD II)	O			O	O	O		O	

TABLE 3-5
Clinically Recognizable Syndromes That Have Had Some Study of the Communicative Component—Cont'd

Syndrome	CLP	NE	LI	A	C	R	V	CHL	SNL
Mulibrey nanism, pericardial constriction, retinal yellow dots				O		F	F		
Multiple synostoses								F	
Myasthenia, congenital, elongated face		F		F			F		
Myotonic dystrophy	O	F		F	F	F		O	
Myotonic myopathy, chondrodystrophy, oculofacial anomalies		F		F					
Nager acrofacial dysostosis				F	O	F		F	
Neurofibromatosis				O	O	O	O		O
Noonan pulmonic stenosis, webbed neck, short stature				F	F	I		O	
Norrie pseudoglioma of retina				F					F
Opitz hypertelorism, hypospadias (G, BBB)	F			F	O	F	F	F	O
Oral-facial-digital (OFD I)				P	F	O		I	
Osteochondromuscular dystrophy						P	F	P	
Osteogenesis imperfecta								F	F
Otopalatodigital syndrome	F			F	F	F		F	
Palatopharyngeal incompetence				F		F			
Pendred hypothyroidism, deafness									F
Pfeiffer acrocephalosyndactyly, broad thumb and hallux				F	O	O		F	
Photomyoclonus, diabetes, deafness, cerebral dysfunction		F							F
Prader-Willi hypotonia, hypogenitalism			F	F	F	O			
Progeroid short stature, pigmented nevi		F					F		F
Pterygium, multiple	F							F	
Pterygium, popliteal	F			F		F		F	
Pycnodysostosis				F					
Refsum hereditary motor and sensory neuropathy		F							F
Rett dementia, loss of purposeful hand movement			F	F	F				
Robinow fetal face, short forearms, hypoplastic genitalia	F			F		F		F	
Rubella embryopathy			F	F	F				F
Rubenstein-Taybi broad thumbs, beaked nose, slanted eyes			F	F	F			P	
Russel-Silver pseudohydrocephalus, short stature				F			F		

Continued

TABLE 3-5
Clinically Recognizable Syndromes That Have Had Some Study of the Communicative Component—Cont'd

Syndrome	CLP	NE	LI	A	C	R	V	CHL	SNL
Saethre-Chotzen maxillary hypoplasia, syndactyly				O	O	O		P	
Schwartz-Jampel myopathy, microstomia				F	F	F	F		
Seckel short stature, prominent nose			F	P	F			P	
Short stature, hyperextensibility, hernia (SHORT)		F	F					F	
Shprintzen-Goldberg craniosynostosis, arachnodactyly				F	F		F		
Sickle cell anemia									F
Simosa elongated craniofacial syndrome				F		F			
Simpson dysmorphia bulldog face, clumsiness, tethered tongue				F			F		
Smith-Magenis brachycephaly, speech and voice disorder		F	F				F		F
Sotos cerebral gigantism				F	F				
Speech development delayed, face, asymmetry strabismus				F					
Spondyloepiphyseal dysplasia	F			F	O	F		F	F
Spondylometaphyseal dysplasia, X-linked		F	F	F					
Stickler flat face, myopia, spondyloepiphyseal dysplasia	F			F		F		F	F
Storage-Glutamyl-5-phosphate			F	F	F		F	F	F
Storage-lysosomal IVB (Generalized gangliosidosis)^c			F	F	F		F	F	F
Storage-lysosomal IVB adult (Gangliosidosis GM1)^c				O	I			F	F
Storage-lysosomal: Gangliosidosis, GM2, A(M)B^c			F	F	F		F	F	F
Storage-lysosomal: Hunter^‡			F	F	F		F	F	F
Storage-lysosomal: Hurler^‡			F	F	F		F	F	F
Storage-lysosomal: Leroy^‡				F	F		F	F	P
Storage-lysosomal: Mannosidosis alpha B^‡			F	F	F		F	F	F
Storage-lysosomal: Mannosidosis B^‡			F	F	F		F	F	F
Storage-lysosomal: Maroteaux-Lamy^‡				F			O	F	P
Storage-lysosomal: Morquio^‡					O		F	F	P
Storage-lysosomal: Pseudo-Hurler^‡				P	F		P	P	P
Storage-lysosomal: Sanfilippo^‡			F	F	F		P	F	P
Storage-lysosomal: Scheie^‡				O	I			F	F
Storage-lysosomal: Schindler (Alpha-galactosidase B)^‡		F	F						

TABLE 3-5
Clinically Recognizable Syndromes That Have Had Some Study of the Communicative Component—Cont'd

Syndrome	CLP	NE	LI	A	C	R	V	CHL	SNL
Storage-Sialic acid‡		F	F						
Syndactyly I, microcephaly, mental retardation		F	F						
Treacher-Collins mandibulofacial dysostosis	F			F	O	F		F	O
Usher retinitis pigmentosa, deafness					O				F
Van der Woude lip pit/cleft lip	F			F		F		F	
Velo-cardio-facial (Shprintzen)	F			F	F	F		F	I
Waardenburg central albinism, hypertelorism, deafness	O			O		O		O	
Weaver macrocephaly, small nose, camptodactyly	O			F	F	O		O	
Williams patulous lips, voice defect, heart malformation				F	F		F		
Wilson hepatolenticular degeneration		F		F	F				

Data from McKusick VA: *Mendelian inheritance in man: catalogues of autosomal dominant, autosomal recessive, and X-linked phenotypes,* ed 12, Baltimore, 1998, Johns Hopkins Press; Jones KL: *Smith's recognizable patterns of human malformation,* ed 4, Philadelphia, 1988, WB Saunders; and Siegel-Sadewitz V, Shprintzen R: The relationship of communicative disorders to syndrome identification, *J Speech Hearing Disord* 47:338, 1987.
Column headings
CLP, Cleft lip/palate; *NE,* neurological abnormalities; *LI,* learning impairment; *A,* articulation impairment; *C,* cognitive impairment; *R,* resonance impairment; *V,* voice impairment; *CHL,* conductive hearing loss; *SNL,* sensorineural hearing loss.
Column codes
F, Frequent; *I,* infrequent; *O,* occasional; *P,* probable. If there is no code in a column, it means that it could not be determined from the data in the literature whether the impairment coded in that column was present or absent.
*Representative of X-linked syndromes of mental retardation with similar speech and language disorders.
†Representative of recessive syndromes of mental retardation with similar speech and language disorders.
‡Characteristics of storage disorders include coarsening features, deterioration of cognition and health.

the milder cases. Perhaps the most insidious of those disorders are the inborn errors of metabolism that can produce relatively few recognizable features and may not be known to exist unless laboratory testing has been done for them.[6] As they are all rare, laboratory testing may not be available through standard hospital and clinical laboratories. Help is often available from the medical geneticist, who can provide the tests or know where they can be obtained. Laboratory testing for these disorders should be considered in any patient in whom a plausible etiology of a communication disorder is lacking.

▼ REFERENCES

1. Foundas AL, Bollich AM, Corey DM, Hurley M, Heilman KM: Anomalous anatomy of speech-language areas in adults with persistent developmental stuttering, *Neurology* 57(2):207–215, 2000.
2. Nopoulas P, Berg S, Canady J, Richmann L, Van Demark D, Andreason NC: Structural brain abnormalities in adult males with clefts of the lip and/or palate, *Genetics in Medicine* 4:1–9, 2002.
3. Thurmon TF: *Mutagens, Radiation, and Teratogens: Modern Witches.* Shreveport, LA: Grand Rounds, LSU Medical Center, 1991.
4. McKusick VA: *Mendelian Inheritance in Man. Catalogues of Autosomal Dominant, Autosomal Recessive, and X-Linked Phenotypes* 10th ed). Baltimore: Johns Hopkins Press, 1992; 251–270.
5. Sever JL, Ellenberg JH, Ley AC, et al: Toxoplasmosis: maternal and pediatric findings in 23,000 pregnancies, *Pediatrics* 82:181, 1988.
6. Thurmon TF: *A Comprehensive Primer on Medical Genetics.* Parthenon Publishing Group, New York, 1999.
7. Carter CO: Multifactorial Genetic Disease. In VA McKusick, R Claiborne (eds), Medical Genetics. New York: Hospital Practice Publishers, 1973.
8. Locke JL, Mather PL: Genetic factors in the ontogeny of spoken language: evidence from monozygotic and dizygotic twins, *J Child Lang* 16:553, 1989.
9. Gilger JW: Genetics in disorders of language, *Clin Commun Disord* 2:35, 1992.
10. Van Camp G, Willems PJ, Smith RJH: Nonsyndromic hearing impairment: Unparalleled heterogeneity, *Am J Hum Genet* 60:758, 1997.
11. Dykens E: Psychologists and geneticists: two cultures, *Am J Hum Genet* 59:29, 1996.
12. Stephens D, Zhao F: The role of a family history in King Kopetzky Syndrome (obscure auditory dysfunction), *Acta Otolaryngol* 120(2):197–200, 2000 Mar.

CHAPTER 4

THE EARLY INTERVENTION TEAM

Giving and Getting the Right Kind of Help

Frances P. Billeaud

W hether services are provided to infants, toddlers, and their families under the traditional clinical model or under the Part C Early Intervention Model, speech-language pathologists (SLPs) are clearly members of a team effort. The team manager, or captain, is always the person (or persons) with the ultimate decision-making authority, that is, the parents. The reality of parents as team managers has always been true, but professionals have sometimes conceptualized themselves as the true leaders, possibly because parents invest the professionals they have chosen with significant authority in the initial stages of the team relationship. During that early period, families are faced with making difficult decisions about their child's care that they never dreamed would be required of them. Simultaneously, they are coping as best they can with the emotional and financial implications for their family's future after having received the news, or confirmation of their suspicion, that their child is in need of specialized care.

Early intervention teams can have many members who represent several professional specialties or can comprise the parents and one or two professionals, depending on the needs of the family. Team functioning is possible across all professional settings; however, making the transition from the traditional clinical operational philosophy, which relies on the collective knowledge and skills contributed by independent practitioners, to one that relies on effective parent-professional partnerships requires a high level of trust among the team members, commitment to implementation of the best practices, willingness to exert the effort, and leadership. Change is never easy, and systems change across and within agencies is extremely difficult, but it is both possible and desirable if undertaken for the right reasons.

Luterman[1] observed that "[p]arents and professionals in speech-language pathology are natural allies. They both want in the most ardent terms the same thing: a child with better communicating skills" (p. 175).

▼ FAMILY AS FOCUS OF THE TEAM EFFORT

The family chooses members of the intervention or treatment team for the primary purpose of getting help for their child. At the outset, they may see the selection of professionals as their only contribution to that end, expecting the professionals they have selected to "fix" or "cure" the problem. As their understanding of the nature of communicative delays and disorders evolves, and it becomes clear that day-to-day activities within the family are part of effective treatment, their roles as team members become more diverse. Under the Individuals with Disabilities Education Act (IDEA) model, in fact, a goal of intervention is to empower the family itself to enhance the child's development. Thus professionals working with infants and toddlers with communicative delays and disorders spend significant amounts of time planning interventions together with the parents; receiving information about the child's activities and behaviors in the home setting, family routines, and cultural and child-rearing practices; and engaging in ongoing evaluation of the effectiveness of intervention and therapy strategies applied in the home setting. Practitioners provide parental guidance, parent education, parent training, and counseling, all as part of the management package. Direct services to the child and consultative services to childcare center personnel and to other practitioners may also be part of the SLP's responsibilities.

Families who contact professionals for assistance come with varying levels of information about their child's condition, which is the reason they are seeking help. On some level (they know it, they suspect it, they were told it), there is knowledge that "something is not right." They expect the professional or team of professionals to offer help. They may have a particular kind of help in mind or may entrust the decision about what kind of help is appropriate to the professionals they have chosen. Just as they have the right to select the professionals on their team, they have the right to add others to the team, terminate services, resume services after a hiatus, seek second opinions, and change service providers. Families have always had such options, but professionals who were trained to believe that their own protocols took precedence over family choices have often judged the exercise of at least some of those options as evidence of "noncompliance" on the part of families. A decade of experience with the Part C approach has modified the thinking of the professional community to some extent, but the advent of managed care may shape philosophies of best practices in a somewhat different direction.

Family Systems Theory in Practice

It is obvious that parent-professional teams are essential in optimizing treatment, management, and intervention outcomes. Practitioners find it useful to consider the family unit from the perspective of family systems theory, because an understanding of the individual child's family helps to formulate effective treatment plans that require family participation. Systems theory can be helpful when thinking about how families operate as they do. Summers and colleagues[2] and Wayman and colleagues[3] suggested that the family system can be considered as interrelationships among the following:

- *Family structure:* the number of people in the family, their respective relationships to each other, and their values and beliefs

- *Family interaction:* the manner in which the individual members interact with the others and their places or roles within the family unit
- *Family functions:* the responsibilities the family unit bears to its members
- *Family life cycle:* those alterations in family structure, function, and interaction that occur as their circumstances change over time and as their children mature

A family is sensitive to the ebb and flow of many events, stresses, pleasures, and challenges that affect both individual members and the collective unit. Professionals must be sensitive both to family members with whom there is direct or indirect interaction and to the stresses, issues, and values that they recognize as influencing their lives and family functioning.

As Luterman[1] pointed out, families of handicapped children are not necessarily dysfunctional families (although some may be), but they are definitely families that are under stress. The presence of a child with special needs affects different families in different ways. It strengthens family bonds for some and, perhaps, places unbearable stress on families that are already fragile. Professionals who provide services to youngsters who have or are at risk for disabilities involving communicative disorders encounter a broad spectrum of coping abilities and responses among the families.

Parents who have looked back on the time at which they first suspected or learned for certain that their child had a significant problem have reported feelings that range from shock and confusion to anger and despair. Some have reported moving through stages of grief much like those that Kubler-Ross[4] described in relation to experiencing a terminal illness or the death of a loved one. On the other hand, some parents reported being readily accepting of the news, especially if there had been other family members affected by the same condition.[5,6]

The personal experience of one family illustrates the importance of being sensitive to the emotional plight of the parents:

When we as parents come to the professionals begging for services, there is an angry little voice inside us that says, "Why does this have to be?" This angry little voice is loud. Behind the anger is fear, big time fear. Fear of the unknown, fear of losing something precious, fear of failure.

My child was diagnosed with a severe language disorder. For well over a year after he was diagnosed, I was devastated. My reaction was completely disproportionate to the reality. It was very hard for me. I had to deal with it on a daily basis. I'm the one who watched as some moms went to the park while we went to therapy. My instinct to protect my child couldn't slow down the ever-widening gap between my child and his friends.

My nightmare was that I would be judged to be unfit and he would be taken away (my nightmare stems from the fact that my older sister who is severely mentally retarded and an epileptic was taken away when I was four).

As I said, not terribly rational, but this is what we [parents] are dealing with. A parent in this state is just trying to defuse the sense of failure, powerlessness, and anger. Even if the service is desperately needed and the parent accepts it, the underlying loss of parental power and self-esteem is there.[7]

Sometimes the presentation of a diagnosis of a significant developmental problem is as hard for the professional to make as it is for the family to hear. Consideration for the feelings of the family as they receive diagnostic information and recommendations about follow-up management should be a concern of professionals whose role it is to interact with families about those matters. Because diagnosis and assessment are often the family's first encounters with "labels" their child may receive, it is also important for the professional to present information to the family about what the diagnostic label implies with respect to eligibility for treatment and management programs, selection of appropriate intervention strategies, and their right to confidentiality of records relating to their child. The amount of information that can be absorbed by a family at one time is limited, especially at a time when diagnosis of a significant disability is presented. Gauging how much information to provide at that time is another responsibility of the practitioner.

Some families may be in crisis when they are first encountered. For example, their child may be suffering from a serious illness or recovering from surgical or medical treatments required to preserve the child's life. They may be preoccupied with financial or logistical problems that require their full energies and resources. Until the crisis is resolved, it will probably be difficult, if not impossible, for family members to participate constructively in the management of their child's needs beyond the provision of basic care. Sometimes even that contribution is beyond the family's ability. In such cases, social welfare agencies or the courts may find it necessary to remove the child from the family for a period of time, so that the primary caregivers can receive appropriate assistance for themselves.

If the family is viewed from the systems perspective, then the child's environment can be considered ecologically. Again, everything within the family environment affects every member of the family in some way to a greater or lesser extent. This concept is useful both from a philosophical point of view and in terms of practical applications of interventions. Because the concept is likely to be a new one to family members themselves, it may be helpful to introduce it early during the formation of the parent-professional team association. The family-needs assessment, required under Part C regulations, can begin with an eco-mapping process that assists the family to recognize its specific strengths (resources); needs (areas of concern); and the interrelationships among activities, agencies, and family functions. The process of eco-mapping is an efficient and practical strategy to help the family select and prioritize the services they desire.

The Eco-Map

Hartman and Laird[8] provided a format for developing the eco-map (Figure 4-1). The family identifies its members (their names are written in the center circle). Connections between the family and its associations and activities (shown in the outer circles) are indicated by different kinds of lines. *Heavy, bold lines* represent strong, positive connections; *narrower solid lines* indicate ongoing positive or neutral connections; railroad-like lines highlight stressful connections; *dotted lines* indicate tenuous relationships or other important connections that the family feels unable to assess accurately. *Arrows* signify the flow of energy, resources, and effort toward or away from the family unit. The resulting picture, the eco-map, becomes a tool created by the family with the professional's guidance, which can be used as a basis for discussing prospective family resources and areas of concern or need. These insights can be useful in planning and shaping components of the intervention program. The eco-map can be modified as conditions within and around the family change over time.

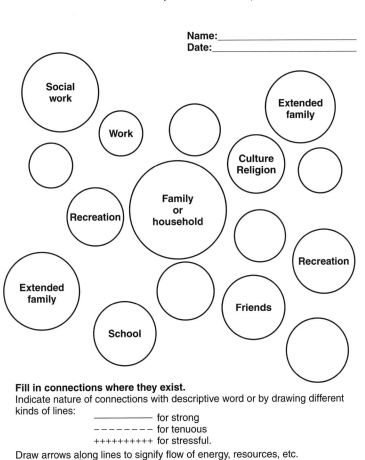

Name:_____
Date:_____

Fill in connections where they exist.
Indicate nature of connections with descriptive word or by drawing different kinds of lines: _____ for strong
          – – – – – – – for tenuous
          ++++++++++ for stressful.
Draw arrows along lines to signify flow of energy, resources, etc.

example: (School)+++++++++––>–>–>–>(Tom)

Identify significant people and fill in empty circles if needed.

▼ **Figure 4-1**   Eco-Map. (From Hartman A, Laird J: *Family-centered social work practice*, New York, 1983, The Free Press, a division of Macmillan, Inc.)

After development of the eco-map, other tools used in the family-needs assessment can then be selected and interpreted in light of knowledge of a particular family system. Questionnaires can be used to identify areas of personal and social resources, service coordination, and time management. Information provided through such tools is more meaningful when considered in light of the family system.

Family Configurations, Demographics, and Cultural Considerations

Families are different in today's world than they were even in the fairly recent past. The demographics of our society speak for themselves.

International adoptions are on the increase, and there are often few facts available to the adoptive parents about their new baby's family health history. One of six children in this country lives in a single-parent home. One of every two black children lives in a single-parent home headed by a woman. In 1986, almost three-fourths of all black infants were born to unwed mothers; half of the mothers were teenagers. Many young women choose to emulate the lifestyle choices of affluent movie stars or music personalities by bearing and keeping babies who have no father figures in the home. Increasing numbers of preterm, very-low-birth-weight, sick infants are being born to women who have had inadequate (or no) prenatal care; most of those babies are being saved by advanced medical technology. Many survive with impairments, and their families require a range of resources. By the year 2000, 38% of all children under the age of 18 were members of ethnic minority families. The fastest growing segment of the country's population is Asian American. Hispanic Americans also represent an expanding portion of the population; in some areas of the country Hispanic Americans already constitute the majority of residents.

In contrast, the professional community continues to be underrepresented by practitioners from minority groups.[9] Clearly, services provided to many segments of the population are influenced by cultural practices and languages that differ from those of the majority of the professional community. Further, the family's cultural perspectives regarding child-rearing practices and interactions with health care providers and educators, handicapping conditions, and appropriate intervention or management strategies can differ significantly from those of the practitioners seeking to provide a child with beneficial services. The practitioner must seek to understand and appreciate the cultural variety of society and be sensitive to the issues that can bring the traditionally trained professional and the family into potential conflict.[10]

Participants at the 1989 conference discussing services to infants and children from culturally diverse backgrounds, conducted by the National Center for Clinical Infant Programs, identified a number of issues of importance to practitioners who serve young children. The conference report[11] is a useful resource for professionals who seek to enhance their knowledge of cultural perceptions and practices. The authors remind us that there are cultural and situational influences that, if ignored, can doom to failure from the outset even the best-intentioned programs for handicapped and at-risk infants and toddlers.

Among the cultural issues that must be considered are (1) how people feel about, manifest, and treat the states of health and illness and physical, mental, and emotional disabilities; (2) the group of people who are considered to be family members and the relationships these people have to one another; (3) child-rearing techniques; and (4) in addition to the language of the home, the various ways in which people communicate. It is important to remember that situational and environmental conditions such as poverty, homelessness, lack of formal education, and other factors that put children and families at grave risk are *not* cultural attributes but are variables that cut across all cultures.

This overview of some of the issues that affect the practitioner's relationship with families from culturally diverse backgrounds is included because of the ecological importance of cultural influences. Competent pediatric practitioners recognize the necessity of being sensitive to potential barriers and possible means of avoiding them in the course of providing services to children with special needs whose family cultures differ from their own.

Tonkovich[12] urges that clinicians "be cognizant of cultural factors that might affect their service delivery to those from multicultural groups. Lack of attention to these factors might lead to mistaken diagnosis or to the risk of offending clients and their families. [They] will appreciate adaptations to testing and treatment procedures to accommodate relevant cultural issues …" (p. 239).

It is possible to develop sensitivity to the factors that are important in working with a given family. Wayman and colleagues[3] developed a useful set of guidelines for early interventionists who have responsibility for home visits. Their approach suggests that it is important to understand family structure, customary patterns of caregiving, child-rearing practices, family schedules, and family responses to the child's behaviors. The family's attitude and perceptions about the child's disability, health, and health care are also important, as are the family's language use (is an interpreter needed?) and interactional styles (is there a designated family spokesperson or leader?). Wayman and colleagues guide practitioners into productive areas of inquiry and observation under each of these areas. The guidelines are equally valuable to practitioners who work with families in settings other than the home. The site of service provision does not diminish the need to understand and respect the family within which the child lives.

Kayser[13] reminds professionals that judgments about a child's language development must be based on assessment of both languages to which the child has been exposed, even if the child speaks only one of them. Assessment conclusions based on competency in English only, especially if it is not the language used in the home, is likely to be erroneous (p. 223). Professionals should look for signs other than lack of understanding of English if it is suspected the young child may have a language disorder (p. 224):

- Inability to discriminate tones, phonemes, morphemes
- Inability to associate sounds with objects or experiences
- Poor vocabulary
- Poor turn-taking
- Inappropriate comments
- Preference for using gestures
- Confused appearance

Such behaviors apply across language contexts and should be considered indicative of the need for thorough assessment incorporating the languages to which the child has been exposed.

Expectations

The expectations of the family and the professional constitute another set of issues about which sensitivity needs to be developed. Luterman[1] emphasized the importance of each party's understanding of the other's expectations of what is to occur during assessment and treatment programs, what each expects the other to contribute, and the outcomes that each expects. *Failure to understand the expectations vested in the process and the people involved is often the root of failure to achieve a successful, collaborative team effort for the benefit of the child with special needs.*

Parents should be provided with information about the practitioner's expectations as the stages of their association advance. For example, it may be helpful to provide the family with information sheets that outline the typical process and sequence of events involved in evaluation and assessment activities. Such information not only prepares them for the unfamiliar series of events but also can help them organize their questions, ideas, and observations, thus enhancing their ability to participate effectively.

Likewise, the professional should seek to discover the family's expectations. This can be done through a number of techniques, but the most successful is probably a face-to-face discussion, which validates the practitioner's interest in the family's concerns and has the advantage of immediacy.

Parents can be active partners in all phases of the assessment and intervention process, not merely signers of informed consents or requests-for-service forms (unless that is the role they choose to play). When this philosophy of parents as active partners is applied, the assessment process itself can become the first step in intervention or treatment. The concept is not a new one, but the means of implementing collaborative parent-professional partnerships can present challenges for which most communication disorders professionals have not been formally trained.

Table 4-1 summarizes some of the means through which a collaborative parent-professional partnership can emerge.

Blosser (p. 34)[14,15] summarized the contributions families make to the SLP's development of management plans appropriate to their particular situation as follows:

TABLE 4-1
Parent-Professional Partnerships: Some Collaborative Activities

Parent and Family Roles	Practitioner Roles
Family assessment of strengths and needs	Selection of tools and approaches (e.g., eco-map, interview, questionnaires)
Identifying priorities for the child concerning communicative development	Eliciting assistance of the family in identifying how the child communicates
	Presenting, clarifying, and exploring treatment options
Acquiring new information about pre-communicative development and emerging communicative skills	Identifying parents' preferred learning methods and providing instruction in an appropriate format
Integrating communicative stimulation into daily routines	Providing information with regard to short-term goals and their connection to targeted priorities
	Showing how play is used as a vehicle for communication
Recording data to track the child's communicative status and development	Training in data-keeping skills
	Selecting appropriate formats
Stimulating, teaching, and modeling language and speech	Modeling, demonstrating, and teaching specific communicative skills
	Coaching, validating efforts, and affirming skills
Accepting and using power to influence child's continuing development	All of the roles listed above
	Talking with (not to or at) the family
Collaborating in evaluation of outcomes and options in ongoing intervention activities	Counseling
	Selecting or providing the forum and means of documentation
Accepting transitions as they become appropriate	Preparing family for service, setting, personnel, program, priority, and relationship changes
Helping the professional to accept transitions as they become appropriate	

- The American family is diverse. *Consider each family's unique state of being when making recommendations and planning treatment.*
- Each person has a unique coping style. *Strive to identify the coping styles demonstrated by your client's family members and select counseling and education techniques accordingly.*
- Family members know their loved one better than you do. They have much to contribute to the assessment, planning, and intervention process. *Develop strategies for incorporating family into every phase of treatment.*
- Technology offers clinicians opportunities to reach family members when they might otherwise be inaccessible. *Be familiar with technological resources; expand your resource library.*
- Families come in all shapes and sizes and are not defined only by blood relationships. *Identify those individuals who share a special relationship with your client and foster their awareness and skills.*

Under the parent-professional team model, the child with special needs is provided with a management program that involves the entire ecosystem (family and community) in which he or she lives. Those who care most about their child with special needs are directly involved in planning and conducting activities that enhance the child's development.

▼ COMMUNICATION DISORDERS SPECIALISTS AS MULTIDISCIPLINARY TEAM MEMBERS

SLPs and audiologists who serve infants, toddlers, and their families must be able to work with very young children whose needs vary widely; whose histories, diagnoses, etiologies, and prognoses differ significantly; and whose families' needs for guidance are equally diverse. It should be obvious that communicative disorders specialists often work together with specialists from many other disciplines to meet the needs of affected children and their families. Sometimes, however, the team is composed of the communicative disorders specialist and the family with only occasional contacts with other professionals. Although children who are identified as "at risk" at or shortly following birth are probably under the care of medical specialists, other professionals may be the first to recognize the need for intervention services, especially among children whose condition is recognized after the first birthday.

Multidisciplinary evaluation and assessment are required to establish eligibility and initiate intervention under federal Part C regulations and companion state statutes. Federal regulations stipulate that at least two professional disciplines be involved in evaluation and assessment activities and allow participation by as many professional disciplines as necessary to complete a thorough assessment and develop an appropriate Individual Family Services Plan (IFSP).

Knowledge, Skills, and Competencies Expected of the Speech-Language Pathologist

The SLP who serves infants and toddlers diagnosed with or at risk for delays, disorders, and disabilities and their families in any setting must have considerable knowledge in a variety of areas. This knowledge must supplement the basic general knowledge acquired by every SLP about communicative development and disorders of communication.

Knowledge

Specifically, SLPs who work with this population must have in-depth information about the following:

- Prenatal development and potential problems associated with the prenatal environment, teratogens, genetic considerations, and maternal health during pregnancy
- Developmental anatomy, physiology, neurological sequences, and the implications of problems that are associated with each area
- Normal infant development across all areas (i.e., physical, neuromotor, social, emotional, and cognitive)
- Sequelae of specific diagnosed conditions with regard to communicative development and the early development that precedes symbolic communication
- Family systems
- Roles, functions, and skills of other professional disciplines that are involved with the care of infants, toddlers, and their families
- Customary treatments and technologies used by related professionals in their work with young children at risk for or diagnosed with delays or disabilities
- Referral criteria and protocols used to secure consultations when there are suspected problems or there is need for specific information
- Pertinent laws, regulations, entitlements, and programs that are applicable and available to the population, and the eligibility requirements for each
- How to access services in the community that may be needed by families of affected children and by the children themselves
- Effective interviewing methods, techniques, and options
- Terminology used by other disciplines so that the professional can (1) understand their reports; (2) be able to interpret information to the family accurately; and (3) communicate effectively with professional colleagues
- The limits of one's own personal and professional practice, referring to other service providers as their expertise is required or appropriate
- How to handle and position infants who require specialized care
- How to conduct feeding and swallowing assessments and perform interventions with infants who exhibit problems in those areas
- The options for multidisciplinary team composition and functioning in various settings

Skills and Competencies

Skills and competencies that the SLP must be able to demonstrate in working with this population likewise are specialized. They represent skills and competencies over and above those the SLP is expected to possess in working with older communicatively impaired individuals and include the following:

- Participating effectively as a multidisciplinary team member
- Conducting screenings to identify atypical communicative development (including presymbolic communicative development and nonverbal forms of communicative development)

- Contributing accurate and clearly worded information to other professionals who work with the child and family and to family members
- Conducting assessments of current levels of communicative development for purposes of developing appropriate treatment, management, or intervention plans
- Exercising effective listening skills with family members and other service providers
- Conducting family interviews to obtain case-history information
- Providing effective family counseling concerning communicative development, referrals, legal rights, community services, and other matters within the scope of professional practice
- Conducting communicative diagnoses separate from or as a part of a larger diagnostic effort
- Conducting examination of the oral mechanism
- Assessing respiratory effort in vocalization
- Assessing receptive communication and expressive communication (including presymbolic and symbolic stages, vocal, verbal, and nonverbal)
- Integrating data supplied by the audiologist and others with regard to its effect on the child's communicative development
- Conducting family-needs assessments (as related to the family's desire and ability to enhance the child's development)
- Participating in planning appropriate management for communicative delays and disorders (per IFSP or other care-plan requirements as appropriate)
- Participating in conducting appropriate management programs, both direct and indirect, and combinations of direct and indirect strategies
- Evaluating outcomes of management programs
- Referring children and their families to appropriate services as needed (e.g., medical: pediatricians, neurologists, ophthalmologists, orthopedists, otorhinolaryngologists, allergists, plastic surgeons, oral surgeons, geneticists, early and periodic screening, diagnosis, and treatment clinics, children's health services, and allied health services such as occupational and physical therapy; dental care; nutrition consultation; social services: financial assistance, transportation, support groups, daycare, respite care; psychological services; and developmental services)
- Interacting with other service providers who conduct portions of the child's total developmental program (e.g., infant interventionists, assessment teachers, noncategorical preschool teachers, daycare providers, social workers, physical therapists, occupational therapists, adapted physical education personnel)
- Collaborating in service provision activities where and when possible (i.e., planning, conducting, and evaluating outcomes)
- Coordinating some or all of the services needed by the child (i.e., family service coordination, formerly designated *case-management services*)
- Planning transitions with the multidisciplinary team, including the family
- Planning transitions before their occurrence
- Choosing and utilizing appropriate interpreters when needed

It is clear that the professional competencies needed by the practitioner do not rest on simple downward extensions of knowledge and skills appropriate to the mature child or adult.[151]

Role of the Speech-Language Pathologist

The SLP practitioner can serve in many roles within and across service-delivery settings. At various times, the SLP serves as a source of information, parent trainer, parent educator, family support professional, diagnostician, communication therapist, researcher, team participant, service coordinator, advisor, counselor, promoter of public awareness, advocate for the child and for early intervention programs, and professional educator. Throughout these activities, the practitioner also remains an individual, who must acknowledge and deal with personal sensitivities, vulnerabilities, biases, values, and the need to continue learning and growing professionally.[1]

It is important that the SLP's roles be recognized by other team members and by family members. Unfortunately, the general public and service providers in other disciplines are often uninformed about the various roles performed by SLPs and audiologists for the target population. Indeed, professionals in related disciplines tend to be underinformed about communicative development in general—an issue that is also of concern to SLPs who serve the infant-toddler population (and an issue that presents ongoing opportunities for offering continuing-education programs designed for professionals as well as family members). There is much work to be done in the area of public awareness and marketing the services of communicative disorders specialists. Chapter 10 addresses this subject.

Speech-language pathology services for the infant-toddler population include several broad categories, within which are clusters of more specific services. The broad service categories are as follows:

- Prevention services
- Diagnosis and assessment services
- Planning of treatment and intervention programs
- Implementation of treatment and intervention programs
- Professional consultation and referral services
- Resource-coordination services (service coordination)
- Parent-training services (individualized to specific needs)
- Parent-education services (group and individual)
- Counseling services
- Transition planning and implementation services

Depending on the type and setting of the SLP's professional practice, services can be offered on a one-time-only basis (e.g., consultation with attending professionals and referral of families to speech-language services or developmental programs nearer their homes), on an intensive short-term basis (e.g., providing services during the infant's stay in the neonatal intensive care unit or intermediate-care nursery before discharge or providing short-term intervention to facilitate language development in late talkers), or on an intermittent basis (e.g., assessment services provided in follow-up clinics when the goal is training, ongoing therapeutic services, and other services to an infant with a diagnosed condition that entails atypical communicative development).

The argument, if there is to be one, is not whether SLPs should be prepared to deliver services in one manner or another, or one setting or another, but rather how the needs of the children and families who seek services can be met effectively in any setting.

The Speech-Language Pathologist and Community Settings

SLPs can be used in a number of settings that bring them in contact with professionals from other disciplines and with at-risk or disabled infants, toddlers, and their families. The SLP is expected to bring to the team specialized knowledge of communicative development and of factors that can interfere with that development or modify its form, the ability to assess capabilities and limitations or barriers involving a particular child and family, and the ability to work with other members of the team to plan and execute appropriate strategies to optimize the child's development.

The settings in which practitioners function influence the array of services provided and their focus. For example, services provided in a neonatal intensive care unit differ from those provided in the home, childcare center, or developmental services program. Whatever the setting, it is essential to remember that SLPs and audiologists who work with infants, toddlers, and families are never solo practitioners. They are always part of a team. The minimum team for the communicatively impaired child is composed of the parent(s), the child, providers of the child's health care, and the communicative-disorders specialist. The team often has other members as well (e.g., other family members, childcare providers, early childhood special educators, psychologists).

▼ SUMMARY

The idea of team functioning is not new in itself, but the importance of thinking of ourselves as team members has recently received renewed emphasis and validation in light of the mandates imposed under IDEA.[15-23] Ultimately, the team is "quarterbacked" or managed by the parents, who make decisions about their child's care and participate in treatment and management programs to the extent that they choose.

▼ REFERENCES

1. Luterman DM.: *Counseling the communicatively disordered and their families,* ed 2, Austin, Tex, 1991, Pro-Ed, p 175.
2. Summers JA, Brotherson MJ, Turnbull AP: The impact of handicapped children on families. In Lynch EW, Lewis RB, editors: *Exceptional children and adults,* Glenville, Ill, 1988, Scott-Foresman, p 504.
3. Wayman KI, Lynch EW, Hanson MJ: Home-based early childhood services: cultural sensitivity in a family systems approach, *Top Early Child Special Educ* 10:56, 1991.
4. Kubler-Ross E: *On death and dying,* New York, 1969, Macmillan.
5. Billeaud FP: Region IV interagency coordinating council needs assessment report, Lafayette, La, 1989, Region IV Interagency Coordinating Council.
6. Borland B: Parents' responses to a child's problems. In Semmler C, editor: *A guide to the care and management of very low birth weight infants,* Tucson, Ariz, 1989, Therapy Skill Builders, p 11.
7. Dawkins C: *Address to the Louisiana Interagency Coordinating Council,* Lafayette, La, November 1990.

8. Hartman A, Laird J: *Family-centered social work practice*, New York, 1983, Free Press.
9. Kayser HR: Bilingual language development and language disorders. In Battle DE, editor: *Communication disorders in multicultural populations*, ed 3, Boston, 2002, Butterworth-Heinemann, pp 205–323.
10. American Speech-Language-Hearing Association: Semiannual counts of the ASHA membership and affiliation for the period January 1 through June 30, 1996, Rockville, Md, 1996, American Speech-Language-Hearing Association.
11. Lynch EW, Hanson MJ: *Developing cross-cultural competence: a guide for working with young children and their families*, Baltimore, 1992, Paul H. Brookes.
12. Tonkovich JD: Multicultural issues in the management of neurogenic communication and swallowing disorders. In Battle DE, editor: *Communication disorders in multicultural populations*, ed 3, Boston, 2002, Butterworth-Heinemann, pp 233–265.
13. Kayser HR: Bilingual language development and language disorders. In Battle DE, editor: *Communication disorders in multicultural populations*, ed 3, Boston, 2002, Butterworth-Heinemann, pp 205–232.
14. Anderson PP, Fenichel ES: *Serving culturally diverse families of infants and toddlers with disabilities*, Washington, DC, 1989, National Center for Clinical Infant Programs.
15. Blosser J: Working with families: making time count, ASHA 38:34, 1996.
16. Peterson NL et al: *Personal training competencies for interventionists serving infants with disabilities and at-risk conditions (birth through age 2)*, Lawrence, Kan, 1988, University of Kansas.
17. Bailey DB et al: *Preparing professionals from multiple disciplines to work with handicapped infants, toddlers and their families: current status and future directions.* Paper presented at the International Early Childhood Conference on Children with Special Needs, Nashville, Tenn, November 1988.
18. Dunst CJ, Trivette C, Deal A: *Enabling and empowering families: principles and guidelines for practice*, Cambridge, Mass, 1988, Brookline Press.
19. Sparks SN: *Assessing infants and toddlers: a family focus.* ASHA Videoconference, Rockville, Md, May 1989.
20. Sparks SN: Assessment and intervention with at-risk infants and toddlers: guidelines for the speech-language pathologist, *Top Lang Disord* 10:43, 1989.
21. Shonkoff JA: Perspective on pediatric training. In J Mulic J, S Pueschel S, editors: *Parent-professional partnerships in developmental disability services*, Cambridge, Mass, 1983, Ware Press.
22. Shonkoff J, Hauser-Cram P: Early intervention for disabled infants and their families: a quantitative analysis, *Pediatrics* 80:650, 1987.
23. Shonkoff J et al: Early intervention efficacy research—what have we learned and where do we go from here? *Top Early Child Special Educ* 8:81, 1988.

CHAPTER 5

THE ROLE OF THE SPEECH-LANGUAGE PATHOLOGIST IN THE NEONATAL INTENSIVE CARE UNIT

Preemies, Micropreemies, and Medically Fragile Infants

Frances P. Billeaud
Donna B. Broussard

The speech-language pathologist (SLP) whose practice includes work in the neonatal intensive care unit (NICU) provides a number of services, each of which requires specialized preparation. Roles can include services provided to and for NICU staff, parents, and families of the infants, as well as direct services to the infants themselves.[1] Services can focus solely on communicative interactions or include consultation and parent education and training in regard to the oral feeding and other oral-motor activities from which the coordinated movements required for speech development evolve.[2,3]

Before detailing the functions of the SLP in executing such specialized roles, it may be helpful to consider the hospital setting in which the services are rendered. The NICU is only one of several units that compose the hospital complex. As a part of the hospital, the NICU must adhere to established standards in terms of physical space, equipment, staff, procedural protocols, and provision of patient care. General requirements for NICUs are prescribed by the Joint Commission on Hospital Accreditation, and maintenance of accreditation depends on ongoing compliance with those requirements.

Once a baby leaves the delivery room, the legal responsibility for care rests with the designated attending physician(s). Depending on hospital policy, the NICU level, the child's needs, and the family's wishes, the physician may be a family practitioner, a pediatrician, a neonatologist, a pediatric subspecialist (e.g., pediatric gastroenterologist, pediatric cardiologist, pediatric neurosurgeon), or a team of specialists. Because of legal and ethical responsibilities, other professionals are called in by the attending physician(s) to provide specific services. No services are provided without orders from the attending physician(s).

If the infant is admitted to the NICU, many professionals participate in caring for the child. Staffing patterns in the NICU usually place one nurse on each shift in charge of from one to four infants. Nurses are responsible for executing the nursing care plan for their assigned infant(s). Other staff typically found in the NICU include neonatologists, occupational and physical therapists, respiratory therapists, case managers, SLPs, social workers, pastoral care providers, dietitians and nutritionists, clinical nurse specialists, educators, and utilization review personnel, all of whom function as part of the multidisciplinary team. The staff also includes technicians who operate specialized equipment (e.g., x-ray and brain-scanning equipment to detect anomalies and intracranial hemorrhages), housekeeping staff who keep floors and other surfaces clean, and maintenance personnel. Parents are also in and out of the unit on a regular basis. Administrative staff make their rounds in the unit on a regular basis. The hub of all the activity, of course, is the infant population, most of whom are connected to a variety of monitors.

Montgomery[4] points out that "NICU patients have an average of 135 caregivers per hospitalization. NICU infants are disturbed nearly 100 times a day for procedures or caregiving events." Lights flash, monitor screens glow with the changing configurations of electronic traces, monitors and alarms hum and buzz to indicate the status of infants' various bodily functions. Beepers page personnel, telephones ring, and incoming and outgoing calls are placed or answered. The NICU is a busy place!

The concept of interdisciplinary developmental care in the NICU is rapidly becoming the norm. VandenBerg[5] summarized the essential knowledge base required of NICU personnel: knowledge of normal infant development, knowledge of atypical infant development, and knowledge of family dynamics and functioning (pp. 163–164). Added specialized knowledge areas cited by VandenBerg include (1) knowledge of fetal and newborn brain development, (2) knowledge of medical conditions of premature and full-term neonates, (3) knowledge of neonatal preterm and full-term infant behaviors and development, (4) knowledge of ecology of the NICU, (5) knowledge of staffing patterns and the cultural patterns in the NICU, and (6) knowledge of parenting in the NICU. These areas of specialized knowledge clearly apply to personnel across all disciplines who function as members of the NICU team. Members of the team should also identify babies and families that will need follow-up care after the baby goes home, especially those who are at risk and are, or may become, eligible for Part C services. If possible, appropriate staff members who are familiar with the baby and family should participate in periodic follow-up visits in the home.

In keeping with hospital policy, detailed charting is maintained of all services provided while the infant is in the facility. Patient records are subject to review by various staff members and hospital committees designated by the hospital (e.g., departmental auditing, quality assurance, institutional review board, infant mortality, infection control, medical ethics) and by representatives of their accreditation bodies. Medical records are also subject to subpoena by the judicial system when disputes arise about legal issues. One of the professional's most important responsibilities is to maintain accurate records in a timely manner.

▼ NEWBORN CARE OPTIONS: NEONATAL INTENSIVE CARE VERSUS OTHER SETTINGS

Many levels of newborn care are available to modern medicine, including at least three levels of intensive care. The condition of the infant at birth generally dictates where neonatal care is provided. There are at least four choices in the hospital system, each level having an increasingly sophisticated capability for dealing with the infant's needs.

Rooming-In Care

Rooming-in allows the mother and her healthy baby to be in the same room throughout the hospital stay, with medical and nursing staff nearby to provide support and care as needed. Rooming-in, with its liberal visiting privileges, provides a home-like environment for the family, while maintaining ready access to medical treatment. Under this option, hospital stay for mother and child is usually brief, usually only 24 to 48 hours.

Level I Nursery Care (Well-Baby Nursery)

Admission to the level I nursery is probably the most common form of newborn care provided in this country. The nursing staff cares for the babies in a common nursery area, which grandparents and friends can view through plate-glass windows. Trips out of the nursery are limited to visiting the mother's room for bottle or breast feedings or periods of nurturing and cuddling. Following delivery, healthy infants and their mothers are usually discharged after a stay of 24 to 48 hours after vaginal delivery and 72 hours after cesarean section delivery (in contrast to the 5- to 7-day confinements common in years past). Treatment for minor problems the infant may develop (e.g., mild jaundice, minor feeding problems) is normally provided in a level I nursery.

Level II and Level III Nursery Care

The level II nursery provides the first level of neonatal intensive care. Level II nurseries were initially designed to serve the needs of preterm infants, or "preemies." Their mission has been expanded to include treatment of other infants who require more attention than is usually available in level I nurseries. The level II NICU is staffed by physicians (pediatricians and staff or part-time neonatologists), nurses, allied health personnel, and technicians with specific skills. Highly sophisticated monitoring equipment is at hand to make certain that infants receive adequate oxygenation and nutrition, maintain adequate body temperature, and are treated promptly for any problem. Isolettes, warming tables, phototherapy lights to treat jaundice, equipment to scan for intraventricular hemorrhages, suctions, feeding tubes, and a wide variety of other equipment are available to provide immediate response to each infant's needs. Babies who require monitoring or treatment for a specific problem may spend only a brief time in the level II NICU, before being discharged or returned to the level I unit. Infants who are significantly preterm (approximately 10% of all pregnancies, according to Reese),[6] or who exhibit problems requiring technological support or extended medical treatment may spend several weeks or even months on the unit. Premature babies are not only smaller than babies born at term but also have immature neurological development, which affects their ability to adjust to life outside the womb (respiration, maintenance of body temperature, regulation of biological state, sleep and wake cycles, and coordination of sucking, swallowing, and breathing). The treatment required to help these fragile infants sustain life sometimes places additional stress on their systems and may result in short- or long-term problems, for which additional intervention is required once the medical condition has stabilized.[7–10]

Level III nurseries provide even more sophisticated care for newborns. Level III NICUs are available in fewer hospitals because of the high costs of maintaining the service (which include the cost of full-time neonatologists, high-tech equipment, and lower staff-to-patient ratios) and the high level of specialized personnel training required to care for very small, very fragile infants. Although level III units are often located in teaching hospitals, it is becoming increasingly common for hospitals to combine level II and III units within a single physical space, allowing babies to move back and forth between levels of care as their needs require. Infants are often transported to level III centers from outlying areas for specialized medical or surgical treatment. Families are often unable to be with their infants during their stay in a level III NICU because of its distance from their homes. Consequently, these sick and fragile babies have a very different start in life than their healthier peers.[11–13]

As soon as the medical crisis is over, and the infant is strong enough to leave the level III NICU, it is customary to transfer the baby to a step-down unit, in which the expenses of providing any needed continuing care are somewhat lower. Babies can remain in the step-down unit—often a level II NICU—as "growers" until they achieve efficient, adequate oral intake and heart rate, attain full-term age, or are otherwise stable enough medically to be released from hospital care.

Level IV Nurseries

The most sophisticated NICUs are rated as level IV NICUs. There are generally only a very few of these in each state. Infants with extremely rare or complex conditions that require highly specialized surgical or medical interventions are often transported to level IV centers for such care.

▼ INVOLVEMENT OF THE SPEECH-LANGUAGE PATHOLOGIST IN NEWBORN CARE

The purpose of all hospitals is to provide treatment for medical and surgical problems presented by their patients, whatever the age, within the role and scope of the institution's mission. The SLP may provide services to children on the pediatric service(s), including the NICU, of a given hospital; provide services across many services (e.g., rehabilitation, out-patient clinics, acute care, pediatrics); or serve only in the NICU, depending on the hospital's structure, mission, administrative philosophy, budget, and staffing patterns. The SLP can serve as a consulting professional, a part-time staff member, or a permanent member of the house staff.

NICU services have developed rapidly as advances in biomedical technology and reliable data on developmental outcomes of an array of management protocols have emerged. The concept of comprehensive neonatal patient care has come to include not only medical treatment but also provision of information, training, and education for family members who now participate in decision making for their infant patients and who are best equipped to provide certain aspects of their care. Other things being equal, infants who are visited regularly by their parents in the NICU tend to do better than those whose families are unable to participate in their care during NICU hospitalization. The primary caregiver's (usually mother's) engagement of the infant through mutual gazing, verbal comforting, early social turn taking, cuddling and stroking, feeding, and rocking all seem to contribute to the baby's biological development and neurobehavioral organization and development.[5,14–17] (Also see the works of T. Berry Brazelton, Heidelese Als, Forrest Bennett, Gretchen Lawhon, and Craig Ramey for specific references in this regard.)

Involvement in the Level III and Level IV Neonatal Intensive Care Unit

Because babies in the level III and IV NICUs are likely to have urgent medical needs that temporarily take priority over their developmental needs, the SLP is less likely to be involved in direct care provision to the baby. However, increasingly, the SLP is directly involved when the baby is medically stable, on room air, at an appropriately corrected gestational age, or developmentally ready for oral nutrition. The SLP is also a regular participant in multidisciplinary team rounds and contributes to the team's ongoing needs assessment and discharge-planning processes.

An active role is likely with babies who have a cleft palate and special feeding needs, especially if they are also preterm, small for gestational age, or have a syndrome of which a palatal cleft is one of several features. For example, infants who have poor tongue control often have significantly improved oral feeding ability when a specialized feeder (i.e., Haberman feeder or specially designed nipple) is used or when the tip of the tongue is sutured to the lower lip, which effectively holds it forward in the mouth and away from the airway (the tack is released as the child gains better oral-motor control). The "tacking" procedure also seems to alleviate episodes of breathing problems associated with the tongue's obstruction of the airway. As a rule, whether or not the tongue has been tacked, these babies should be held in a nearly upright position for oral feedings to facilitate gravitational assistance in fluid intake.

Families are encouraged to visit and gradually participate in the care of their infants in the level III and IV settings. In the initial stages, they too may be limited to bedside visits, talking to their babies, and being physically near them. As the baby's health improves, and tolerance for a bit more involvement is evident, parents are encouraged to take on more direct caregiving roles.

Involvement in the Level II Nursery

Babies in the level II nursery are more likely to be available to developmental care in general, especially when they "graduate" to room oxygen and are considered by the medical staff to be growers. The SLP evaluates and provides therapy and other direct services to the baby and also may serve the infant's needs in the role of consultant to NICU staff and family members, providing information about oral stimulation; reducing tactile defensiveness in and around the baby's mouth; giving information on the benefits of nonnutritive sucking for babies who are tube fed; recognizing the baby's signs of stress and reducing interactional demands on the child during those periods; teaching the significance of eye contact between child and caregiver; and emphasizing the importance of talking to the child in a soothing, reassuring, pleasant manner. The SLP also may play the part of coach to the parent or designated caregiver, encouraging appropriate interactions or teaching about and demonstrating feeding techniques or strategies designed to build oral-motor coordination in preparation for oral feedings. The SLP may also participate in discharge planning by providing the family with lists of community contacts through which follow-up developmental monitoring and assessments are available and assisting in the design of a plan that assures a smooth transition from the structured world of the NICU to the home and community.

Obviously the SLP who works in the hospital setting needs a basic understanding of preterm infants and their problems. Likewise, it is the responsibility of the SLP to provide staff education that helps other members of the team understand the important relationship between an infant's very earliest experiences and subsequent communicative development.[18] Participation in staff-development seminars, on-site training provided by other members of the team, and participation in continuing-education programs to acquire and enhance skills are also required of the SLP.

The SLP is likely to be involved in developmental feeding or positioning program strategies and may provide other direct therapy to the infant in keeping with developmental care practices. In any case, the SLP's role will involve the processes of team functioning and the principles of adult education and interaction with parents and members of the professional staffs.

▼ OTHER CONSIDERATIONS

There are some general considerations regarding work in the NICU with which the SLP must be familiar. These include information about infection control, characteristics of preterm infants, signs of infant stress, and roles of other members of the multidisciplinary team.

Infection Control

The NICU staff must observe strict infection-control protocols. Although the requirements vary somewhat from site to site, universal infection control precautions are common to all sites.

It is imperative that staff who contact the infants know and use appropriate hand-washing procedures. Before or upon entering the unit, hands are washed thoroughly, using a germicidal soap or solution and a scrub brush or pad (paying special attention to the nails). Scrubs of 2 to 5 minutes are usually required. Rings should be removed (pinning them to scrub suit, apron, or undergarment with a safety pin to avoid potential loss or theft). Hands should be carefully washed between contacts with different infants and before a subsequent contact with a child if the staff member has handled equipment. Some hospitals require that clean cloth gowns or disposable aprons be worn by staff and visitors to the unit. Depending on hospital policy, sterile gloves may be required; they always should be used by workers who have a cut, burn, or other wound on the hand. Gloves should be changed between contacts with different babies and after handling equipment. Those SLPs who provide oral stimulation or participate in therapeutic feeding activities must be especially alert to the potential for spreading infection through improper hand washing and lax sanitary precautions.

The advent of congenital acquired immunodeficiency syndrome (AIDS) among newborn infants has made it imperative that certain additional precautions be taken by personnel. Some hospitals require masking and eye protection as a precaution against unanticipated exposure to urine, blood, or other body fluids. Although the SLP is less likely than the medical staff to have high-risk exposure, many AIDS babies have neurological involvement that affects their developmental progress. Exposure to the virus is possible during assessment and intervention activities. The practitioner should be familiar with universal precautions for health care providers.[19]

Characteristics of Preterm Infants

Preterm infants (those born before 40 weeks' gestation by some definitions, or earlier than 38 weeks by the World Health Organization's definition) possess a number of common characteristics that have a bearing on development. An infant's gestational age can be established by a combination of means. The most commonly used measures include (1) date of birth from conception (9 months plus 1 week is a common reckoning of term); (2) birth weight (i.e., average, small, or large for gestational age); and (3) physical characteristics (i.e., presence or absence of lanugo [body hair], skin color and transparency or opaqueness, and reflexes). Preemies are often low birth weight (LBW = <1500 g; i.e., less than 3 lb 4 oz) or very low birth weight (VLBW = <1000 g, i.e., less than 2 lb 4 oz); and micropreemies can have birth weights under 800 g (i.e., just over $1\frac{1}{2}$ lb). The organ systems of preterm infants are immature, especially the respiratory system.

Preterm infants can require immediate—and sometimes heroic—treatment to sustain life. It is not uncommon for preterm infants with respiratory problems to receive surfactant therapy (prophylactically to prevent development of respiratory distress or therapeutically to treat established respiratory distress) and then to be on oxygen therapy for a period of time. Some infants experience bronchopulmonary dysplasia (BPD), a condition linked with developmental problems.[20] Depending on the circumstances, the oxygen requirements to sustain life can have deleterious effects on the child's hearing or vision, which, in turn, place the child at risk for subsequent difficulties in communicative development.

Many preterm infants suffer from hypoxia (inadequate supply of oxygen). They may also have episodes of apnea (cessation of breathing for 15 seconds or longer) for a short or prolonged period of time. These and many other conditions may require supplemental oxygen treatment that may involve insertion of an endotracheal tube for ventilation, continuous positive airway pressure (CPAP) supplementation via a nasal canula or an oxyhood. Babies with "upper airway abnormalities … including conditions such as cleft lip and palate, choanal atresia, and tracheoesophageal fistula" are not candidates for CPAP, because "these conditions make it technically difficult or impossible to pass the [endotracheal] tube and establish a secure airway …" (p. 10).[21] Those who work with preterm infants and with infants who are admitted to the NICU for other reasons need to know that a bluish tinge to the lips, skin, or nails can be a sign that the child needs medical attention immediately.[11] However, these signs can be present in babies who are long-term oxygen dependent and are being treated for chronic hypoxia.

Other problems often seen in the NICU and implicated in developmental delays or disorders include (1) intraventricular hemorrhages (grades III and IV being significant), (2) prenatal drug exposure (cocaine and crack cocaine being especially important), (3) perinatal asphyxia (which may require "blow-by" oxygen supplementation at feedings, continuous oxygen saturation monitoring, provision of an apnea monitor at discharge, or any combination of these), (4) seizures, (5) fetal alcohol syndrome, (6) anatomical anomalies involving the head and neck, (7) congenital or perinatal infections, and (8) frank neuromotor impairment.

Chapter 2 provides more detailed information regarding causes of later communication disorders that may be identified very early in infancy.

Signs of Infant Stress

Babies are adept at signaling their need to discontinue interactions with their caregivers. Unfortunately, not all caregivers are adept at reading the signals. The communicative disorders specialist should be alert to the infant's attempts to communicate a need to rest from the current activity, regardless of how passive the activity seems to the adult. The baby may exhibit one or a combination of the following signals that indicate stress:

- Yawning
- Averting eye contact
- Straightening the arms
- Stiffening the body
- Covering the face with a hand
- Spitting up
- Sneezing
- Spreading the fingers
- Arching the back
- Crying
- Saluting (arms up in the air)
- Coughing
- Changing color
- Abrupt changes in muscle tone
- Abrupt changes in respiratory rate
- Abrupt changes in heart rate
- Bradycardia (slowing)
- Tachycardia (racing)
- Apnea

The SLP needs to be aware of the superficial physical signs that are considered significant by the medical staff. McKenzie[22] suggested a useful framework for identifying the level of behavioral organization in newborns, which is shown in Table 5-1.

Sometimes the staff inadvertently creates stressful conditions for the fragile infant. For example, difficulty in maintaining appropriate body temperature is a common problem for preterm infants. Newborns do not shiver to maintain body temperature, and a great deal of energy is expended in reestablishing an adequate temperature after it has been lost. Preterm babies need their energy for other purposes. As simple as it may seem, the SLP (or other staff member) with cold hands should warm them before handling, positioning, or initiating stimulation activities with the infant.

Another inadvertent cause of infant stress can be related to excessive auditory stimulation of the preterm infant. Montgomery[23,24] notes that "[i]n utero, infants are exposed to rhythmic continuous sounds of <72 dB. In NICU, the average sound is 60–90 dB with peaks up to 120 dB." Although a number of researchers have confirmed that appropriate auditory stimulation can have positive effects, cautions against overstimulation of any kind is a paramount consideration. Unless there is a current contraindication, it can be appropriate to suggest talking and singing to the baby, playing tape recordings of the mother's voice, and playing soft music. Babies who can tolerate these types of auditory stimuli have been shown to have higher scores on infant assessment tests and improved physical growth.[25-27]

The SLP must coordinate efforts with medical staff, other allied health professionals, and parents, who all interact with the infant at various times. Ongoing

TABLE 5-1
Infant Cues to Behavioral Organization

Element	Organized	Disorganized
Color	Even Pink Stable	Uneven Pale, blue, or labile
Gaze	Focused Connected Intense	Glazed Dull Stunned
Alertness	Peaceful Content Bright	Irritable Fussy Grunting
Motor	Smooth Ballet-like Quiet	Jerky Erratic Staccato
Breathing	Regular	Irregular Colic

Modified from McKenzie M: *How do you say CCMDFFSDS?* Keynote address at Region IV Interagency Coordinating Council's Multi-disciplinary Conference on Handicapped Infants and Toddlers, Lafayette, La, October 1990.

communication with the nursing staff assists the SLP in becoming acquainted with each infant's general condition, current status, temperament, feeding schedule, schedule of procedures or tests ordered for the day, and other important procedural information.

▼ Specialized Teams in the Neonatal Intensive Care Unit

The preceding discussion provides an overview of the many people and specialty areas represented in the NICU in general. Each member of the team is important to optimizing care for children admitted to the NICU, and each member works in conjunction with the other members of the staff, contributing unique expertise and experience. In addition to the team in general, there are also smaller teams designed to meet specialized needs of the patients and their families and comprised of a smaller number of practitioners who usually also serve on the total NICU team.

Composition, Styles, and Roles for the Speech-Language Pathologist on Specialized Teams Within the NICU

In addition to the highly trained team constituted by the NICU staff, specialized teams often bear titles that reflect the functions they perform. Examples of such teams include the following:

- Feeding teams can be composed of an occupational therapist, nurses, physician, nutritionist, SLP, and parents.
- Developmental assessment teams' members include specialists with expertise in sensorimotor, neurobehavioral, social, emotional, and communicative development. A growing number of multidisciplinary developmental assessment teams have been established as a result of implementation of early-intervention legislation. Under the Part C model, parents are team members, along with professionals, serving as decision makers and contributing to the fund of knowledge about their child's individual development.
- Parent and family support teams sometimes exist for the purpose of providing information, support, and technical training to parents and other family members who are caregivers of infants discharged from the NICU. During the infant's hospital stay, parents may be introduced to families of unit "graduates," who assist them in anticipating what to expect when they take their baby home.
- Discharge planning teams provide the family with information and recommended procedures to implement the infant's care following release from the hospital. Discharge planning is often handled by a designated individual, generally a social worker or a nurse, but team planning is becoming more common. In some hospitals, all discharge planning for the NICU is handled through the multidisciplinary team.
- Follow-up teams conduct regular follow-up monitoring of NICU graduates. Though more often conducted in a clinic format, follow-up monitoring is sometimes provided in the home by an outreach team from the NICU. Studies indicate that developmental follow-up care is useful for preterm babies whose only problem is prematurity.[28]

Because communicative development is dependent on and interrelated with development in other modalities, the SLP has much to offer as a member of many specialized teams. The present focus on prevention and habilitation, as opposed to the rehabilitative focus of the recent past, encourages a proactive approach in identifying and using the infant's developing skills in one area to build skills in related areas. Recalling the concept of brain plasticity in the young child, developmental intervention gives families defined objectives to work toward and emphasizes establishing positive outcomes, rather than waiting to implement remedial activities designed to undo established behaviors at a later time.

Infant Assessment in the Neonatal Intensive Care Unit

Infants admitted to the NICU are assessed constantly. The purposes of the assessments vary, but they usually analyze the child's physical state in relation to survival and wellness. As noted earlier, babies in the NICU are exposed to a great deal of stimulation. Their schedules are not the same as those followed by infants who spend a brief period of time in the hospital and then go home to the rhythms of family life. They must undergo treatments that in many cases are aversive. They live in an environment in which the lights may always be on and the hustle and bustle of activity is constant. All of this must be taken into consideration as the SLP participates in assessments, just as it is taken into account by nurses who utilize the Neonatal Individualized Developmental Care and Assessment Program (NIDCAP).[29]

The SLP can provide or participate in providing at least two major assessments in the NICU: feeding assessments and developmental assessments, both of which are performed as part of the team effort.

Feeding Assessment

Once the immediate medical problems have been resolved, concern shifts to the child's ability to take in sufficient calories for growth and development. Many infants initially receive nourishment via nasogastric or gavage feedings. Oral feeding is the normal and preferred means of feeding as soon as neuromotor development has advanced enough to make it feasible. Some infants have great difficulty managing the motor coordination required to feed from bottle or breast, and it is those children who require a feeding assessment. There are any number of reasons a child can fail to develop a normal suck-swallow-breathe pattern. Included on the list of possible reasons are the following:

- Prematurity
- Poor general health
- Lack of motor coordination
- Respiratory complications
- Cerebral palsy
- Unilateral vocal cord paralysis
- Paresis
- Hypotonia
- Neuromotor impairment
- Cardiac problems

- Cleft palate
- Other craniofacial anomalies
- Sensory (tactile) anomalies

Because vegetative functions of the oral mechanism predate developmentally and form the foundation for later functions of oral communication, it is entirely appropriate for a knowledgeable SLP to be a part of the feeding assessment and management team. Good nutrition promotes growth and development in all areas, including cognitive, social, and communicative development. Overt and submucous palatal clefts and other craniofacial anomalies that are associated with poor oral feeding can also lead to communicative impairment.

Suggestions for conducting feeding assessments for infants and toddlers along with selected techniques to assist in development of appropriate oral motor and feeding skills are included in Appendix A. It must be reiterated that the SLP who participates in or conducts feeding and swallowing assessment must have adequate training to do so.

The knowledgeable SLP may make recommendations about the type of nipple a given infant should use to minimize spillage during feedings, the pacing and frequencies of feedings to avoid overly expending the baby's energy reserves— signs of which may be reflected in the baby's oxygen saturation levels, heart rate, respiratory patterns, and/or state of alertness. Additionally, the SLP may make recommendations regarding whether oral stimulation should be used, or delayed, with a particular infant based on knowledge of whether the baby's neurological organization suggests one option or the other at any point in time. If nonnutritive sucking is appropriate, it may be advisable (again depending on the infant's stage of oral-motor organization) to use the same type of nipple used in oral feedings rather than using a stimulation device such as the Nuk, which is often recommended for infants with more advanced oral-motor coordination. Attention to such details can result in better tolerance of the feeding nipple and improved oral nutritional intake. When it is appropriate for a given infant, the SLP may document contraindications for specific feeding procedures (such as chin support). Any recommendation(s) made should be recorded both in the medical chart and in the form of a note alerting the nursing staff and parents of the recommendation(s), along with a brief note telling why it is being made with respect to developmental issues. It is also wise to discuss the recommendation(s) with the nurses assigned to the infant and with the parent(s), if they are available.

A major contribution to optimizing feeding skills is knowledge of whether to select and implement sensory strategies or motor strategies for a given infant. Clues to that selection are found in the practitioner's knowledge of primitive oral reflexes. Successful oral feedings are one of the major goals in optimizing infant development.

Once the baby is discharged from the hospital, it is wise to conduct follow-up consultations with the parent(s) and/or caregivers to answer any questions they may have about feeding practices and to be certain that the infant is gaining weight and not experiencing problems related to feeding. Such follow-ups might take the form of telephone contacts at appropriate intervals (the intervals are determined by the history of the individual child with feeding experiences in the hospital) while the child is on bottle feedings and at the point of transition to baby foods and, later, to table foods. A child who tolerates bottle feedings may not tolerate changes in texture as well or may have difficulty managing the oral-motor and sensory aspects of manipulating a substantial bolus of food or of chewing and swallowing. If problems are identified, the child's physician should be advised so that appropriate management or referral can occur.

Developmental Assessment

A discussion of the general nature of multidisciplinary developmental assessment is provided above. The present discussion is designed to provide additional information pertinent to working with medical and allied health specialists on what has historically been their turf, that is, the hospital. Remembering that their primary orientation and training have focused on sustaining life and curing disease, the developmental assessment will probably be approached by the medical staff from an orientation toward physical growth and development and gross neurological functioning. There may be an established protocol for conducting such assessments, using developmental assessment tools that are familiar to the medical staff. Increasingly, developmental assessments are being performed by physical therapists, occupational therapists, or both, and nursing staff trained to conduct the assessments. Suggested changes in their usual methods of completing evaluations may not be received well and should be initiated with caution. It may be more appropriate to suggest including an additional element in the assessment to address early communication development. Modifications in the interdisciplinary assessment procedure can emerge as mutual recommendations after the SLP becomes a trusted member of the team.

Developmental tests with which the medical community is most likely to be familiar are shown in Table 5-2.[30–32] It is essential to know how the norms were

---

TABLE 5-2
Assessment Instruments Commonly Used in Infant Assessments

Tool	Reference	Comments
The Neonatal Behavioral Assessment Scale (NBAS)	22	This is a widely used tool recommended for full-term newborns or preterm infants 37 weeks postconception and in stable medical condition. Administration time is approximately 30 minutes.
The Assessment of Preterm Infant Behavior	23	This tool was designed to be a downward extension of the NBAS. Examiners must be carefully trained in its administration. Assessment time is approximately 30 minutes.
Naturalistic Observation of the Preterm Neonate	24	This is an observation method that focuses on preterm newborns' responses to stress and adjustments in response to environmental supports. System requires observing the infant in 2-min time segments, and reports require anecdotal notes of the examiner.

developed for the tests in use in a particular unit. For example, for the Bayley Scales, under revision at this writing, typically developing children between 2 and 30 months living at home were the "norming" population. Healthy newborns were also used in developing the Neonatal Behavioral Assessment Scale. Instruments normed on infants not known to have disabilities and who were born at term have obvious limitations in their application to other populations.

Many hospitals' and some individual states' early-intervention systems (e.g., Louisiana, see Appendix A, Figure A-2) have adopted protocols based on the philosophical and procedural protocols of several instruments that their practitioners find particularly useful.

Observation of the child's patterns of development over a period of time and review of chart entries, medical information, and specific neurodevelopmental assessments, in addition to discussions with staff and parents, make it possible to gather assessment information without being intrusive or disturbing the baby.[33] If the baby appears to be having problems with markers of communicative development, discussions with the staff can include seeking technical information from them with regard to the possible causes of the problem and management options, as well as providing information for their consideration from the perspective of speech-language pathology.

Participation in continuing education activities and offering to conduct some of the in-house sessions on developmental care can serve the dual purposes of providing useful information to professional colleagues in related professions and of building an effective team of practitioners devoted to achieving optimal outcomes through developmental care in the NICU.

The SLP should be familiar with formal statements published by various professional organizations that outline the roles of practitioners who work with neonatal populations, including but not limited to the policy statement of the American Academy of Pediatrics (AAP) on the role of the primary care physician in the management of high-risk newborn infants[34] and the AAP's position on advanced neonatal nursing.[35] Taking the time to be familiar with what is recommended by the professional organizations of NICU colleagues is a gesture of respect for their training and professional endeavors and also goes a long way toward building trusting relationships among team members.

Working With Families in the Neonatal Intensive Care Unit

The necessity of dealing with families and their feelings in an empathetic and constructive way is stressed throughout this book. Very few families anticipate having an infant with problems. Parents struggle with their feelings of grief over the loss of the perfect child whom they were prepared to receive, feelings of concern and anxiety about the survival or appearance of the child who was born, feelings of helplessness and concern about lacking basic information on their child's condition, feelings of apprehension about the decisions they are required to make (often under extreme pressure to make them quickly), and the anxieties and stress brought about by the financial aspects of their situation.[36,37] In 2001, the average cost of the NICU stay was $2000/day, and the stay often extends to several weeks or even months. Montgomery[38] reported that "[i]npatient care provided to preterm infants … accounts for about one-third of the health care dollars spent on children." Robinson[39] noted that "[i]n 1987 the cost of treating a child in the NICU was between $12,000 and $39,000 and in some cases even exceeded $1,000,000."

However, babies born weighing less than 1200 g are identified by the Social Security Administration as being "disabled" and are automatically eligible for Medicaid benefits *while they are in the hospital and until they are at least a year old,* regardless of parental income. Thus the hospital bill will be covered. Babies weighing between 1200 and 2000 g at birth may also be considered disabled if they are small for their gestational age and have serious medical problems.[40] After discharge, parental income *is* considered in determining whether the infant will continue to be eligible for benefits. Such benefits, if they are determined to be appropriate, are incremental and tied directly to the family's income level. Keeping such information in mind, it is counterproductive to flood the family with information that they are not ready to deal with. The best-intentioned SLP who approaches the family too soon and overwhelms them with information or suggestions about behavioral or attitudinal changes is doomed to failure. Moreover, the family may erect emotional barriers that have an adverse effect on future interactions and make it difficult to develop an effective intervention plan.

The family's desire for additional information, their ability to process new knowledge, and their interest in pursuing developmental enhancements becomes clear to the SLP who employs active listening techniques and is appropriately responsive to the family's needs as *they* express them. The family's priorities change, sometimes several times in a single day, as they process the information they are receiving from a myriad of sources. There are always primary and secondary issues about which they are concerned.

The NICU staff will not have answers to all the questions a family may have but should be able to refer the family to sources from which reliable information can be obtained. For example, there are over 6000 genetic conditions and diseases known to affect several million persons in this country alone.[41] In an effort to provide reliable information about such disorders, the Genetic and Rare Diseases Information Center provides a free service that can be accessed by phone (888-205-2311), TTY (888-205-3223), e-mail (gardinfo@nih.gov), fax (202-966-5689), or mail (P.O. Box 8126, Gaithersburg, MD 20989-8126). Other sources that can be accessed by the Internet are listed in Appendix D.

Individual members of the family vary in their levels of acceptance, capacity to cope with the various stresses connected with their infant's care and nurturing, and in their desire for specific guidance from professionals. Appreciating the dynamics of each family's situation and dealing with each situation individually is a team effort.

If the SLP has physician orders to provide direct feeding therapy, it will be possible to provide direct information to the family in connection with the procedures being used. If that is *not* the case, questions such as "How may I help you today?" or "Is there anything I can do to help with that?" are always preferable to statements such as "Let me tell you what I think you should focus on next" or "Let me show you how to get your baby to do [or stop doing] that." Rossetti[1] suggested asking "What has changed since we last talked?" as a way of obtaining information, conveying genuine interest, and orienting the interaction toward issues about which the parents, rather than the SLP, are concerned.

Assisting parents in knowing what to expect is another way to help them focus their questions about their interactions with the infant. For example, the SLP can tell the parents that consistent interactive responses from their baby are unlikely to appear before 28-weeks gestational age. That knowledge, combined with an understanding that an otherwise healthy, premature baby who is held and talked to generally gains weight faster[1,41] and can recognize the mother's voice can cause parents to increase their visits and time spent holding the baby. The infant's early passivity is less worrisome when parents know that it is expected.[42]

As Rocco[43] observed,

[A]ssessments shape expectations. That is why they are so powerful. Assessments of infants and toddlers have a profound effect on how parents view their children's future and how they view their own competence as parents. Professionals who are involved in the assessment of very young children's development need to be aware of the power of the process and must be careful not to abuse it (p. 55).

Payment for Services Rendered

Billings for services rendered can be indirect (i.e., billed to an insurer or state agency) or direct (i.e., charged to the parent responsible for paying the baby's hospital bill). Billing can be done automatically as part of the NICU package provided by the hospital or can be accomplished through itemized charges submitted by a consulting professional who renders service.

It is important that the SLP find out what is reimbursable under the various mechanisms and the appropriate codes or terminology used to access the reimbursement source. For example, neurodevelopmental assessments, usually conducted by the physical or occupational therapist, are commonly reimbursable. Communication assessments, less familiar to insurers of children in this age group, may or may not be considered reimbursable as a unitary billing item. They have, however, traditionally been an appropriate portion of the pediatric developmental assessment (see the communication or oral language assessment sections of standardized developmental assessment tools) and, as such, are regularly reimbursed. Wording is often critical to whether a claim is reimbursed or denied—a fact of life in any area of health care—but one with which the SLP who is inexperienced in reimbursement practices may lack familiarity. Standard medical and psychological codes pertinent to SLP practice and that are contained in the ICD-10, DSM-4, or CPT (see Chapter 1 for references) are important to know for billing purposes.

Many early-intervention services are now covered under Medicaid, which has also recently revised its eligibility requirements to include families with higher income levels than were eligible before. Familiarity with Medicaid reimbursement policies is important for practitioners who work in any hospital or other setting that serves Medicaid-eligible families.

▼ SUMMARY

Specialized skills and evolving roles for the SLP in the NICU constitute a relatively new and challenging aspect of professional practice. Those SLPs who deal with infants after their hospital discharge must also have an appreciation for the NICU experience that was so recently an important part of the life of both baby and family.

▼ REFERENCES

1. Rossetti LM: *Speech-language pathologists in the NICU.* Paper presented at ASHA Conference, St. Louis, November 1989.
2. Brazelton TB: A window on the newborn's world: more than two decades of experience with the neonatal behavioral assessment scale. In Meisels SJ, Fenichel E, editors: *New visions for the developmental assessment of infants and young children*, Washington, DC, 1996, Zero to Three, p 127.
3. Gottwald WR, Alper BS: *Neonatal intensive care: the speech-language pathologist's role.* Paper presented at ASHA Conference, St. Louis, November 1989.
4. Montgomery LA: Implementing the neonatal individual developmental care and assessment program (NIDCAP) in a special care nursery [University of Iowa School of Nursing web site]. Available at http://www.nursing.uiowa.educ/gnirc/5thabstracts/ru98-g3.htm. Last revised July 12, 2001.
5. VandenBerg MA: Basic competencies to begin developmental care in the intensive care nursery, *Infant Young Child* 6:52–59, 1993.
6. Reese J: Pregnancy, parturition and premature birth [Bioethics web site]. Available at http://www.ajobonline.com;. Created Oct 17, 2000.
7. Kulinski J: Hoping for the best [Bioethics web site]. Available at http://www.ajobonline.com;. Created Oct 17, 2000.
8. Piecush RE, et al: Outcome of infants born at 24–26 weeks' gestation: II. Neurodevelopmental outcome, *Obstet Gynecol* 90:809–814, 1997.
9. Halsey CL, Collin MF, Anderson CL: Extremely low birthweight children and their peers: a comparison of school-age outcomes, *Arch Pediatr Adolesc Med* 150:790–794, 1996.
10. Wood NS, et al: Neurologic and disability after extremely preterm birth, *N Engl J Med* 343(6):378–384, 2000.
11. Hack M, Klein N, Taylor HG: Long term developmental outcomes of low birth weight infants, *The Future of Children*, Spring 5(1), 1995, The David and Lucile Packard Foundation.
12. Harrison H, Kositsky A: *The premature baby book: a parents' guide to coping and caring in the first years*, New York, 1983, St. Martin's Press.
13. Goodman DC, et al: Are neonatal intensive care resources located according to need? Regional variations in neonatologists, beds, and low birthweight newborns, *Pediatrics* 108:426–431, 2001.
14. Clark DL, et al: Effects of rocking on neuromuscular development in the premature, *Biol Neonate* 56:306, 1989.
15. Gorski PA: Premature infant behavioral and physiological responses to caregiving interventions in an intensive care nursery. In Call J, Galenson E, Tyson R, editors: *Frontiers of infant psychiatry*, New York, 1982, Basic Books, p 256.
16. Mouradian LE, Als H: The influence of neonatal intensive care unit caregiving practices on motor functioning of preterm infants. Special issue: neonatal intensive care unit, *Am J Occup Ther* 48:527, 1994.
17. Rauh VA, et al: The mother-infant transaction program: the content and implications of an intervention for the mothers of low-birthweight infants, *Clin Perinatol* 17:31, 1990.
18. Miller RM, Groher ME: *Medical speech pathology*, Rockville, Md, 1990, Aspen.
19. American Speech-Language-Hearing Association, Committee on Quality Assurance: AIDS/HIV: implications for speech-language pathologists and audiologists, *ASHA* 31:33, 1989.
20. Landry SH, et al: The social competence of children born prematurely: effects of medical compilations and parent behaviors, *Child Dev* 61:1605, 1990.

21. Berends SK: Nasopharyngeal CPAP: a nursing art, *J Neonatal Nurs* 20(6):9–16, 2001.
22. McKenzie M: *How do you say CCMDFFSDS?* Keynote address at Region IV Interagency Coordinating Council's Multidisciplinary Conference on Handicapped Infants and Toddlers, Lafayette, La, October 1990.
23. Montgomery LA: Making a multidisciplinary neonatal developmental care team a reality, *Neonatal Network* 18(4):47–49, 1999.
24. American Academy of Pediatrics Committee on Environmental Health: Policy statement—noise: a hazard for the fetus and newborn, *Pediatrics* 100(4):724–727, 1997.
25. Leib SA, Benefield DG, Greidubaldi J: Effects of early intervention and stimulation of the preterm infant, *Pediatrics* 66:83, 1980.
26. Katz V: Auditory stimulation and developmental behavior of the premature infant, *Nurs Res* 20:196, 1971.
27. Kramer LI, Pierpoint ME: Rocking waterbeds and auditory stimuli to enhance the growth of preterm infants, *J Pediatr* 88:297, 1976.
28. Ramey CT, et al: Infant health and development program for low birth weight premature infants: program elements, family participation, and child intelligence, *Pediatrics* 89:454, 1992.
29. Als H: Reading the premature infant. In Goldson E, editor: *Developmental interventions in the neonatal intensive care nursery*, New York, 1999, Oxford University Press, pp 18–85.
30. Brazelton TB: *Neonatal behavioral assessment scale clinics in developmental medicine*, No. 88, London, 1984, Spastics International Medical Publisher.
31. Als H, et al: Manual for the assessment of preterm infant behavior (APIB). In Fitzgerald HE, Lester BM, Yogman BM, editors: *Theory and research in behavioral pediatrics*, vol 1, New York, 1983, Plenum.
32. Als H: *A manual for the naturalistic observation of the newborn (preterm and fullterm)* [rev], Boston, 1984, Harvard Medical School, Department of Psychiatry.
33. American Academy of Pediatrics, Committee on Practice and Ambulatory Medicine and Committee on Fetus and Newborn: Policy statement: the role of the primary care physician in the management of high-risk newborn infants, *Pediatrics* 98(4): 786–788, 1996.
34. Ferrari F, et al: Cramped synchronized movements in preterm infants as an early marker for cerebral palsy, *Arch Pediatr Adolesc Med* 156(5):422–423, 460–467, 2002.
35. American Academy of Pediatrics, Committee on Fetus and Newborn: advanced practice in neonatal nursing, *AAP News* 8(7), 1992.
36. Minde K, et al: Mother-child relationships in the premature nursery: an observational study, *Pediatrics* 61:373, 1978.
37. Popper BK: Achieving change in assessment practices: a parent's perspective. In Meisels SJ, Fenichel E, editors: *New visions for the developmental assessment of infants and young children*, Washington, DC, 1996, Zero to Three, p 59.
38. Montgomery LA: Implementing the Neonatal Individualized Developmental Care and Assessment Program (NIDCAP) in a special care nursery [University of Iowa, School of Nursing web site]. Available at http://www.nursing.uiowa.educ/gnirc/5thabstracts/ru98-g3.htm. Dated July 12, 2001.
39. SSI can help pay for cost of care for smallest infants, *Social Security Courier* June/July; 4, 1993.
40. Robinson K: Ethical issues in the neonatal intensive care unit. Babies get a new chance at life [University of Pennsylvania web site]. Available at http://www.med.upenn.edu/bioethic/Museum/Robinson/NEO~1.HTM
41. Genome research institute launches information center, *Adv Speech-Lang Pathologists Audiologists* 12(10):22, 2002.
42. Moore ML: *High-risk mothers and infants.* Presented at the seminar sponsored by the Woman's Foundation, Inc, Lafayette, La, March 1988.
43. Rocco S: Toward shared commitment and shared responsibility: a parent's vision of developmental assessment. In Meisels SJ, Fenichel E, editors: *New visions for the developmental assessment of infants and young children*, Washington, DC, 1996, Zero to Three, p 55.

CHAPTER 6

IDENTIFICATION AND ASSESSMENT OF HEARING-IMPAIRED INFANTS AND TODDLERS

Thomas G. Rigo
Shalini Arehole

Hearing evaluation of infants and toddlers is one of the most challenging aspects of the practice of audiology. Many of the test procedures are unique to this population and must be tailored to the child's particular capabilities. The audiologist's primary goal is the identification and comprehensive assessment of the infant's hearing impairment at as young an age as possible. This is because it is necessary to obtain an accurate and detailed description of the degree and nature of the hearing loss before optimal hearing aid fitting and aural habilitation procedures can be initiated. As in adult assessment, the examiner must rely on a battery of test results to form a meaningful picture of the child's auditory capabilities. This battery includes both behavioral and objective tests that, when used in combination, provide information concerning the extent, site, and perceptual effect of the auditory pathology. This chapter reviews the procedures that are commonly used in test centers today and will provide the reader some insight into the capabilities and limitations of the techniques described. Chapter 10 discusses the effects of early hearing loss on communication ability and reviews the remediation procedures that are used to facilitate the development of speech and language.

▼ BEHAVIORAL THRESHOLD ASSESSMENT

Neonates

Behavioral assessment of neonates is limited to observations of overt reflexive responses to sound. Optimally, the infant is tested in a light-sleep state to minimize the false positives that occur with awake babies and the false negatives likely with infants in deep sleep.[1] However, in light of the reality of the test situation and the transitory nature of states of arousal, evaluation should be attempted regardless of the initial state observed.

The neonate is most responsive to complex, wide-band, sudden-onset stimuli.[2] White noise, narrow-band noise, speech bursts (e.g., *buh-buh-buh*), and premeasured noisemakers (e.g., squeeze toys or horns) are good examples. Suprathreshhold stimulation is necessary to elicit observable and reliable responses. During the first several weeks of life, responses to sound include arousal from sleep, eye widening, eye blinks, startling, changes in respiratory pattern, and initiation or cessation of the sucking reflex.[3] The type of response demonstrated by the infant depends on the prestimulus state. Quiet and sleeping babies show increases in activity; active babies display reductions or cessation of prestimulus behaviors.[4]

The probability and validity of response are highest when testing is conducted in a sound-treated audiometric booth. Examinations can be administered in a quiet room, provided ambient noise levels do not exceed 60 dB SPL.[1] Testing is usually conducted with the child in the parent's arms. The tester and parent should ensure that the child's ears remain unobstructed. The stimulus should be presented briefly (for 2 seconds), and the response must be seen within 2 seconds of stimulus presentation. If noisemakers are used, they should be held motionless next to the child for several seconds before stimulation, and any airstream emitted from the noisemaker should be directed away from the child. Repeat testing should be conducted to validate the initial response. Most examiners conclude testing by introducing an intense stimulus; the clear startle response that is usually seen serves to substantiate the more subtle responses observed with softer stimuli. Testing with frequency-specific stimuli (e.g., warble tones, narrow-band noise) can be attempted, but the examiner should be aware of the infant's relatively low responsiveness to these stimuli and the probability of the response ceasing to manifest on repeated stimulation. Information relative to type of hearing loss can be obtained by repeating the above procedures with a bone-conduction receiver placed high on the infant's forehead and comparing these responses to those observed in response to air-conducted stimuli.

Older Infants

By 3 months of age, the infant's developing auditory experience and motoric maturation allow for more elaborate orienting responses to sound. At 3 to 4 months, orientation is limited to a horizontal head turn towards the sound source. Initially, infants localize horizontally to sounds originating at, above, and below their eye level. As motor control improves, more accurate localizations emerge. Direct localizations to sounds below eye level are seen by 9 to 13 months and above eye level by 13 to 16 months.[1]

The signal intensity necessary to elicit a behavioral response decreases in a systematic fashion as the infant grows. Two trends are of particular importance. First, the growing infant responds to decreasing sound intensities irrespective of the type of stimulus presented. Second, at any age, the infant remains most responsive to complex, relevant stimuli, such as speech.

The child's increased responsiveness to sound provides the examiner with the opportunity to acquire more detailed sensitivity data. Of prime importance is the determination of behavioral threshholds for frequency-specific stimuli. Use of wide-band inputs provides little information about hearing sensitivity as a function of frequency. An infant's audiometric configuration can be established only with frequency-specific inputs such as warble tones or, to a lesser extent, narrow-band noise. For example, an infant who suffers from high-frequency hearing loss responds to a simple speech stimulus, such as *buh-buh-buh*, at normal threshold by receiving and reacting to the low-frequency energy contained within the syllable *buh*. The response indicates that at least some portion of the child's hearing is within normal range but does not rule out the presence of hearing loss.

The use of frequency-specific stimuli in infant testing presents a problem of response habituation. A significant number of stimuli must be introduced during a test session to acquire sensitivity data across a meaningful range of frequencies. Unfortunately, inputs such as warble tones are abstract and nonmeaningful, and an infant's response to these types of sounds extinguishes quickly. This difficulty can be overcome by using a test technique most often referred to as *visual reinforce-ment audiometry* (VRA).[5] In this operant conditioning procedure, a visual stimulus serves to reinforce the infant's localization response to sound. Reinforcers can range from blinking lights to animated toy animals. In effect, the entertaining visual event following a response to an auditory signal sustains the continued reaction to that signal.

The VRA procedure is best conducted with the infant facing forward on the parent's lap. Stimuli are presented from one of two speakers located 45 to 90 degrees to each side of the child's position and introduced at descending inten-sity levels until a threshhold is reached. Some infants, particularly those younger than 12 months, respond inconsistently to warble tones despite the best attempts of the examiner. In these cases, introduction of narrow-band noises, music, noise-makers, or speech can provide better results. It must be remembered, however, that these types of inputs limit, to varying degrees, one's ability to determine audiometric configuration because of the loss of frequency specificity.

Soundfield testing is generally considered the most appropriate method of evaluating children under 2 years of age. The great majority of children in this age group do not tolerate placement of earphones, and their attempted use often results in aggravated test situations. Soundfield procedures, however, impose several limitations on test interpretation. First, depending on age, infants with severe and profound hearing loss may not show any response in a soundfield test environment, thus limiting the examiner's ability to differentiate these degrees of impairment. This is because of the output limitations of soundfield systems, which, for example, can range from 90 to 105 dB HL for speech inputs. Second, conclusions concerning individual ear sensitivity can be reached only when test-ing is conducted with earphones. It is incorrect to assume that the observation of accurate localizations during soundfield testing implies bilateral sensitivity. It follows that the examiner can only assume that the better ear is being tested when assessment is limited to soundfield procedures. Finally, the inability to determine bone-conduction thresholds in soundfield prevents the examiner from ascertaining whether a measured hearing loss is conductive, sensorineural, or mixed in nature.

Modification of the standard soundfield procedure can be attempted with headphones and the bone vibrator. The success of these procedures is, of course, dependent on the child's willingness to allow placement of these devices. Localizations can be successfully generalized from soundfield to headphone conditions.[6] When testing with the bone vibrator, however, the examiner should accept any visual response observed because localizations can be difficult or impossible to achieve or, in some cases, can be reversed because of the occlusion effect.

2- to 3-Year-Old Children

By 2 years of age, children may begin to respond successfully to more conventional threshold procedures. The technique of choice for the 2- to 3-year-old child is conditioned-play audiometry. In this procedure, the child is conditioned to respond to an auditory signal with some form of play activity, such as putting pegs in a hole, throwing blocks into a bucket, stacking rings on a stick, or putting pieces of a puzzle together. Conditioned play should be attempted on all children older than 2 years of age, but the procedure may not be entirely successful for many children between the ages of 2 and 3 years. Levels of success are highly dependent on the child's disposition, manageability, social maturity, and cognitive and language abilities. By 3 years of age, however, the procedure is usually effective for all but the most difficult-to-test children.

Play audiometry begins with a conditioning period in which the child is trained to perform the play activity in response to the suprathreshold presentation of a pure tone. Most children respond appropriately to verbal instruction and encouragement; for younger children and those with cognitive or receptive language limitations, however, it is usually necessary for the examiner to shape the response. After conditioning, testing is conducted with earphones and the bone vibrator using conventional threshold-seeking techniques.

▼ Speech Audiometry

Speech audiometrics should be considered a routine component of the pediatric hearing evaluation. For children younger than 3 years of age, procedures are restricted in scope and usually are conducted in an informal and subjective manner because of the infant's limited responsiveness, short attention span, and restricted receptive vocabulary. Despite these constraints, speech testing is often the only procedure that can be administered successfully to a young, difficult-to-test child. Speech materials are more meaningful and interesting than inputs such as warble tones and bands of noise and usually hold a child's attention for a longer period of time.

Speech Detection Threshhold

Speech detection threshhold refers to the lowest intensity at which a listener can detect the presence of a speech stimulus. It is an awareness measure and does not necessarily imply recognition or comprehension of the stimulus. It is usually the sole speech measure obtainable for infants younger than 1 year because of their limited linguistic development.

Speech Reception Threshold

Speech reception threshold (SRT) is generally thought of as the softest intensity at which speech can be recognized. It is defined operationally as the lowest intensity level at which a listener can repeat 50% of speech stimuli presented. The SRT is usually determined by presenting spondee words (composed of two long or stressed syllables) in isolation. It has been found to be highly correlated to midfrequency pure-tone average in cases of flat and mildly sloping hearing loss.[7] SRT can be acquired in older infants after some degree of receptive language has been established.

Word Recognition

Word recognition (also referred to as *speech discrimination*) is the ability to identify monosyllabic words when presented in isolation. The specific test procedure depends on the type of information that is being sought. Testing is usually conducted to determine the listener's maximum intelligibility score. In this procedure, a list of 25 or 50 stimulus items is presented at a sensation level of 40 dB (re: SRT), and a percent-correct recognition score is obtained. The test results can be helpful in determining lesion site, predicting the benefits to be obtained from using a hearing aid, and identifying the specific linguistic confusions caused by the impairment.

Standardized word-recognition tests for children younger than 2.5 years of age are not generally available. The assessment of word intelligibility for these children is informal, with the stimulus items and response tasks shaped to meet the child's level of function. Standardized tests include the Northwestern University—Children's Perception of Speech test[8] for children older than 2.5 years of age, the Auditory Numbers Test[9] and the Pediatric Speech Intelligibility test[10] for children at least 3 years of age, and the Word Intelligibility by Picture Identification test[11] for children between 4 and 6 years of age. These ages refer to receptive language age. Most standardized tests use closed-stimulus sets and picture-identification response modes.

▼ IMMITTANCE TESTING

The immittance battery consists of two tests: tympanometry and acoustic reflex testing. These tests are designed to evaluate the status and function of the middle ear and the acoustic reflex arc, respectively. The main feature of the immittance meter is the probe assembly and its three measurement systems. The first system, consisting of a sound generator and loudspeaker, emits a low-frequency pure tone (referred to as the *probe tone*) of fixed intensity and frequency. High-frequency probe tones can also be used to gain additional information about certain types of middle-ear pathologies. The second system is composed of an air pump and manometer, which serve to alter and measure the air pressure within the ear canal. Most immittance meters provide for pressure variations within the range of +300 to –600 dekapascals (daPa). The third system consists of a microphone that measures the SPL within the external meatus. Before testing, a pliable probe tip is placed over the end of the probe assembly and inserted into the ear canal so that an airtight seal is obtained.

The central measure in immittance testing is middle-ear admittance. In practice, admittance refers to the mobility, or vibratory efficiency, of the middle-ear structures. It is derived from the measurement of the SPL contained within the sealed meatal cavity and is expressed in cubic centimeter (cc) or milliliter (ml) units of equivalent volume. The relationship among these three measures is complex and is best explained within the context of the tympanometric test technique.

Tympanometry

Normal transmission of sound through the conductive system depends on the vibration of the tympanic membrane and ossicles of the middle ear. The admittance of the middle-ear system is greatest when air pressure is equal on each side of the tympanic membrane. Any pressure imbalance between the outer and middle ear displaces the tympanic membrane from its normal position. This displacement reduces the membrane's ability to vibrate in response to sound energy, resulting in a reduction in the admittance of the conductive system. Other factors that can affect middle-ear admittance include the presence of fluid or other material in the middle-ear space, a stiffening or a disarticulation of the ossicular chain, and structural damage to or changes in the elasticity of the tympanic membrane.

In tympanometry, the admittance of the middle ear is measured as air pressure is varied in the external meatus. A normal tympanogram and the way in which it is derived are shown in Figure 6-1. Tympanometry begins by inducing a positive pressure of 200 daPa in the external meatus (Figure 6-1, point *a*), creating a pressure imbalance across the tympanic membrane. The imbalance displaces and stiffens the membrane, reducing middle-ear admittance. As a result, a large proportion of the acoustic energy of the probe tone is reflected from the tympanic membrane and back into the ear canal. Under this condition, the probe microphone measures a

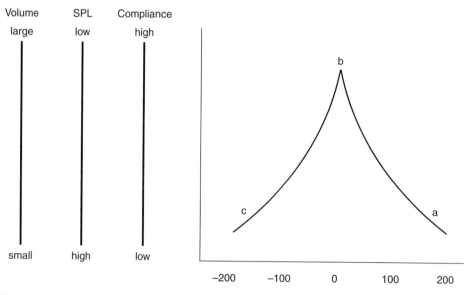

▼ **Figure 6-1** The relationship among the measures of middle-ear admittance, sound pressure level (SPL) in the external meatus, and equivalent volume in a normal middle ear.

high SPL within the external meatus. The air pressure is then reduced, lessening the imbalance across the tympanic membrane. When the air pressure in the external meatus is equal to that in the middle ear (Figure 6-1, point *b*), the admittance of the middle ear system is maximized. A large proportion of the acoustic energy of the probe tone is transduced and passed through the middle ear, minimizing the level of reflected sound in the ear canal. At this point, the microphone measures a low SPL within the external meatus. As the pressure is reduced further (Figure 6-1, point *c*), a pressure imbalance is created again across the tympanic membrane. The membrane stiffens, and admittance is reduced. The amount of reflected energy increases, and, again, a high SPL is measured in the ear canal. As can be seen, the examiner can make inferences about the admittance of the middle ear by measuring the SPL within the external canal. The relationship is an inverse one; a high SPL is measured when middle-ear admittance is low, and a low SPL is measured when the admittance of the middle ear is high.

Middle-ear admittance is expressed in ml or cc units of equivalent volume. Under conditions of reduced admittance, the high SPL measured by the probe microphone is equivalent to that expected for a small cavity. When middle-ear admittance is high, the low SPL measured is equivalent to that expected for a larger cavity (see Figure 6-1). It is important to remember that changes in equivalent volume during tympanometry represent changes in the admittance of the middle-ear system, not in the physical volume of the external meatus. Equivalent volume measures correspond to actual cavity size only when the middle ear is noncompliant.

Two primary measures are used to classify and interpret tympanometric configurations: middle-ear pressure and static admittance. Middle-ear pressure is derived from the location of the admittance peak. Because admittance is maximal when pressure is equal in the outer and middle ear, pressure in the middle ear can be deduced as equal to that contained in the outer ear when peak admittance is reached. Middle-ear pressure is considered to be normal when it is ±100 daPa (0 daPa represents ambient pressure). Static admittance is computed by subtracting the volume reading at +200 daPa (point of lowest admittance) from the volume reading at the admittance peak (point of highest admittance). This is simply a way to quantify the mobility of the middle-ear system. A small static admittance value suggests a stiff middle ear, whereas a high value indicates a hypermobile, or flaccid, system. Normal static admittance values generally range between 0.3 ml and 1.6 ml for most instruments.

The most common tympanometric classification system is that described by Jerger.[12] The various configurations are shown in Figure 6-2. Included in the figure is an unclassified tympanogram that is usually referred to as *transitional* or *intermediate*. It is characterized by a shallow, rounded admittance peak occurring within or outside of the normal pressure range. Table 6-1 outlines the interpretive measures and associated conditions for each tympanometric configuration.

Tympanometry is of limited diagnostic value for infants younger than 7 months of age, because of high false-negative findings.[13] For these children, a flat configuration is strongly associated with a pathological condition, but a normal result does not necessarily imply the absence of middle-ear involvement. Despite this limitation, tympanometry should be administered to this population in light of the incidence and consequence of middle-ear pathology during the first year of life.

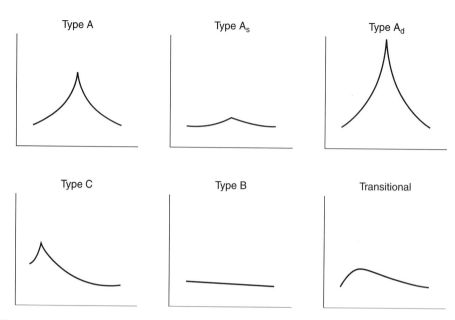

▼ **Figure 6-2** Classification of tympanometric configurations.

TABLE 6-1
Tympanometric Classifications and Associated Pathologic Conditions

Classification	Interpretive Measures	Associated Conditions
Type A	Normal pressure Normal admittance	Normal middle ear Otosclerosis
Type A$_s$	Normal pressure Reduced admittance	Otosclerosis Adhesions Tympanosclerosis Cholesteatoma
Type A$_d$	Normal pressure Elevated admittance	Disarticulation Flaccid tympanic membrane
Type C	Negative pressure Normal admittance	Eustachian tube dysfunction
Type B	No discernible peak Reduced admittance	Effusion Cholesteatoma Foreign bodies Impacted cerumen Tympanic membrane perforation (with high volume) PE tubes in situ
Transitional	Shallow, rounded peak Normal or reduced admittance	Effusion Cholesteatoma

Acoustic Reflex Testing

The *acoustic reflex* refers to the contraction of the stapedius muscle of the middle ear in response to an intense auditory stimulus. The action of the stapedius muscle is controlled by the facial nerve (cranial nerve VII) and a central network, or arc, located in the lower brain stem. The ipsilateral and contralateral pathways of the reflex arc give the acoustic reflex a bilateral character. That is, auditory stimulation to one ear elicits a stapedial contraction in both ears.

Contraction of the stapedius muscle causes a stiffening of the ossicular chain and a reduction in the admittance of the middle-ear system. Consequently, the acoustic reflex can be identified indirectly by the probe system as a change in the admittance of the middle ear on auditory stimulation. Because the reflex occurs bilaterally, it can be measured in the ear being stimulated (ipsilateral measurement) or in the ear contralateral to stimulation (contralateral measurement).

In acoustic-reflex assessment, the examiner measures the reflex threshold at octave frequencies of 500 to 4000 Hz. The acoustic-reflex threshold is found normally at sensation levels of 70 to 100 dB. It is important to note that reflex thresholds are documented in HL values but are interpreted according to the sensation levels (re: audiometric threshold) at which they occur. Pathology is indicated when reflexes are absent or when their thresholds are found at sensation levels lower or higher than the normal range of 70 to 100 dB. By analyzing findings across test conditions, lesion sites can be localized to the conductive system, cochlea, auditory nerve, or facial nerve.

Reflex results are broadly classified into two groups: probe effects and stimulus effects. A *probe effect* refers to the presence of abnormal findings when the probe is placed in a particular ear, regardless of the ear being stimulated. A probe effect indicates either the presence of middle-ear pathology in the probe ear or the presence of a facial-nerve lesion medial to stapedial innervation.

A *stimulus effect* is indicated when reflex abnormalities are associated with stimulation to a particular ear, regardless of the ear in which the reflex is measured. Stimulus effects suggest pathology of the ascending (auditory) portion of the reflex arc and can be reliably determined only when measurement is made from a normal middle ear. The site of lesion within the auditory system can be established by analyzing the sensation levels at which the reflex thresholds occur.

Reflex thresholds at reduced sensation levels (less than 70 dB) indicate cochlear site of pathology. Reflex thresholds at elevated sensation levels (greater than 100 dB) suggest neural pathology. In conductive losses, reflex thresholds occur at normal sensation levels, but the hearing levels may be higher than expected for a normal ear, as a result of the elevation of audiometric thresholds. Reflexes are absent under all test conditions in cases of bilateral conductive pathology, because the bilateral involvement prevents the measurement of reflexes in either ear.

▼ OTOACOUSTIC EMISSIONS

Otoacoustic emissions (OAEs) are sounds generated by a normal cochlea during auditory processing. The emissions are soft and occur at subthreshold levels. It is believed that OAEs are produced by the electromotility of the outer hair cells. The

OAEs generated within the cochlea travel through the middle ear and into the ear canal, where they can be measured with an insert microphone. Any pathology that affects normal outer hair-cell activity reduces or abolishes the OAE response. This allows OAEs to be used to assess cochlear function.

There are two basic categories of OAEs being measured for clinical purposes: transient evoked otoacoustic emissions (TEOAEs) and distortion-product otoacoustic emissions (DPOAEs). TEOAEs are generated by introducing a short-duration stimulus to the ear.[14] DPOAEs are generated by a simultaneous presentation of two different tonal stimuli to the ear. Both OAE measures are well-suited to the infant population because they are reliable, rapid, cost-effective, and noninvasive.[14,15]

Transient-Evoked Otoacoustic Emissions

TEOAEs are recorded by presenting repeated click stimuli to the ear in a quiet environment. A click is a short, broadband stimulus with an instantaneous rise and fall time. The clicks are introduced through an eartip at a high intensity level (around 80 dB SPL). A microphone enclosed in the eartip records both ambient noise and the emissions generated by the cochlea. The amplitude of the emissions are extremely small compared to that of the noise. The repeated presentation of the click stimulus, however, increases the amplitude of the emissions and decreases the amplitude of the noise, allowing the visualization of the TEOAE. Typically, the TEOAE is seen over and above the background noise across the frequency range of 500 to 5000 Hz.

TEOAEs are larger in infants than in adults.[16] Generally, infants' emissions are seen across a wider range of frequencies and at higher amplitudes. The differences in the response between infants and adults have been attributed to the difference in the dimensions of the ear canal, the angle of the tympanic membrane with respect to the ear canal, and the tissue composition of the ear canal.[17]

It is well established that TEOAEs are present in nonpathological ears with hearing thresholds better than 20 to 30 dB HL.[15,18] In contrast, emissions are absent in listeners with hearing loss ranging from mild to profound.

In evaluating the TEOAE, the examiner takes into consideration the following factors: (1) the amplitude of the TEOAE versus that of ambient noise (signal-to-noise ratio); (2) the frequencies at which the emissions are present; and (3) the reproducibility of the response. Figure 6-3, *A*, shows the TEOAE test results of a normal-hearing patient. The emissions are clearly visible above the noise floor across frequencies of +500 to 5000 Hz. Figure 6-3, *B*, shows the TEOAE results of a patient with a sensorineural hearing loss at frequencies above 2000 Hz. The absence of emissions above 2000 Hz is indicative of hearing thresholds greater than 20 to 30 dB HL at these frequencies. However, the degree of hearing loss at these frequencies cannot be determined from TEOAE testing.

Distortion-Product Otoacoustic Emissions

DPOAEs are produced by the simultaneous presentation of two pure tones (called *primary tones*) that differ in frequency.[19] When the primary tones are introduced to the ear at a moderate intensity level, they produce an emission whose frequency is different than that of the two primary tones. This emission is referred to as the *distortion product*. The presence of the distortion product indicates normal cochlear

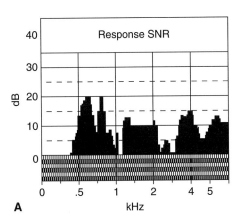 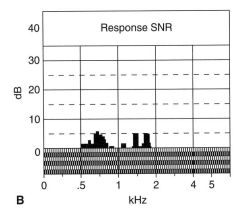

▼ **Figure 6-3** Transient evoked otoacoustic emissions (TEOAE) of a normal-hearing patient (**A**) and a patient with sensorineural hearing loss above 2000 Hz (**B**). TEOAE response is shown in black; noise floor is shown in gray. *SNR*, signal-to-noise ratio.

function in the frequency area of the higher primary tone or at the geometrical mean frequency of the primary tones. By shifting the frequencies of the primary tones and measuring the resultant distortion products, a measure of cochlear function across a range of frequencies can be obtained. A response is said to be present if DPOAE amplitudes are greater than the noise floor by at least 3 dB.[20] DPOAEs are present at frequencies whose hearing thresholds are within normal range. Emission amplitudes are reduced when hearing thresholds are between 15 and 50 dB HL. DPOAEs are not detected when hearing thresholds are greater than 50 dB HL. Figure 6-4, *A*, shows the DPOAE test results of the same patient as shown in Figure 6-3, *A*. The emissions are seen to occur at least 3 dB above the noise floor across frequencies of 1500 to 6000 Hz. Figure 6-4, *B*, shows the DPOAE results of the same patient as shown in Figure 6-3, *B*. The absence of emissions above 2000 Hz indicates sensorineural hearing loss at these frequencies.

Although evoked otoacoustic emissions (EOAEs) show great promise as an objective and reliable test of cochlear function, there are several limitations to the procedure: (1) External or middle ear involvement can interfere with measurement of emissions, and therefore, abnormal results under these conditions do not necessarily indicate cochlear pathology; (2) a high level of ambient noise, such as that found in nurseries or neonatal intensive care units, can interfere with the measurement of emissions, particularly in the lower frequencies; and (3) neural involvement can adversely effect cochlear function, and consequently, the use of OAEs in differentiating cochlear versus neural lesion sites can be limited.

▼ AUDITORY BRAIN STEM RESPONSE

The auditory-evoked potential (AEP) consists of a series of neuroelectrical responses generated throughout the auditory pathway. It is seen as a transient neuroelectrical pattern that is time-locked to an auditory stimulus and superimposed on the larger electroencephalographic (EEG) waveform. Components of the AEP occur as late as 500 msec after stimulus onset. Classification of the AEP is not yet standardized, but

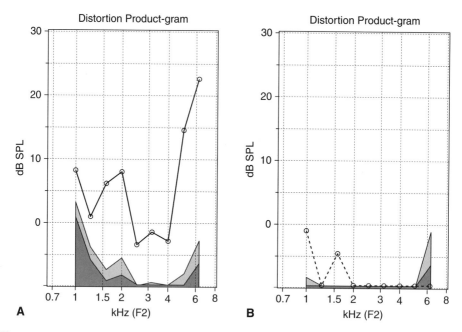

▼ **Figure 6-4** Distortion-product otoacoustic emissions (DPOAE) of a normal-hearing patient (**A**) and a patient with sensorineural hearing loss about 2000 Hz (**B**). (F2 = second [higher] frequency.)

its components are usually organized according to their site of generation and latency. For example, responses can be categorized as "fast" (1 to 10 msec), "middle" (8 to 50 msec), "slow" (50 to 300 msec), and "late" (300+ msec).

The AEP that has received the greatest clinical attention is the "fast" response, referred to as the *auditory brain stem response* (ABR). The adult ABR is composed of seven wave peaks occurring within the first 10 msec after stimulus onset. The wave peaks are designated as roman numerals I through VII in the order of their latency of occurrence.[21] The wave peaks are products of graded postsynaptic potentials and action potentials from different locations along the auditory nerve and brain stem. The latency from stimulus onset to the wave peaks (absolute latency) and latency from peak to peak (interpeak latency) represent axonal conduction time to and between generator sites, respectively.

The ABR of an infant is different from that of an adult. The waveform is usually limited to three wave peaks that correspond to the adult waves I, III, and V. Absolute and interpeak latencies are longer than adult values, and amplitudes of the wave peaks are markedly different. Variations between the infant and adult responses are attributed to several factors related to peripheral and central maturation. These include myelination, cochlear development, middle-ear condition, synaptic efficiency, and synchrony of neuronal firing.[22] Adult values are normally reached between 12 and 18 months of age.

Measurement of the ABR response presents a problem akin to that of finding a needle in a haystack. Stimulus-related potentials, including the ABR, are extremely small in amplitude when compared to that of the spontaneous EEG and other nonauditory physiological potentials. The instrumentation used is designed to extract the ABR by maximizing its signal and minimizing extraneous physiological and external "noise." This is accomplished by the use of specific electrode arrays, differential preamplification, filtering, analog-to-digital conversion, and repeated sampling and summation of the neuroelectrical activity that is time-locked to auditory stimulation.

Successful measurement of clear and reliable ABR waveforms requires the use of acoustic inputs that produce a high degree of neural synchrony. In this context, synchrony refers to the degree to which simultaneous neuroelectrical responses occur across a population of neural fibers. The greater the neural synchrony, the larger the magnitude of the ABR and the greater the time relationship of the ABR components to the signal onset. The highest degree of neural synchrony is achieved with a click stimulus because of its short duration and fast rise time. The use of the click, however, limits the interpretive power of the ABR because it is a broadband sound. Thus, in an effort to achieve neural synchrony, frequency specificity is lost. With the click stimulus, neural synchrony is greatest at the basal region of the cochlea, and it is generally assumed that the ABR response to click stimuli is correlated to behavioral threshold in the high-frequency region of 2000 to 4000 Hz. Other inputs having greater frequency specificity can be used during testing and are discussed in the following sections.

Clinical application of the ABR can be categorized into three major areas: (1) evaluation of the neural integrity of the auditory nerve and brain stem; (2) estimation of hearing threshold; and (3) determination of site of peripheral pathology. ABR testing is of particular value when assessing an infant because the measure does not require a voluntary, behavioral response and is unaffected by patient state and level of consciousness. Clear waveforms do require, however, that the child be relaxed, quiet, and unmoving. Most children between the ages of 8 months and 5 years are sedated before testing, usually with chloral hydrate. Neonates and infants younger than 8 months of age can be tested while in a natural sleep state. This state can be encouraged through sleep deprivation and feeding before testing. Children older than 5 years of age and adults can be tested in an awake state, provided they can remain relaxed and unmoving during test runs.

Evaluation of Neural Integrity

The ABR test is the most powerful tool in the audiological battery for the identification of tumors of the eighth nerve and brain stem. The measure is also useful in identifying vascular lesions and the effects of demyelinating diseases. Neurological assessment is conducted by presenting click stimuli at a suprathreshold intensity level. Most examiners test at levels between 75 and 95 dB nHL. (Zero dB nHL denotes average normal-hearing threshold for a click stimulus.) A normal ABR obtained from the right ear of a 32-month-old girl is shown in Figure 6-5. In normal patients, wave I is found to occur between 1.4 and 2.0 msec after stimulus onset, with each successive wave occurring at intervals of approximately 1 msec. Waves I, III, and V are generally the most prominent wave peaks and are used to interpret test findings. Hearing loss can have a significant effect on the absolute latencies of the ABR wave components. Wave I can be delayed or missing, or in cases of severe hearing loss, the entire response can be absent. Although absolute latencies can be prolonged, interpeak latencies are not affected by conductive or cochlear hearing loss.

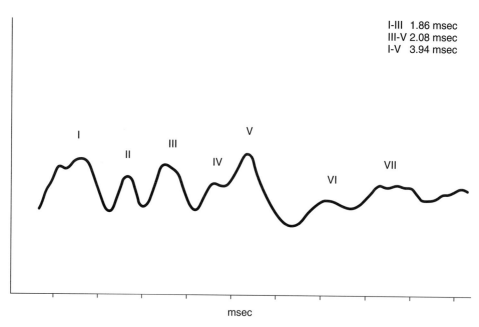

▼ **Figure 6-5**   Auditory brain stem response obtained from the right ear of a 32-month-old female patient (acquired at 95 dB nHL).

The most useful interpretive measure in neurological assessment is interpeak latency, specifically, I to V, I to III, and III to V latencies. A normal I to V latency is approximately 4.0 msec, whereas normal I to III and III to V latencies are about 2.0 msec. Standard deviations are generally between 0.1 and 0.2 msec. Interpeak latencies are considered abnormal and indicative of neurological abnormality when their values are greater than two standard deviations beyond the normal mean. When wave I is absent, interpeak latencies cannot be calculated. In these cases, the absolute latency of wave V or the interaural latency difference of wave V can be used for interpretive purposes.

A second indicator of neurological pathology is the partial or complete absence of wave peaks in patients who possess significant residual hearing. For example, in cases of eighth nerve or low brain stem lesions, all waves beyond wave I may be missing. For lesions affecting higher portions of the brain stem, waves I and III may be present with wave V absent.

Other measures that indicate neurological involvement include abnormal V to I amplitude ratios, "noisy" or poorly formed waveforms, and abnormal wave V latency shifts with increases in stimulus repetition rate.

Threshold Estimation

Stimulus intensity has a predictable and measurable effect on the ABR waveform. As stimulus intensity is decreased, wave components decrease in amplitude and increase in latency. Wave V is the most robust wave component and remains detectable at levels as low as 10 to 20 dB nHL. Other waves disappear at higher levels. For this reason, wave V is used as the basis for threshold estimation.

The threshold estimation procedure consists of obtaining ABR waveforms at decreasing stimulus intensity levels until wave V is no longer discernible. Wave V increases in latency on an average of 0.3 to 0.4 msec per 10 dB decrease in stimulus intensity within the range of 90 to 20 dB nHL. The lowest level at which wave V is detectable is referred to as *ABR threshold*. The exact relationship between ABR and behavioral threshold varies across test centers. Generally, when using a click stimulus, ABR threshold is reached 10 to 20 dB above behavioral threshold in the 1000- to 4000-Hz frequency range. Threshold estimation results for the previously described 32-month-old girl (see Figure 6-5) are shown in Figure 6-6. As can be seen, wave V decreases in amplitude and increases in latency as stimulus intensity is reduced from 95 to 25 dB nHL. Wave V is visible to 25 dB nHL, suggesting normal hearing sensitivity in the 1000- to 4000-Hz region. Bone-conducted click stimuli can also be used to determine sensorineural reserve and, when compared to air-conducted click responses, can provide information concerning site of lesion (see Figure 6-6).

A 500 Hz toneburst stimulus can be used to obtain low-frequency sensitivity data. With this stimulus, the ABR waveform usually appears as a single, relatively

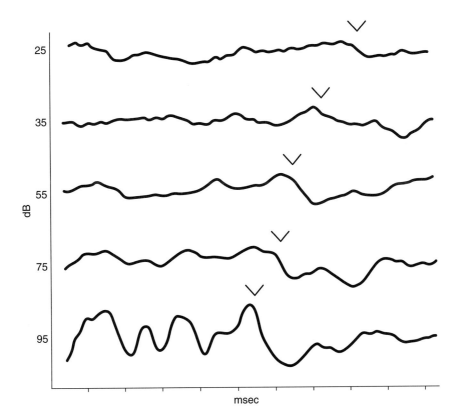

▼ **Figure 6-6** Threshold estimation results showing auditory brain stem response waveforms as a function of decreasing stimulus intensity.

broad wave peak. Its threshold is generally reached 30 to 40 dB above behavioral threshold at 500 Hz. This measure is useful for estimating the degree of low-frequency residual hearing and, when used in conjunction with the click stimulus response, can provide an approximation of the audiometrical configuration.

Determination of Site of Peripheral Pathology

By determining wave V latency across a range of stimulus intensities, a latency-intensity function (LIF) can be constructed. An LIF is a graphic plot that shows wave V latency changes as a function of intensity. The LIF for the patient discussed above (see Figures 6-5 and 6-6) is shown in Figure 6-7. The unlined area represents the normal latency-intensity relationship. By plotting a particular patient's LIF and comparing its slope to that of normal results, information concerning site of pathology can be obtained. Cochlear losses often display a steeper LIF slope than normally seen. That is, wave V latencies increase at a faster rate with decreases in stimulus intensity when compared to noncochlear lesions and normal ears. Often,

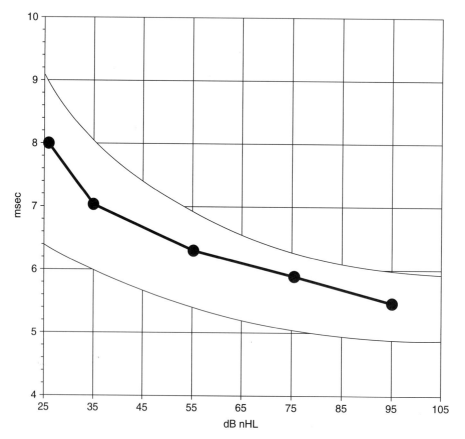

▼ **Figure 6-7** A wave V latency-intensity function. (Wave V latencies taken from Figure 6-6.)

normal latencies are seen at high intensity levels. In conductive losses, the LIF is shifted to the right but demonstrates a slope similar to that seen for normal results (see Figure 6-7).

▼ NEONATAL SCREENING

Optimal habilitation of the hearing-impaired requires identification of their disorder at the earliest possible age. Under ideal conditions, a congenitally hearing-impaired infant should be evaluated, fitted with hearing aids, and enrolled in an aural habilitation program by 6 months of age. This requires the existence of effective and efficient neonatal screening programs and procedures.

The routine hearing screening of all newborns, referred to as *universal screening*, is the best way to identify children with hearing impairment at birth. Universal hearing screening has been endorsed by professional associations and infant-hearing task forces[15,23,24] and is in effect at many birthing facilities. For a significant number of centers, however, the cost of universal screening programs is prohibitive. In cases where universal screening is not possible, guidelines have been developed for the hearing screening of neonates and infants who are at risk for hearing impairment.[23,24] The risk factors apply to neonates (birth to 28 days) and to infants (29 days to 2 years) who develop particular health conditions that require (re)screening. Those children who manifest one or more of the risk factors should be referred for hearing screening. Although risk-factor screening is less costly than universal programs, it must be recognized that this approach identifies only 50% of children born with significant sensorineural hearing loss.[23,24] The risk factors included within the guidelines are as follows.

Neonates (Birth Through 28 Days)

1. An illness or condition requiring admission of 48 hours or more to an NICU
2. Stigmata or other findings associated with a syndrome known to include a sensorineural and or conductive hearing loss
3. Family history of permanent childhood sensorineural hearing loss
4. Craniofacial anomalies, including those with morphological abnormalities of the pinna and ear canal
5. In-utero infection such as cytomegalovirus, herpes, toxoplasmosis, or rubella

Neonates or Infants (29 Days Through 2 Years)

1. Parent or caregiver concern regarding hearing or developmental delay
2. A family history of hereditary childhood sensorineural hearing loss
3. Stigmata or other findings associated with a syndrome that is known to include a sensorineural or conductive hearing loss
4. Postnatal infections associated with sensorineural hearing loss including bacterial meningitis
5. In-utero infection (e.g., toxoplasmosis, other agents, rubella, cytomegalovirus, herpes simplex [TORCH])

6. Neonatal indicators—specifically hyperbilirubinemia at a serum level requiring exchange transfusion, persistent pulmonary hypertension of the newborn associated with mechanical ventilation, and conditions requiring the use of extracorporeal membrane oxygenation (ECMO).
7. Syndromes associated with progressive hearing loss, such as neurofibromatosis and Usher's syndrome
8. Neurodegenerative disorders, such as Hunter syndrome, sensory motor neuropathies, such as Friedreich's ataxia and Charcot-Marie-Tooth syndrome
9. Head trauma
10. Recurrent or persistent otitis media with effusion for at least 3 months

Test procedures are identical for universal and risk-factor screening programs. Neonates should undergo hearing screening before being discharged from the hospital. The procedures of choice for neonates and infants to 6 months of age are EOAE or ABR. Most centers use one or the other test, although the National Institutes of Health (NIH)[15] recommends that both tests be used under certain conditions. Under the NIH protocol, the use of EOAEs alone is sufficient if the screening is passed; if it is failed, it should be followed by ABR screening. This two-stage procedure is recommended because EOAE is a more rapid and cost-effective test but lacks the degree of specificity of the ABR test.

The pass criteria for EOAEs is the presence of emissions bilaterally at an acceptable signal-to-noise ratio in response to suprathreshold clicks in TEOAE screening or in response to a series of suprathreshold primary tones in DPOAE screening. The pass criterion for ABR is the presence of wave V bilaterally in response to click stimuli presented at 35 dB nHL or lower.[24]

For children between the ages of 6 months and 3 years, behavioral screening techniques can be used. VRA is the procedure of choice for children between the ages of 6 months and 2 years. Conditioned play audiometry can be attempted when screening the 2- to 3-year-old child. The pass criteria for these techniques are reliable responses to 1000-, 2000-, and 4000-Hz pure tones presented bilaterally at 30 dB HL for VRA and at 20 dB HL for conditioned play audiometry. In cases where soundfield testing is necessary because earphone placement is not possible, parents should be advised that the existence of unilateral hearing impairment is not ruled out.[24]

Screening failures should be referred for audiological evaluation to include behavioral testing, additional electrophysiological testing, and immittance measures. Follow-up and management systems for children identified as hearing-impaired should include medical, otological, and diagnostic and habilitative audiological services.

▼ REFERENCES

1. Northern JL, Downs MP: *Hearing in children*, ed 4, Baltimore, 1991, Williams & Wilkins, p 139.
2. Bench J, et al: Studies in behavioral audiometry. III. Six-month-old infants, *Audiology* 15:384, 1977.
3. Eisenberg RB: *Auditory competence in early life*, Baltimore, 1976, University Park Press.
4. Bench J: The law of initial value: a neglected source of variance in infant audiometry, *Int Audiol* 9:314, 1970.

5. Liden G, Kankkunen A: Visual reinforcement audiometry, *Acta Otolaryngol* 67:281, 1969.
6. Haug O, Baccaro P, Guilford F: A pure-tone audiogram on the infant: the PIWI technique, *Arch Otolaryngol* 86:435, 1967.
7. Carhart R: Observations on relations between thresholds for pure tones and for speech: *J Speech Hear Disord* 36:476, 1971.
8. Elliot L, Katz D: *Development of a new children's test of speech discrimination*, St. Louis, 1980, Auditec.
9. Erber NP: Use of the auditory numbers test to evaluate speech perception abilities of hearing-impaired children, *J Speech Hear Disord* 45:527, 1980.
10. Jerger S, et al: Pediatric speech intelligibility test. I. Generation of test materials, *Int J Pediatr Otorhinolaryngol* 2:217, 1980.
11. Ross M, Lerman J: A picture identification test for hearing-impaired children, *J Speech Hear Res* 92:311, 1970.
12. Jerger J: Clinical experience with impedance audiometry, *Arch Otolaryngol* 92:311, 1970.
13. Paradise JL, Smith C, Bluestone CD: Tympanometric detection of middle ear effusion in infants and young children, *Pediatrics* 58:198, 1976.
14. Kemp DT: Stimulated acoustic emission from within the human auditory system, *J Acoust Soc Am* 64:1386, 1978.
15. National Institutes of Health: *Consensus statement: early identification of hearing impairment in infants and young children*, Bethesda, Md, 1993, NIH, p 11.
16. Bray P, Kemp DT: An advanced cochlear echo technique suitable for infant screening, *Br J Audiol* 21:191, 1987.
17. Norton SJ: Applications of transient evoked otoacoustic emissions to pediatric populations, *Ear Hear* 14:64, 1993.
18. Prieve BA, Gorga MP, Neely ST: Otoacoustic emissions in an adult with severe hearing loss, *J Speech Hear Res* 34:379, 1991.
19. Kemp DT: Evidence of mechanical non-linearity and frequency selective wave amplification in the cochlea, *Arch Otorhinolaryngol* 244:37, 1979.
20. Lonsbury-Martin BL, et al: Clinical testing of distortion-product otoacoustic emissions, *Ear Hear* 14:11, 1993.
21. Jewett DL, Williston JS: Auditory-evoked far fields averaged from the scalp of humans, *Brain* 94:681, 1971.
22. Cox LC: Infant assessment: developmental and age-related considerations. In Jacobson JT, editor: *The auditory brainstem response*, San Diego, Calif, 1985, College-Hill Press, p 297.
23. Joint Committee on Infant Hearing Year 2000 position statement: principles and guidelines for early hearing detection and intervention programs, *ASHA* 21(suppl): 29–32, 2002.
24. Audiologic Assessment Panel: *ASHA desk reference*, Rockville, Md, 1997, American Speech-Language-Hearing Association.

CHAPTER 7

AUTISTIC SPECTRUM DISORDER

Special Considerations in Assessment and Intervention with Infants and Toddlers

Frances P. Billeaud

A utistic spectrum disorder (ASD) represents a special and unique concern for parents and professionals. There is an urgent need for early diagnosis of the condition and for immediate intervention when the diagnosis has been made.[1–3] Autistic spectrum disorder is one of several conditions that fall under the broader category of pervasive developmental disorder (PDD) in the diagnostic reference *The Diagnostic and Statistical Manual-IV*[4] published by the American Psychiatric Association, which is used by a wide range of professionals as the standard criteria for specifying this diagnosis.

As Scambler, Rogers and Wehner[5] point out, "[w]hile it was formerly considered to be a low-incidence disorder, it is now recognized to be more prevalent in childhood than diabetes, cancer, spina bifida, and Down syndrome." Some believe the increasing numbers of identified cases constitute an epidemic; others ascribe the increased prevalence figures to increased vigilance and better diagnosis at earlier ages.

The families of children with ASD face difficult social issues, educational management issues, and behavioral issues that present themselves in the course of raising their children. Early and appropriate management has proven to be beneficial for both the families and affected children.

▼ PERVASIVE DEVELOPMENTAL DISORDERS AND AUTISTIC SPECTRUM DISORDER

The general category of pervasive developmental disorders includes ASD, Rett's disorder, Asperger syndrome, childhood disintegrative disorder, and PDD not otherwise specified (PDD-NOS). The term *PDD* is often used in the literature as a synonym for ASD, especially before a differential diagnosis is possible, but the presence of certain atypical communicative and behavioral characteristics common to the spectrum of disorders is documented in a given child. ASD is a neurological disability of unknown origin in most cases; in some cases, it is the result of a genetic problem. It is presumed by most to be present from birth, although some assert that it can be acquired through an intolerance for certain elements that occur in the environment. A criterion for ASD is that it must be present before the age of 3 years. ASD affects 1 in 500 children in this country,[2] and there are an estimated 5 million total cases across age groups.[6–8] Prevalence rates are reportedly similar in the United Kingdom and in India. Nearly all studies report that about four boys are affected by ASD for every girl so diagnosed.[9–10]

Because several other syndromes and conditions mimic the characteristics of ASD, it is imperative that a differential diagnosis be established as soon as possible. For example, tuberous sclerosis complex, certain severe emotional disorders, Landau Kleffner syndrome, Fragile X, and Smith-Magenis syndrome[11] may either coexist with or be mistaken for ASD; the importance of early differential diagnosis is that appropriate treatments for the various conditions differ from what is an appropriate treatment program for ASD. Unfortunately, reaching a differential diagnosis usually takes time. Therefore, when the triad of symptoms clusters characteristic of the PDDs is present, very young children—for example, those who have not yet developed oral language—who may be suspected of having ASD are "temporarily labeled" as having PDD. The triad of symptoms clusters necessary for the definition of ASD includes (1) qualitative impairment in reciprocal social interaction; (2) qualitative communication impairment; and (3) a narrow, restricted range of interests and insistence on "sameness" (sometimes referred to as *idiosyncratic behaviors*). For the reason cited, Tsai[12] prefers the term *autistic continuum disorder*, which would allow children to move up or down on the continuum as symptoms emerge or disappear over time. Despite the complexities of arriving at a differential diagnosis—or even agreement on what to call the problem—recent research and clinical practice have made it possible to identify children with ASD as early as 12 to 18 months of age. Newer research is pointing in the direction of the possibility of identifying symptoms of risk in infants as early as 8 or 9 months.[13–17]

Bauman [18] points out that:

During infancy, autistic children may be extremely passive babies requiring little attention, or they may be very irritable, difficult to feed, have irregular sleep patterns, and resist cuddling. As young children, they appear to be socially aloof, seemingly unaware of the presence or feelings of others. Alternatively, some autistic children can be overly and inappropriately affectionate, even with strangers. They can become excessively attached to and clingy with one parent and tolerate separation poorly (p. 690).

Many autistic children appear to have difficulty in modulating the input of sensory information. Some appear to be particularly sensitive to auditory stimuli, such as mechanical noises, school bells, a baby's cry, or the subtle noises made by fluorescent lighting. Some are particularly sensitive to light touch, such as tags in their shirts, seams in their socks, haircuts, and new unwashed clothing.... Alternatively, these same children may appear impervious to pain, failing to cry even when severely hurt.

Some seek comfort from the sensation of pressure ... some autistic children also appear to be excessively sensitive to odors and others to food textures... (p. 691).

In their 2001 editorial in the *Journal of the American Medical Association*, Hyman, Rodier and Davidson[19] summarized the findings of Short and Schopler[20] and Stone and colleagues[21]: "More than 75% of children with autism who have language delays and differences in social interaction and behavior are identified by their parents as being 'different' by age 2 years."

Box 7-1 shows the DSM-IV criteria for making the diagnosis of autistic spectrum disorder. Early signs of ASD have been identified and are discussed later in this chapter.

Children with ASD, like all other children, have their own individual personalities and behaviors, although many of the behaviors found among children with ASD are commonly observed (e.g., hand flapping, aversion of eye-contact, behaviors indicative of tactile sensitivity or vestibular disturbances). Children with ASD exhibit the full range of intellectual functioning; some have various levels of mental retardation, some possess normal intelligence, and some are extremely bright.

Although ASD has been presumed to be a lifelong condition—and certainly is among those individuals whose ASD is traceable to a genetic marker—some children are said to have grown to be considered "normal" with appropriate care. Early intervention, provided from the time the child is suspected of having ASD, has proven to ameliorate the sequelae of the condition and to enable affected children to achieve significantly improved social, communicative, and academic skills.[2,3] Early intervention consists of a coordinated program of strategies to promote appropriate behaviors, communicative development, and social interactions. Recent research indicates that between 20 and 25 hours of such programming is the minimal requirement to produce optimal results.[2,22]

▼ DIAGNOSIS, ASSESSMENT, AND PROCEDURAL PROTOCOLS FOR VERY YOUNG CHILDREN

It is quite possible that a child with ASD may be referred first to a speech-language pathologist (SLP) because of parental concern for delayed onset of speech or atypical speech and language development. Children with ASD are often physically healthy, growing normally, and not a particular concern to the medical community. Parents are, in fact, often reassured by busy pediatricians or family practitioners that speech will emerge in due time and that the time to be concerned about a delay might be around age 24 to 36 months. Physicians are, however, becoming more attuned to parental concerns in terms of delayed or atypical communicative and behavioral development as a result of two articles published in the medical literature: "Practice Parameter: Screening and Diagnosis of Autism" (published by the American Academy of Neurology in 2000)[1] and "The Pediatrician's Role in the Diagnosis and Management of Autistic Spectrum Disorder in Children" (published by the American Academy of Pediatrics in 2001)[3]. A less widely circulated work, *ICDL Clinical Practice Guidelines*, published by The Interdisciplinary Council on Developmental and Learning Disorders in 2000 addresses clinical guidelines for physicians as well as SLPs, pediatric occupational therapists, physical therapists, child psychiatrists, ophthalmologists, social workers, and early childhood educators.[23]

Box 7-1
DSM-IV Criteria, Pervasive Developmental Disorders

299.00 Autistic Disorder

A. A total of six (or more) items from (1), (2), and (3), with at least two from (1), and one each from (2) and (3):
  (1) qualitative impairment in social interaction, as manifested by at least two of the following:
    (a) marked impairment in the use of multiple nonverbal behaviors, such as eye-to-eye gaze, facial expression, body postures, and gestures to regulate social interaction
    (b) failure to develop peer relationships appropriate to development level
    (c) a lack of spontaneous seeking to share enjoyment, interests, or achievements with other people (e.g., by a lack of showing, bringing, or pointing out objects of interest)
    (d) lack of social or emotional reciprocity
  (2) qualitative impairments in communication, as manifested by at least one of the following:
    (a) delay in, or total lack of, the development of spoken language (not accompanied by an attempt to compensate through alternative modes of communication such as gesture or mime)
    (b) in individuals with adequate speech, marked impairment in the ability to initiate or sustain a conversation with others
    (c) stereotyped and repetitive use of language or idiosyncratic language
    (d) lack of varied, spontaneous make-believe play or social imitative play appropriate to developmental level
  (3) restricted, repetitive, and stereotyped patterns of behavior, interests, and activities as manifested by at least one of the following:
    (a) encompassing preoccupation with one or more stereotyped and restricted patterns of interest that is abnormal either in intensity or focus
    (b) apparently inflexible adherence to specific, nonfunctional routines or rituals
    (c) stereotyped and repetitive motor mannerisms (e.g., hand or finger flapping or twisting or complex whole-body movements)
    (d) persistent preoccupation with parts of objects
B. Delays or abnormal functioning in at least one of the following areas, with onset prior to age 3 years: (1) social interaction, (2) language as used in social communication, or (3) symbolic or imaginative play.
C. The disturbance is not better accounted for by Rett's disorder or childhood disintegrative disorder.

299.80 Pervasive Development Disorder, Not Otherwise Specified

This category should be used when there is a severe and pervasive impairment in the development of reciprocal social interaction or verbal and nonverbal communication skills, or when stereotyped behavior, interests, and activities are present, but the criteria are not met for a specific pervasive developmental disorder, schizophrenia, schizotypal personality disorder, or avoidant personality disorder. For example, this category includes "atypical autism"—presentations that do not meet the criteria for autistic disorder because of late age of onset, atypical symptomatology, or subthreshold symptomatology, or all of these.

299.80 Asperger's Disorder

A. Qualitative impairment in social interaction, as manifested by at least two of the following:
  (1) marked impairment in the use of multiple nonverbal behaviors, such as eye-to-eye gaze, facial expression, body postures, and gestures to regulate social interaction
  (2) failure to develop peer relationships appropriate to developmental level

Box 7-1
DSM-IV Criteria, Pervasive Developmental Disorders—Cont'd

    (3) a lack of spontaneous seeking to share enjoyment, interests, or achievements with other people (e.g., by a lack of showing, bringing, or pointing out objects of interest to other people)

    (4) lack of social or emotional reciprocity

B. Restricted, repetitive, and stereotyped patterns of behavior, interests, and activities, as manifested by at least one of the following:

    (1) encompassing preoccupation with one or more stereotyped and restricted patterns of interest that is abnormal either in intensity or focus

    (2) apparently inflexible adherence to specific, nonfunctional routines or rituals

    (3) stereotyped and repetitive motor mannerisms (e.g., hand or finger flapping or twisting, or complex whole-body movements)

    (4) persistent preoccupation with parts of objects

C. The disturbance causes clinically significant impairment in social, occupational, or other important areas of functioning.

D. There is no clinically significant general delay in language (e.g., single words used by age 2 years, communicative phrases used by age 3 years).

E. There is no clinically significant delay in cognitive development or in the development of age-appropriate self-help skills, adaptive behavior (other than in social interaction), and curiosity about the environment in childhood.

F. Criteria are not met for another specific pervasive developmental disorder or schizophrenia.

299.80 Rett's Disorder

A. All of the following:

    (1) apparently normal prenatal and perinatal development

    (2) apparently normal psychomotor development through the first 5 months after birth

    (3) normal head circumference at birth

B. Onset of all of the following after the period of normal development:

    (1) deceleration of head growth between ages 5 and 48 months

    (2) loss of previously acquired purposeful hand skills between ages 5 and 30 months with the subsequent development of stereotyped hand movements (i.e., hand-wringing or hand washing)

    (3) loss of social engagement early in the course (although often social interaction develops later)

    (4) appearance of poorly coordinated gait or trunk movements

    (5) severely impaired expressive and receptive language development with severe psychomotor retardation

299.10 Childhood Disintegrative Disorder

A. Apparently normal development for at least the first 2 years after birth as manifested by the presence of age-appropriate verbal and nonverbal communication, social relationships, play, and adaptive behavior.

B. Clinically significant loss of previously acquired skills (before age 10 years) in at least two of the following areas:

    (1) expressive or receptive language

    (2) social skills or adaptive behavior

    (3) bowel or bladder control

    (4) play

    (5) motor skills

Continued

Box 7-1
DSM-IV Criteria, Pervasive Developmental Disorders—Cont'd

C. Abnormalities of functioning in at least two of the following areas:
  (1) qualitative impairment in social interaction (e.g., impairment in nonverbal behaviors, failure to develop peer relationships, lack of social or emotional reciprocity)
  (2) qualitative impairments in communication (e.g., delay or lack of spoken language, inability to initiate or sustain a conversation, stereotyped and repetitive use of language, lack of varied make-believe play)
  (3) restricted, repetitive, and stereotyped patterns of behavior, interests, and activities, including motor stereotypes and mannerisms
D. The disturbance is not better accounted for by another specific pervasive developmental disorder or by schizophrenia.

Diagnostic and Statistical Manual, 4th Edition, ©1994, American Psychiatric Association, reprinted with permission.

Differential Diagnosis

Because characteristics of ASD may be present in other genetic and neurological disorders, it is becoming increasingly important to rule out those other conditions when they are suspected and to provide appropriate treatment for them. The differential diagnosis of ASD, therefore, is a diagnosis of exclusion, that is, ruling out all the other known causes of the symptoms. The process of differential diagnosis involves a team effort, and the SLP may be the one to make the initial referral(s) to institute the process. This step should not be undertaken without considerable preparation and thought, because the process is very expensive for families and because preliminary assessment may indicate that the step is not necessary. Differential diagnosis may include consultations with developmental pediatricians, neurologists, geneticists, endocrinologists, psychologists, physical therapists, and occupational therapists; it may involve laboratory tests, electrophysiological testing, neuroimaging, and other specialized procedures *when indicated*.[3,5,6]

Why might such an extensive protocol be required? The goal is to determine whether the characteristic behaviors of the child might be caused by some problem other than ASD. Some of the possible problems that could be identified through differential diagnosis include the following:

• Mental retardation
• Seizure disorder
• Affective disorder
• Other serious psychiatric disorder
• Metabolic disorder
• Genetic disorder
• Brain malformation or damage

Treatments for such disorders require a different approach than treatment for ASD, and the ASD-like behaviors may be resolved by successful treatment of the underlying disorder.

A referral for specialized examinations or tests may be made at any time, but the SLP who initiates referral(s) for a differential diagnosis must do so only after having gathered and analyzed a substantial amount of reliable information. The decision to make a referral for specific or extensive testing must be made in consultation with the child's family. The written referral should be addressed to the child's primary physician in the form of a one- or two-page letter that contains (1) the request for specific evaluations or for referral to appropriate specialists; (2) the reason(s) for making the referral, along with a brief description of observed behaviors that support the concerns on which the referral is being made; (3) a list of conditions that need to be excluded or confirmed (based on clinical symptoms reported or observed); and (4) either a complete report prepared by the SLP, a one-page synopsis of the procedures completed and the outcome thereof *or* a statement that a complete report is available on request. If the complete report is forwarded, be certain to include a copy of the permission form signed by the child's parent or legal guardian.

The SLP bears a significant amount of responsibility in the process of diagnosis. As Tsakiris[24] points out, "Because speech-language and communication skills (and lack thereof) are among the defining features and earliest diagnostic indicators of children on the autistic spectrum, this is one of the most important functional developmental areas in this syndrome" (p. 736). In most cases, assembling sufficient information to make a judgment about whether a child has ASD and/or should be referred for other services requires the SLP to complete a thorough evaluation.

Case History

First, a thorough case history must be obtained from the family. The SLP should establish that family members are essential members of the team serving the child and that they alone have certain knowledge and insights about their child that can aid in achieving the best outcome for the child's development. In addition to the information obtained from the case history (a model form is provided in Appendix A), the SLP must collaborate with the parents to obtain information relating to possible signs of a variety of potential problems. A time-saving strategy is to send the case history form(s) to the family ahead of the appointed time to meet with them. If that is done, efforts should be made to have the information returned before the appointment (providing the family with a self-addressed envelope and/or making a follow-up phone call to remind them of the need to have the information before the appointment could facilitate cooperation). The supplementary form might request information regarding the following:

- Have other family members been diagnosed with PDD, ASD, or other exceptionality?
- Does the child have extreme aversions to or preferences for any foods?
- Does the child have extremely atypical responses to sensory stimuli (touch, sound, motion)?
- Is the development of the child significantly different from that of other children in the family? If so, how?
- Is it possible the child has seizures?
- Does the child have physical characteristics that are of concern to the family or the child's physician?
- What behaviors of the child are of concern to the family? Be specific.
- Are there times of the day or night when the child's behavior is of concern?
- Are the routines of daily living or caregiving of particular concern?
- Has the child experienced regression in development of skills that were emerging or once were established?

A study done in Japan that evaluated the speech abilities of 99 individuals whose ages ranged from 3 years 6 months to 29 years 9 months found that the age of onset for single word utterances was between just over 12 months and 48 months. Few of the subjects had two-word utterances. One-third of the group had lost their words within 12 to 36 months of the onset of speech.[25]

Obtaining a case history that includes this sort of information may seem beyond the province of the SLP, but it provides clues to behaviors that may be observed by an experienced practitioner. For example, seriously disturbed sleep patterns are common among children with ASD; persistent and severe resistance to diapering or dressing are sometimes associated with tactile hypersensitivity;[26] peculiar eating patterns or rejection of significant numbers of foods may be associated with oral defensiveness, food allergies (common among ASD children), or more severe problems with metabolic processes. When combined with other information to be gathered, the case history can validate or contraindicate going on to the next level of investigation of the problem.

Parent/Family Interview

After reviewing the information provided by the family in the case history, the SLP should provide sufficient time to complete a conversation with family members about their present concerns. If the SLP is the first professional they have consulted, it is probable that their concerns will center on the child's atypical or delayed acquisition of speech or language and possibly on the child's unusual social behaviors as well. The conversation should allow for parental questions of the SLP as well as parental responses to questions raised by the SLP. Family members should be reassured that their input is critical to the professional's understanding of the child's situation.

Review of Reports by Other Professionals

If the family has consulted other professionals about their concerns for the child, any resulting reports of their findings should be reviewed by the SLP. Of special interest are reports from psychologists, early childhood educators, and medical personnel. Sometimes families feel that findings with which they do not agree are not suitable to be shared by subsequent individuals who might see the child, because they fear the possible bias that might be developed by the next professional. That is their privilege. However, if the family is willing to permit review of pertinent reports that they may view negatively, provided they are permitted to submit a confidential statement reflecting their doubts or disagreements, it may be possible to obtain them for review.

Observation of the Child

It is imperative that the SLP observe the child in one or more natural environments (i.e., environments with which the child is familiar—the home, childcare setting) and with people in whose care the child is comfortable. Not only is observation in the natural environment a requirement of Part C legislation,[27] it is also best practice protocol for all professionals involved with assessment and management of children with delays or disabilities. Children with ASD do not adapt easily to new situations or to changes in their routines. Many children in the toddler age group without ASD also have difficulty with unfamiliar situations. Serial observations, rather than a one-time observation, are imperative to prevent formulating professional judgments that may not be based on the child's usual behaviors. Direct observations should document the child's responses to people and conditions of the environment in which the observation takes place. Responses to stimuli provided (bids for attention by others, tactile stimulation, auditory stimulation, visual stimulation); the child's initiation of actions; and levels of alertness, curiosity, bids for attention, and play should also be documented. "Best practice" guidelines published in the Division of Early Childhood (DEC) of the Council for Exceptional Children (CEC) outline useful skills and competencies of early interventionists that relate to the issue of observing very young children.[28]

If it is impossible to observe the child directly on more than one occasion, analysis of videotapes made by the family (contemporary and/or from past family occasions or events) can also be used to obtain valuable information about the child in a familiar surrounding. The parents should confirm that the behaviors represented on the tape are typical of their child. Written records of such videotape analyses should be made a part of the records kept by the SLP.

Earliest Indications of PDD and ASD

By whatever means the following social behavior and communication indications are discovered, the SLP must know that a *combination* of items listed points to a possible (if not probable) diagnosis of ASD. The listing below synthesizes behaviors commonly seen in young children with ASD.

- Absent or poor monitoring of gaze or pointing of communicative partner
- Absent or poor pretend play expected at age of development
- Absent or scant use of declarative pointing at expected age of development
- No babbling by age 12 months
- No single words by age 16 months
- Absent or poor orientation to social stimuli
- Absent or abnormal shift of attention between people and objects
- Absent or infrequent seeking attention of communicative partner to share information or an experience
- Any loss of language or social skills at any age

Direct Testing and Assessment Approaches

Although protocols involved with processes of diagnosis and evaluation of young children suspected of having ASD are time consuming, the gravity and implications of making the diagnosis of ASD justifies the care, time, and caution required.

Every child with delayed or atypical language development must have an audiological examination. In addition to identifying hearing losses, audiological examinations can establish the presence of hyperacusis when present among young children with ASD.

When a child is suspected of having ASD, it may not be possible to use the direct assessment routines and testing protocols designed to analyze delayed onset of speech or delayed/disordered language described in the next chapter. Some of them may be used with higher functioning children suspected of having ASD, but specialized tools and procedures may be needed instead. Practitioners should be aware that some states require the use of standardized instruments in assessing infants and toddlers for the purposes of Part C enrollment, whereas other states allow for expert professional judgment as a criterion and do not require utilization of standardized instruments. The "lead agency" for each state can provide the applicable and current Part C eligibility rules (a list of lead agencies appears in Appendix C).

▼ SELECTED TOOLS AND PROCEDURES

A wide range of tools and procedures that are used in diagnosing PDD and ASD are listed in the literature. Many of them are appropriate for older children but do not apply to the infant-toddler population. A few of them may be used to assess children not suspected of having ASD as well as infants and toddlers who *are* likely to be on the ASD spectrum. This discussion of tools and procedures is limited to those that may be of some use to in evaluating children under the age of 3 years.

Some of the tools require direct testing or interaction with the child, whereas others are based on observation of the child while engaged in daily activities or play with a familiar caregiver, and still others rely on questionnaires completed by parents or primary caregivers. Table 7-1 provides a listing of selected instruments and procedures applicable to the infant-toddler population.

Stability of a diagnosis of ASD in very early childhood is considered to be quite reliable. Lord[43] indicated that 94% of children diagnosed at age 2 years remained on the autism spectrum at age 3 years, with 75% of that group retaining the diagnosis of autistic disorder and the remaining 25% moving to a diagnosis of PDD-NOS. A more recent study by Lord and Risi[44] indicates that 74% of children diagnosed at age 2 years remained on the spectrum at age 3 years.

▼ WHAT FOLLOWS A DIAGNOSIS OF ASD?

Once it has been determined that a child has ASD, follow-up care includes a number of strategies that involve both the family and the child. Family members, especially those who will make decisions for the affected child, will need information about the condition and its causes and about treatment options for the child. They may also need counseling services, including but not limited to genetic counseling.

Information About the Condition and Its Causes

Information that helps family members understand the condition and its causes should come from reliable sources. Initially practitioners may want to supply the family with fact sheets available on the Internet from the Autism Society of America and the National Institutes of Health. After the family has received basic information provided in the fact sheets, further information will be needed for the family to make crucial decisions about choosing among the various treatment options. A wealth of Internet resources available to families of children with ASD appears in Appendix D under the heading "Autistic Spectrum Disorders." Excellent books are available that cover the categories of ASD; bibliographies of these are readily available on the Internet. The writer suggests going to http://www.google.com and entering the search phrase "autism spectrum disorder bibliographies" for further information that is updated frequently.

TABLE 7-1
Useful Tools in Determining a Diagnosis of Autistic Spectrum Disorder in Very Young Children

Type and Name of Tool	Source/Reference	Description	Authors
Screening Tools			
Ages and Stages Questionnaire, ed 2[29]	Paul H. Brookes Publishing Co. P.O. Box 10624, Baltimore, MD 21285-0624 Ph: 800-638-3775	30-item questionnaires completed by parents at 2-mo intervals (4–24 mo) and 3-mo intervals (27–36 mo); assess skills in communication, gross motor, fine motor, problem solving, personal-social development; also available in Spanish and French	Bricker D, et al
Autism Diagnostic Interview-R (ADI-R)[30]	Lord C, Rutter M, LeCouteur A: *J Autism Dev Disord* 24: 659–685, 1994; contact Western Psychological Services for pending publication information.	Takes about 3 hr to administer and requires specific training to administer properly	Lord C, Rutter M, LeCouteur A
Autism Diagnostic Observation Schedule (ADOS)[31]	Lord C, et al: *Autism diagnostic observation schedule,* WPS edition, Los Angeles, 1999, Western Psychological Services	Geared to children younger than 6 years old who are not yet using phrase speech; takes about 30 min to administer; linked to diagnostic constructs associated with ICD-10 and DSM-IV criteria	DiLavore PC, Lord C, Rutter M (see *J Autism Dev Disord* 25(4):355–379, 1995)
Childhood Autism Rating Scale[32] (CARS), 1988	Western Psychological Services Ph: 1-800-648-8857 http://www.wps.com	2 yr and older, widely used, but not adapted to DSM-IV diagnostic criteria	Schopler E, et al
Social Communication Questionnaire[33] (SCQ; formerly Autism Screening Questionnaire—ASQ)	Contact Western Psychological Services for more information on anticipated publication date and developmental research Ph: 1-800-648-8857 http://www.wps.com	0-item questionnaire based on the ADI-R; in preliminary research stages for use with children under 4 yr (Research at University of Michigan)	Berument SK, et al (see *Br J Psychiatry* 175:444–451, 1999)

Continued

**TABLE 7-1
Useful Tools in Determining a Diagnosis of Autistic Spectrum Disorder in Very Young Children—Cont'd**

Type and Name of Tool	Source/Reference	Description	Authors
Screening Tools			
Childhood Development Inventories (CDIs),[34] 1994	Behavior Science Systems P.O. Box 580274 Minneapolis, MN 55458 Ph: 612-929-6220	Infant inventory—0 to 21 mo; early childhood inventory—15 to 36 mo; completed by parental report in about 5–10 min; screens for language, motor, cognitive, preacademic, social, and self-help problems	Ireton H
Checklist for Autism in Toddlers (CHAT)[35]	Baron-Cohen S, Allen J, Gillberg C: *Br J Psychiatry* 168:158–163, 1996.	Designed for ages 18 mo and older; 14 questions and simple risk-rating check-off; parent questions: 9 items and 5 quick observation items; not sensitive to milder ASD cases	Baron-Cohen S, Allen J, Gillberg C
Modified Checklist for Autism in Toddlers[36]	Robins DL, et al Available at http://www.firstsigns.org/downloads/m-chat_scoring.PDF	18–24 mo; 23-item checklist for parents; takes 10 min to complete; failure of 3 items suggests follow-up	Robins DL, Fein MA, Barton M, Green JA
Detection of Autism by Infant Sociability Interview[37] (DASI)	Wimproy DC, et al: *J Autism Dev Disord* 30(6):525–536, 2000.	Geared to first 24 mo; 16 of 19 items distinguish between autistic and nonautistic children	Wimproy DC, Hobson RP Williams JM, Nash S
Pervasive Developmental Disorders Screening Test (PDDST),[38] 1996 AND Pervasive Developmental Disorders Screening Test II (in development at this writing)	Bryna Siegel, PhD Langley Porter Psychiatic Institute University of California San Francisco, CA 94143-0984	Parent-completed checklists in which parents compare their child to experiences with other children, the child's siblings, or what they expected their child to be like; ratings on items are "Yes, usually true" or "No, usually not true"	Siegel B

Tool	Contact	Description	Author
Screening Tool for Autism in Two-Year-Olds[39] (STAT) (unpublished; available from author)	Wendy Stone, PhD Vanderbilt Child Development Center Medical Center South, Rm 426 2100 Pierce Ave Nashville, TN 37232-3573 Ph: 615-936-0249 E-mail: wendystone@mcmail.vanderbilt.edu	Stage I: 0–36 mo; stage II: 24–35 mo; 20 min play activities, sample reciprocal play, motor imitation, and nonverbal communication; differentiates between autism and other developmental disabilities	Stone W

Language Assessment Tools

Tool	Contact	Description	Author
Communication and Symbolic Behavior Scales[40]	The Speech Bin 1965 Twenty-Fifth Ave Vero Beach, FL 32960 Ph: 1-800-4-SPEECH Also available from Brookes Publishing P.O. Box 10624 Baltimore, MD 21285-0624 Ph: 1-800-638-3775 www.brookespublishing.com	8–24 mo; uses 22 five-point rating scales: communicative functions/means, reciprocity, verbal/nonverbal symbolic behavior, social/affective signaling	Wetherby A, Prizant BM
Communication and Symbolic Developmental Profile[41]	See CSBS source above	Identifies children at risk; consists of a caregiver questionnaire, a behavior sampling protocol, and a pre-referral checklist; takes 30 minutes to complete	Wetherby A, Prizant BM
The Rossetti Infant-Toddler Language Scale, A Measure of Communication and Interaction,[42] 1990	LinguiSystems 3100 4th Ave East Moline, IL 61244-9700 Ph: 1-800-776-4332 www.linguisystems.com	0–36 mo; consists of a parent questionnaire and a series of items that assess interaction-attachment, pragmatics, gesture, play, language comprehension, and language expression; items may be scored by parent report, observation, or elicitation; though not designed specifically for detection of autism, unusual responses to items may implicate ASD behaviors	Rossetti L

In addition to information specific to ASD, families need information relating to applicable laws (federal and state) that apply to eligibility requirements and services available through public resources. Readers are referred to the list of "Internet Resources" in Appendix D for more information about accessing information on Individuals with Disabilities Education Act (IDEA) and other pertinent statutes.

Counseling

Various types of counseling may be needed by families whose children have been diagnosed with ASD. Not every family needs every type of counseling, but many—if not most—families are in need of some type of counseling as time progresses. The various forms of counseling include but are not limited to genetic, medical, educational, family, financial, and psychological counseling. Additionally, counseling with respect to communication and language development is in order.

Genetic counseling may be needed because there is a known risk of recurrence of ASD in 3% to 7% of children born to these families subsequent to the child who has been diagnosed with ASD.[3] With the increased frequency of more and more reports appearing in the medical literature as more is learned about the human genome, the risk statistics may be revised in the future. Medical counseling may be needed by families whose children have co-morbid conditions for which medical treatment is appropriate. It is also known that children with ASD appear to have a high prevalence of allergies; some need special diets that should not be undertaken without medical consultation.

Educational counseling is probably needed to assist families in choosing educational settings and programs that are appropriate for the needs of their individual children as they grow older. Such needs should be anticipated and investigated well in advance of the time these educational decisions have to be made. Some children with ASD require special education classroom settings, whereas others do well in regular classrooms with specific supports. Given the differences between medical diagnoses and disability categories recognized by the educational system as criteria for specific services, getting a head start on acquiring information and counseling by knowledgeable professionals is wise.

Family counseling may encompass all members of the family or only a segment of the family unit. For example, counseling for siblings of children with disabilities is available and often can be quite helpful.

Financial counseling has been offered to families of children with disabilities, including ASD, for a number of years through parent support organizations. When a child has severe mental limitations, behavioral disorders, or other problems common in the ASD population, parents and other family members are often concerned about what will become of the child when they are no longer able to care for the child in their home. Estate planning is an area of financial counseling that can be helpful in such circumstances. Counseling with respect to insurance coverage is another area of financial counseling that many families need, especially as new governmental benefits for the disabled emerge and requirements for health care coverage, caps on benefits, and managed care considerations change over time.

Individual psychological counseling may be needed from time to time to cope with the stresses of raising a child with ASD. Marital stresses, coping with the time requirements of caring for a child with ASD, and even the burden of making decisions about forms of treatment may take their toll on parents and other family members. Certain elements of psychological counseling relating to physical, emotional, and social development also may be beneficial to the child with ASD.[3]

Communication and language counseling is a role for SLPs and audiologists. Because children with ASD are extremely variable in their communication skills and deficits, it is impossible to predict a typical developmental course for all children with the diagnosis. Guidance is needed from professionals who are familiar with determining where a given child currently is in terms of linguistic development at any point in time, what the next level of achievement should be, and how to promote activities that will enhance the probability that the child will achieve the next and subsequent levels of communicative competency.

Support for the family is a recognized element of the pediatrician's role in diagnosis and management of ASD.[3] It is an element of the role of *every* professional who deals with the families of children with ASD.[23]

Treatment/Intervention/Management Options

One of the most difficult series of decisions facing families of children diagnosed with ASD is what course of treatment/intervention/management to pursue. Professionals play a significant role in assisting families to come to terms with the necessary decisions. For example, although the American Academy of Pediatrics asserts that a pediatrician "should not delay referral to early intervention program while waiting for a definite diagnosis," it acknowledges that "[e]ven when programs are locally available, the pediatrician may be unaware of them."[3]

Greenspan[45] concludes, "At present and for the foreseeable future, clinical experience together with research is necessary to provide the clinical knowledge needed to individualize approaches to the child and family's functional assessment …[and]… the formulation of a child-and-family-specific comprehensive intervention program" (p. 5). In other words, there are no one-size-fits-all recommendations to be made; every child and family must be viewed as having unique needs. There is general agreement, however, that treatment should begin early (as soon as the diagnosis is made) and that it should be intensive (at least 25 hours a week, year round).[46] Prizant and Rubin[47] suggest five principles for guiding decisions about which program(s) to select for a given child:

1. The program should be matched to individual needs based on the child's developmental level.
2. The program should be based on what is known about child development.
3. The program should ensure that the intervention addresses core deficits in autism.
4. Implementers of the program should match valued outcomes and the process used to achieve them.
5. Implementers of the program should understand the basis of the interventions used (e.g., theory-based, data-based, knowledge of best practice).

With those conditions in mind, parents face a wide array of choices in determining which program is best suited to the needs of their child. Fortunately, some excellent choices are available; also some promising, but as yet experimental, programs are emerging from research efforts. Unfortunately, some treatments that have been scientifically discredited are also still being promoted by some groups. To further confound the matter, some programs of proven worth may not be readily available to families for a variety of reasons (e.g., no trained personnel to implement the programs are in or near the area where the family lives, the cost of a particular program may be prohibitive for the family, insurance coverage may be denied, the family is unable to take on the responsibilities of the program that call for substantial time commitments). A useful resource for the family is a professional who is familiar with the statutory requirements of Part C of IDEA and with the somewhat checkered successes of some families across the country who have turned to legal remedies to pay for services they believe will benefit their child. Because the goals of many treatment programs are to establish functional language and social skills, it is often the SLP, a developmental psychologist, an early interventionist, or a social worker who will have such knowledge or know how to access it.

Approaches That Have Proven Helpful With Infants and Toddlers

Very few "programs" (i.e., formal, published, curricula or protocols) *per se* are available for use primarily with infants and toddlers who have been diagnosed with ASD. However, there are a few. Intervention procedures exist that meet the criteria for selecting an appropriate management or treatment approach with very young children. "Floor Time" is an approach that has been written about at some length by Greenspan;[48] it is based on adapted play activities that are enjoyable to young children and on an adult's adaptation to expanding experiences based on the child's demonstrated interest (or lead). It is practical, requires a minimum of parental education on what to look for and how to adapt activities to the child's interest, and it can be employed over the course of the child's ordinary activities during the day. Applied behavioral analysis (ABA) is a highly structured program developed by Smith and Lovaas[49] that requires special training of those who participate in its implementation. Implementation is recommended at a level of about 40 hours per week. It stresses a stimulus-response-consequence model through which, after a series of trials that are tightly controlled, the child's response to a given stimulus or set of stimuli is shaped or modified. This program has many adherents and promoters, and its founder has published accounts of a number of successes—sometimes even labeled as "cures." Its drawbacks, if one views it in that light, are the cost and the time commitment required of the families who are engaged in its implementation. In an effort to reduce the cost associated with this form of treatment, some professionals have adopted a modified ABA approach in which 20 to 25 hours of treatment are implemented. Some practitioners and researchers have reported positive results with the shortened treatment regimen.

Some approaches used by professionals from many disciplines involve an eclectic mix of strategies that are designed to address the needs of an individual child with ASD. They utilize techniques of speech-language therapy (language development in the case of infants and toddlers), occupational therapy (often sensory integration strategies), family education and family training, environmental modification (to reduce the number or intensity of stimuli with which the child must deal), and transition planning (anticipating upcoming changes that will occur as a result of the child's progress in therapy, advancing age, or changes in family circumstances—such as the birth of another child). Collaborative teaming among the participants is essential when this approach is used. It is helpful to the family if these services can be provided under one roof, but that is not always possible or practical. In that case, it is recommended that the family and professionals maintain a communication journal in which entries related to treatment strategies, questions, and observational information can be shared on an ongoing basis among all the professionals who are involved. In that way, for example, the occupational therapist's recommendations about using positioning or pressure to calm the child and enhance attention to task can be shared with the other professionals and family members. Families can share information about the child's interests in the home; SLPs can enter information about language goals and seek the assistance of other team members in providing opportunities during their treatment or interaction sessions for the child to be exposed to the targeted concepts or skills.

Wetherby and Prizant[41] have proposed an organized treatment plan based on the outcome of administration of the communication and symbolic behavior scales (CSBS). It proposes "outcomes" for the caregiver and for the child and focuses attention on prelinguistic and linguistic behaviors that are key to communication development. This methodology, described in the next chapter, can be easily combined with an eclectic team treatment approach as described above and has yielded excellent results in terms of providing caregivers with easily understood information about language development and with practical strategies to use in their respective settings.

Experimental and Emerging Treatment Elements

The nature of ASD and its apparent increase in prevalence have spurred efforts to devise treatments that address physical, educational, and social aspects of the problem. Some of these approaches are extremely controversial, whereas others have gained support among certain segments of the professional community. Among these treatments are several with which the SLP should become familiar because reports about them have appeared in the national media, and parents are likely to have questions about them. The SLP also should know where to refer parents who have questions to reliable sources of information. Fortunately, most—if not all of the treatments—are designed for use with children who are older than 3 years. However, as parents hear about them and as they look forward to their child's advancing age, they may inquire about them.

Some of the experimental treatments fall under the umbrella of "Complementary and Alternative Medicine" (CAM).[50,51] At this writing, some of the treatments under study include the use of secretin,[51,52] chelation therapy to remove mercury from the body,[53] and specialized diets (e.g., gluten-free diet, casein-free diet). Most of these treatments are not accepted at this time by the American medical community as a whole.

At this writing, gene therapy for ASD has not been undertaken. Practitioners should be alert to studies that may emerge in this area.

Unproven Therapies

Some therapies have been touted over time as being applicable to individuals with ASD. They have often had large groups of adherents who have applied political pressure for their adoption in school systems and by professionals in private practice. Like the experimental treatments, most of the unproven therapies were designed for use with children older than 3 years, but at least one (the patterning approach advocated by Doman and Delacato of the Better Babies Institute) has been offered to younger children as well. Among the unproven therapies with which the SLP should be familiar are patterning, facilitated communication, auditory integration therapy, nutritional supplements, and immunoglobulin therapy.[54] Information about each of these approaches is available in the professional literature and on the Internet.

As a member of the ASD assessment and management team, the SLP plays many important roles. Every SLP who is an ASD team member will participate in the following:

- Collaborating with other professionals and families to provide optimal services and outcomes for the child
- Screening and early identification of children suspected of having ASD
- Evaluation, assessment, and diagnosis of the condition and the characteristics of each child so diagnosed
- Referral, when needed, to complete the differential diagnosis and evaluation for implementation of other treatment or management that may be indicated
- Communication intervention: prelinguistic and early language development
- Providing communication counseling, parent information, and parent training in specific techniques
- Keeping the professional knowledge base current through the literature
- Conducting clinical research

The next chapter deals with assessing and examining infants and toddlers who may have communication delays or disorders but who are not suspected of having ASD.

▼ REFERENCES

1. Filipek PA, et al: Practice parameter: screening and diagnosis of autism—report of the Quality Standards Subcommittee of the American Academy of Neurology and the Child Neurology Society, *Neurology* 55(4):468–479, 2000.
2. Lord C, McGee JP, editors: Committee on Educational Interventions for Children with Autism, Division of Behavioral Sciences and Education, National Research Council, *Educating children with autism*, Washington, DC, 2001, National Academics Press, p 219.
3. American Academy of Pediatrics, Committee on Children with Disabilities: Technical report: the pediatrician's role in the diagnosis and management of autistic spectrum disorder in children, *Pediatrics* 107(5):1221–1226, 2001.
4. American Psychiatric Association: *Diagnostic and statistical manual*, ed 4, Washington, DC, 1994, APA.
5. Scambler D, Rogers S, Wehner EA: Can the checklist for autism in toddlers differentiate young children with autism from those with developmental delays? *J Am Acad Child Adolesc Psychiatry* 40(12):1457–1463, 2001.
6. Giddings S: Seizing opportunities: researchers are taking advantage of imaging technology to unlock the secrets of brain disorders that profoundly affect children, *Adv Imaging Radiat Ther Profess* 15(10):26, 27–29, 2002.
7. American Academy of Neurology: Practice parameter: screening and diagnosis of autistic spectrum disorders (a multi-society consensus statement, 02/25/00). Summary statement prepared by PA Filipek, corresponding author and project chair (E-mail: filipek@uci.edu).

8. Dunlap G, Bunton-Pierce MK: Autism and autism spectrum disorder (ASD). ERIC Digest #E583. Available from ERIC Clearinghouse on Disabilities & Gifted Education, CEC (E-mail: ericec@cec.sped.org).
9. Chakrabarti S, Fombonne E: Pervasive developmental disorders in preschool children, *JAMA* 185(24):3093–3099, 2001.
10. Chandrasekaran B: Detection of autism delayed in India, *Adv Speech-Lang Pathologists Audiologists* 11(38):18, 2001.
11. Solomon BI, Sonies BC: *Oral-motor, speech and swallowing functions in three rare genetic syndromes*. Seminar presented at the Conference of the American-Speech-Language-Hearing Association, New Orleans, La, Nov 16, 2001.
12. Tsai L: *Autistic spectrum disorder: new definition, advances in neurobiological research, and treatment implications*. Keynote address at the Woman's Foundation, Inc, Conference on Autistic Spectrum Disorders, Lafayette, La, Oct 21, 2000.
13. Osterling J, Dawson G: Early recognition of children with autism: a study of first birthday home videotapes, *J Autism Dvmtl Disord* 24(3):247–257, 1994.
14. Mars AE, Mauk JE, Dowrick P: Symptoms of pervasive developmental disorders as observed in prediagnostic home videos of infants and toddlers, *J Pediatr* 132(Pt 1): 500–504, 1998.
15. Brown E, et al: *Early identification of 8- to 10-month-old infants with autism based on observation from home videos of infants and toddlers*, Atlanta, Ga, 1998, International Society of Infant Studies.
16. Osterling J, Dawson G: Early identification of 1-year-olds with autism vs. mental retardation based on home videotapes of first birthday parties. Proceedings of the Society for Research in Child Development, Albuquerque, NM, 1999.
17. Baranek GT: Autism during infancy: a retrospective videoanalysis of sensory-motor and social behaviors at 9–12 months of age, *J Autism Dev Disord* 29(3):213–224, 1999.
18. Bauman ML: Autism: clinical features and neurobiological observations. In *ICDL clinical practice guidelines*, Bethesda, Md, 2000, Interdisciplinary Council on Developmental and Learning Disorders, pp 689–703.
19. Hyman SL, Rodier PM, Davidson P: Editorial: Pervasive developmental disorders in young children, *JAMA* 285(24):3141–3142, 2001.
20. Short B, Schopler E: Factors relating to age of onset in autism, *J Autism Dev Disord* 18(2):207–216, 1988.
21. Stone WL, et al: Early recognition of autism, *Arch Pediatr Adolesc Med* 148(2):174–179, 1994.
22. Prelock P: Understanding autism spectrum disorders: the role of speech-language pathologists and audiologists in service delivery, *ASHA Leader* 6(17):5–7, 2001.
23. Interdisciplinary Council on Developmental and Learning Disorders: *ICDL clinical practice guidelines*, Bethesda, Md, 2000, Author. [Free download available at http://icdl.com/ICDLguidelines]
24. Tsakiris ET: Evaluating effective interventions for children with autism and related disorders: widening the view and changing the perspective. In *ICDL clinical practice guidelines*, Bethesda, Md, 2000, Interdisciplinary Council on Developmental and Learning Disorders, pp 725–866.
25. Uchino J, et al: Development of language in Rett syndrome, *Brain Dev* 23(Suppl): S233–S235, 2001.
26. Grandin, Temple: Interview with Stephen Edelson, Feb 1, 1996. Available online at http://www.autism.org/interview/temp_int.html.
27. U.S. Department of Education: Assistance to states for the education of children with disabilities and early intervention program for infants and toddlers with disabilities. 34CFR Part 303: Early intervention program for infants and toddlers with disabilities, *The Federal Register* 64(48):12505–12554, 1999. [Full text of final regulations for IDEA available at http://www.icase.org/idea/regulations/12416.htm]
28. Sandall S, McLean M, Smith B, editors: *DEC recommended practices in early intervention/ early childhood special education*, Longmont, Colo, 2000, Sopris West.
29. Bricker D, et al: *Ages and stages questionnaire*, ed 2, Baltimore, Md, 1999, Brookes Publishing.
30. Lord C, Rutter M, LeCouteur A: Autism diagnostic interview-R : a revised version of a diagnostic interview for caregivers of individuals with possible pervasive developmental disorders, *J Autism Dev Disord* 24(5): 659–685, 1994.

31. Lord C, et al: *Autism diagnostic observation schedule,* WPS edition, Los Angeles, Calif, 1999, Western Psychological Services.
32. Schopler E, et al: *Childhood autism rating scale,* Los Angeles, Calif, 1988, Western Psychological Services.
33. Brument SK, et al: Autism screening questionnaire: diagnostic validity, *Br J Psychiatry* 175:444–451, 1999.
34. Ireton H: Childhood development inventories, Minneapolis, Minn, 1994, Behavior Science Systems.
35. Baron-Cohen S, Allen J, Gillberg C: Checklist for autism in toddlers. In Psychological markers in the detection of autism in infancy in a large population, *Br J Psychiatry* 168:158–163, 1996.
36. Robins DL, et al: *Modified checklist for autism in toddlers, 2001.* Available at http://www.firstsigns.org/downloads/m-chat_scoring.PDF.
37. Wimproy DC, et al: Are infants with autism socially engaged? A study of recent retrospective parental reports, *J Autism Dev Disord* 30(6):525–536, 2000.
38. Siegel B: *Early screening and diagnosis in autistic spectrum disorders: the pervasive developmental disorders screening test.* Paper presented at the State of the Science in Autism: Screening and Diagnosis Working Conference, June 15–17, 1998, Bethesda, Md. [The Developmental Disorders Screening Test and the Developmental Disorders Screening Test II, 1996 are available from author: Bryna Siegel, PhD, Langley Porter Psychiatric Institute, University of California at San Francisco, CA 94143-0984.]
39. Stone W: *Screening tool for autism in two year olds* (STAT). n.d. Available from author at Vanderbilt Child Development Center, Medical Center South, Room 426, 2100 Pierce Ave., Nashville, TN 37232-3573.
40. Wetherby A, Prizant BM: *Communication and symbolic behavior scales,* Baltimore, Md, 1993, Brookes Publishing.
41. Wetherby A, Prizant BM: *Communication and symbolic development profile,* Baltimore, Md, 2002, Brookes Publishing.
42. Rossetti, L: *The Rossetti infant-toddler language scale: a measure of communication and interaction,* East Moline, Ill, 1990, LinguiSystems.
43. Lord C: Follow-up of two-year-olds referred for possible autism, *J Child Psychol Psychiatry* 36:1365–1382, 1995.
44. Lord C, Risi S: Early diagnosis in children with autism spectrum disorders, *Advocate* 33:23–26, 2000.
45. Greenspan SI: Introduction. In *ICDL clinical practice guidelines,* Bethesda, Md, 2000, Interdisciplinary Council on Developmental and Learning Disorders, pp 1–5.
46. Lord C: *The earlier the better: interventions that benefit children with autism,* The ERIC/OSEP Special Project News brief. Available at http://ericec.org/osep/newsbriefs/new21.html.
47. Prizant BM, Rubin E: Contemporary issues in interviews for autism spectrum disorders: a commentary, *J Assoc Persons Severe Handicaps* 24(3):199–208, 1999.
48. Greenspan SI: A developmental approach to problems in relating and communicating in autistic spectrum disorders and related syndromes, *SPOTLIGHT Top Dev Disabilities* 1(4):1–6, 1998.
49. Smith R, Lovaas OI: Intensive, early behavioral intervention with autism: the UCLA young autism project, *Infant Young Child* 10:67–78, 1998.
50. Hyman SL, Levy SE: Autistic spectrum disorders: when traditional medicine is not enough, *Contemp Pediatr* 17:101–116, 2000.
51. Eisenberg DM, et al: Trends in alternative medicine use in the United States, 1990–1997: results of a follow-up national survey, *JAMA* 280(18):1569–1575, 1998.
52. Sandler AD, Bodfish JW: Placebo effects in autism: lessons from secretin, *J Dev Behav Pediatr* 21(5):347–350, 2000.
53. Dunn-Geier J, et al: Effect of secretin on children with autism: a randomized controlled trial, *Dev Med Child Neurol* 42(12):796–802, 2000.
54. Holmes, Amy: *New directions in autism.* Presentation at The Woman's Foundation, Inc, Seminar on Autism, Lafayette, La., September 20–21, 2000.

CHAPTER 8

ASSESSMENT: EXAMINATION, INTERPRETATION, AND REPORTING

Frances P. Billeaud

▼ IDENTIFICATION OF ATYPICAL COMMUNICATIVE DEVELOPMENT

Communicative *forms* and *means* among very young children can be plentiful in the absence of severe disabling conditions or quite limited in the presence of such conditions. In typically developing children, acquisition of communicative skills progresses along a reasonably predictable path, and specific components of communicative competence are commonly measured by comparing a given child's status with sequences typically expected for the child's developmental age. For many children, however, individual circumstances require more intensive efforts to identify whether there is a problem with communicative development and, if a problem is present, to describe its nature, determine an appropriate treatment plan, and interpret the findings and recommendations to the child's family. This process can be undertaken either under a traditional clinical format or, usually more productively, with full participation of family members in each phase of the assessment.

Earlier chapters have explored the many possible causes and risk factors for compromised or atypical communicative development. Significant communicative delays or disorders require specialized investigation by professionals experienced in working with infants and toddlers.

The basic elements of conducting such an investigation are as follows:

1. The speech-language pathologist's (SLP's) knowledge of normal developmental patterns across modalities, against which a particular child's communicative development can be compared
2. The SLP's knowledge of factors known to cause or be associated with atypical development that may apply to a particular child

141

3. A complete history of the child's prenatal course, birth, and subsequent development through which clues to the child's condition can be obtained
4. Information provided by the parents and usual caregivers about the child's development and communicative abilities
5. Evaluation of the child's hearing
6. Examination of the oral mechanism and related physical characteristics
7. Assessment of the child's communication patterns
8. Serial observation and analysis of the child's interactions with familiar caregivers and others
9. Play assessment
10. Inventory of typical and atypical child behaviors

Using these 10 approaches in combination, professionals are able to determine which children are at risk for or are already demonstrating atypical communicative development. There are, of course, tools that can assist the practitioner in conducting infant and toddler assessments. See Tables 8-1, 8-3, and 8-4 for information on these tools. Giving attention to each of the 10 assessment elements is essential to achieve the goal of constructing a valid profile of a child with suspected communicative development problems.

The Triage Concept in Assessment

The task that is before the professional at this point in the assessment process can be considered a triage process similar to the three-level process described by Lewis and Fox.[1] Usually, it is possible to place communicatively at-risk infants and toddlers in one of three distinct groups by the end of the assessment process:

1. Children who have obvious handicapping conditions that have predictable effects on communicative development and that may (or may not) require consideration of alternative or augmentative communication
2. Children who can be identified as being at medical or biological risk for conditions that affect communicative development and for whom referral to other professionals along with periodic monitoring or specific SLP interventions are appropriate
3. Children who are at risk because of environmental factors that are known to affect communicative development and for whom other interventions, especially modification of the environment or of interactions with significant adults, are appropriate

This categorization is important to families and may determine access to services that their children may require or benefit from. Policies that govern services provided by a given agency or institution often affect the specification of treatment groups (see Chapter 1 for detailed discussion), making the triage concept useful.

The triage concept is not perfect. Many factors affect a child's development. Further, transactional processes *among* those factors can be more important than a given set of specific conditions in and of themselves. For example, a very low birth weight (VLBW) child with significant impairment, born to a family with little education and low socioeconomic status (SES), is at far greater risk than other VLBW infants who are physically resilient and are discharged to situations where ongoing medical care and appropriate stimulation are available. In fact, when biologically at-risk infants have access to early and ongoing medical care and appropriate environmental stimulation, some studies indicate that even those VLBW babies who experience respiratory distress syndrome and intraventricular hemorrhage can be expected to have typical communicative development "as long as there are no long-lasting health problems that follow from this experience" (p. 193).[2] A word of caution, however, must also be included: there are infants for whom tolerance for seemingly insignificant or marginal physical insults or environmental factors is so low that a single factor in and of itself is the critical element that affects subsequent development.[3]

With reference to low birth weight babies, Sherman and Shulman[4] stated, "[t]he presence of short-term effects does not necessarily mean that there will be long-term effects, and, conversely, just because no short-term effects are evident does not mean there will be no long-term effects" (p. 83).

Family Assessment

As SLPs undertake the task of assessing the child, it must also be acknowledged that the "history" of the child and family are constantly "under construction" with the passage of time and experiences of life. It is impossible to separate the experience of the child from the experience of the entire family. It is essential to understand the basic dynamics of the child's family to provide effective guidance and engage the family in effective planning and habilitation efforts that fit their individual circumstances. If the family grants permission, Part C requires that a family assessment be completed and that such an assessment be family-directed. Balancing the timing of the family assessment with the requirements of obtaining other information essential to the process of identifying parameters of the child's developmental problem(s) is an issue for the practitioner and the family to work out together. Dictates of reimbursement schedules, constraints of time within the professional's practice setting, and the family's ability to make time for (and possibly bear the cost of) additional visits are factors in arriving at the appropriate time to undertake this facet of the assessment process.

A tool to facilitate the family assessment, the eco-map, is described in Chapter 4 (see Chapter 4, Figure 4-1). Completion of the eco-map can be done in less than 1 hour. Another approach is to explain what it is, how it is used, begin the process of completing the instrument, and then send the parents home with the form to be completed at their leisure and before the next appointment. This method allows the parents more time to contemplate not only the many factors they deem important in their family dynamics but also the elements that they deal with from day to day. This adds to their perception that the practitioner truly believes that they are the experts on their own family.

Each child and family present a unique set of circumstances with which the practitioner must deal. The case history is indispensable for those who work with the infant and toddler population. The eco-map can be considered part of the case history.

Information Provided by the Parents About the Child's Communicative Abilities

Parental concerns are acknowledged by most professionals to be a valid screening tool. Even the two-question Parents' Evaluations of Developmental Status,[5] which takes less than 3 minutes to complete, is reliable in correctly identifying at least 73% of children who are later diagnosed with communicative disorders through speech and language testing.[6] The two questions included on the questionnaire are (1) "Please tell me any concerns about how your child is learning, developing, and behaving" and (2) "Do you have any concerns about how he or she understands what you say? . . . talks? . . . makes speech sounds? . . . uses hands and fingers to do things? . . . uses arms and legs? . . . behaves? . . . gets along with others? . . . is learning to do things for himself or herself? . . . is learning preschool and school skills?"

As the SLP and parents engage in exchanges of information relating to the child's personal history, information is likely to be provided that opens the discussion to parental interactions with the child. Such interactions are generally not viewed as "communication encounters" by the parents, especially if the child is in a preintentional or preverbal developmental stage. Such discussions provide optimal opportunities for the SLP to discuss communicative means (e.g., eye-gaze shifts, gestures, facial expressions, vocalizations) and communicative functions. The examiner can then provide a list of functions appropriate to the child's estimated developmental level. The emergence of communicative intent can be determined and, if necessary, pointed out to the family as a step in the sequence of communicative development. A list of some of the more popular and useful parent questionnaires is provided in Table 8-1.

The family and other caregivers are invaluable sources of information about what the child has done and is currently doing. Because parents know the child best and have observed and interacted with the child across time and across experiences, they are the experts on that child. Professionals need to affirm that fact in interactions with the family.

Examination of the Oral Mechanism and Related Physical Characteristics

The oral mechanism is inspected for integrity of structure and function in the usual manner. If the child's voice is hoarse, weak, or nasal, the SLP should be particularly alert to potential palatal (e.g., frank clefting, velopharyngeal insufficiency) and craniofacial anomalies as referenced on pages 155–156 of this chapter. The examiner also notes symmetry of facial features at rest and during movements. Although a baby is unlikely to follow the directive "pucker your lips," it is quite likely that the infant will mimic the examiner or parent's model of that movement to allow observation of motor function during the act.

Special attention to uncoordinated motor sequences in swallowing, biting, and chewing should be undertaken, especially if there is a reported history of feeding problems. Early signs of possible developmental apraxia of speech (DAS) may be present and should be noted. Early signs of DAS may include the following:

- Lack of babbling in infancy
- Delayed onset of speech
- Inconsistent use of phonemes in words that are used often
- Use of relatively few different consonants appropriate to the child's developmental age.

Family history of DAS, which may be called by as many as 20 other names,[7,17,18] is strong and should be of special note if reported. This disorder

TABLE 8-1
Questionnaires Intended for or Adaptable to Parent Use in Determining Levels of Communicative Development in Infants and Toddlers

Questionnaire	For Ages	Description
CSBS Developmental Profile (CSBS-DP) (Research Edition)[7]	8–24 mo	Caregiver questionnaire is one part of the CSBS-DP (others are behavior sampling protocol and a pre-referral check list); quickly identifies children at-risk for language problems
Denver Developmental Screening Questionnaire[8]	0–6 yr	
Infant/Child Monitoring Questionnaire of Assessment, Evaluation, and Programming System (AEPS)[9]	44–36 mo	30-item questionnaires for use at 2-mo intervals from 4–24 mo and 3-mo intervals from 30–36 mo; versions in English, Spanish, and French
Infant-Toddler and Family Instrument (ITFI)[10]	6 mo–3 yr	35-question interview with caregivers; covers gross and fine motor, social and emotional, language, coping and self-help areas of development
MacArthur Communicative Development Inventory: Infant Form and Toddler Form[11]	10 mo–3 yr	Questions relate to words the child understands and says; toddler form also includes phrases that the child says
Language Development Survey[12]	2 yr	Designed for use in a variety of settings; can be completed in 5 min or less
The Rossetti Infant-Toddler Language Scale: Parent Form[13]	0–3 yr	Covers attachment, gestural, receptive, and expressive language components
Cue Questions (intended for use with children who have developmental disabilities)[14]	Adaptable to infants and toddlers	Checklist format draws attention to a wide range of verbal and nonverbal communication skills and habits
Receptive-Expressive Emergent Language Scale-2 (REEL-2)[15]	1 mo–3 yr	Though not very detailed, clearly worded and quickly completed; resembles *Vineland Social Maturity Scale* format
Semantic/Pragmatic Communication Report Form[16]	Symbolic stages	Designed for use with families of children with developmental disabilities

rarely exists in isolation. It has been diagnosed in children as young as 20 months, although it is more likely to be diagnosed in children of $2\frac{1}{2}$ years (if they are highly verbal) or 3 years of age.[8] Jakielski[19] suggests using the label "childhood apraxia of speech" rather than DAS, because insurance coverage is more likely to be available under that term for reimbursement purposes.

The presence of a biological concern or an atypical vocal tract, although the structures are not visible on cursory examination, may be deduced if the child's voice or cry is unusually high pitched, weak, hoarse, or if there are obvious problems with respiration. The possible implications of vocal anomalies are discussed in Chapter 5 of this book.

Communication Patterns Typical of the Child

Communication patterns of very young children can be described. Early interactions in which turn-taking occurs can be observed. The child's ability to localize to sounds and voices, affective responses to the adult's tone of voice and loudness level, and development of intentional communicative acts to attract the attention of others or to engage in vocal play are also available for description.

The child's spontaneous vocalizations (e.g., coos, cries, babbling) can be used to assess characteristics of phonation (i.e., quality, pitch, loudness).[20] Resonance characteristics are more easily detected in toddlers, but hypernasality and hyponasality can be discernible in babbling patterns of older infants. If either is noted, further investigation of the cause is warranted as indicated in the preceding section. Assessment of respiratory function for vocalization (and verbalization in older babies) is also rated by the examiner.

Articulatory function is assessed as soon as it is possible to do so. Variety in babbling is expected to emerge in predictable patterns with random sound production preceding reduplicative and canonical babbling. The phonemes of the language of the home gradually emerge as the preferred sounds for babbling. A method for analyzing infants' babbling patterns is outlined by Mitchell.[21] Such detailed analysis is not necessary if the SLP determines that babbling patterns are within expectations for the child's developmental age; however, the method described by Mitchell is useful when that is not the case. Children who do not exhibit variety in their babbling or whose babbling is discontinued after what appeared to be normal onset should alert the examiner to the possibility of a hearing impairment or other problem that results in delayed or disordered expressive language and speech at a later time. The possibility of one of the pervasive developmental disorders (PDDs) should also be considered if communicative development has been interrupted in a toddler.

As spoken words emerge, it is possible to determine the child's phonemic inventory for consonant and vowel production. Wetherby[22] suggested that production of different phonemes should approximate the following sequences for the ages given: 8 to 12 months (prelinguistic stage), average of three; 12 to 15 months (early one-word stage), average of five; 15 to 18 months (late one-word stage), average of seven; and 18 to 24 months (multiword stage), average of twelve. Scant vocal and verbal output are considered signs of possible problems with development of communication skills.

Physical characteristics to be observed include those that have their origins early in fetal development. These characteristics are sometimes referred to as *soft neurologic signs*, for they can be associated with some syndromes or conditions that are known to be related to communication difficulties. Bell[23] and Superneau[24] suggested making special note of the following traits, especially if they occur in combination:

- Head circumference out of the normal range on growth charts
- More than one hair whorl (cowlick) (consider whether this is a family trait.)
- Very fine, electric hair
- Epicanthus
- Upslanted palpebral fissures in individuals not of Asian descent (less than 1% occurrence)
- Downslanted palpebral fissures (less than 1% occurrence)
- Hypertelorism (widely spaced eyes) (beware of mislabeling this feature.)
- Malformed ears, absent ear lobe, microtia, atresia, skin tags
- Low-set ears (be certain that you are not observing slight posteriorly rotated, rather than low-set ears.)
- High-steepled palate
- Furrowed or "geographic" tongue
- Curved fifth finger
- Single palmar crease (palm creases are laid down at 12 to 14 weeks' gestation.)
- Webbing (syndactyly) of the fingers or toes
- Third toe longer than the second
- Splotchy pigment of the skin
- Absent or malformed fingernails and toenails
- Cafe-au-lait spots, which can be associated with neurofibromatosis

Bell[23] asserted that:

as early as the first year of life there is an indication that infants with a high count of minor physical anomalies are not processing information properly, either having difficulty forming a schema from what is presented to them or forming a hurried, imperfect schema. They appear to shift from ponderous attention to flitting when they become fatigued (p. 29).

Such behavior has serious implications regarding communicative development, especially language development, which relies heavily on the child's ability to focus and maintain attention.

Superneau[24] reiterated the caution that diagnosis of syndromes and medical conditions should be matters entrusted to experienced physicians. Suspected problems should be referred; and families should be counseled by experts in the field. However, the SLP must be alert to early identification of syndromes and medical conditions because of their implications for formulation of appropriate communication management plans.

Serial Observation and Analysis of the Child's Interactions With Familiar Caregivers and Others

Infants and toddlers are unique in that their endurance, attentiveness, and interests vary considerably with their caregiving requirements and routines, sleep and wake cycles, their sensitivity to new situations and people (e.g., the examiners), their attachment to the accompanying adult, and other factors that are not necessarily applicable to older children who have developed more mature patterns of behaviors and activities. It is crucial that practitioners who work with infants and toddlers have several opportunities to observe them and assess their behaviors and interactions rather than drawing conclusions based on observations obtained at a single visit. The potential for accumulating incomplete behavioral data leading to unfounded conclusions or misdiagnosis is high with this population.

To the extent possible, it is also imperative that the assessment of very young children be conducted in settings the children are accustomed to and in the company of familiar people—family members or regular caregivers. The dual evaluation tasks of the team or individual practitioner are "shopping for skills" (p. 65)[25] and identifying impediments to acquisition of communicative skills. It would be ideal if it were possible in every case to identify the source of the communicative delay or disability and to provide curative treatments. Unfortunately, that is seldom the final outcome of the assessment process because of the complexities of the variables involved and of their interrelationships.

Serial assessments of young children should include observation of their behaviors during routine daily activities, interactions with familiar people, manipulation of objects, and development of play. Videotaping the activities is highly recommended, as it frees the professional from the immediate need to document observations with paper and pencil and enables participation in—or at least undistracted observation of—the activity in progress. The videotapes can then be used to verify observed behaviors, detail or quantify the occurrence of specific communicative events, illustrate observations to the parent(s) by replaying pertinent sections of the tape, and contrast communicative behaviors in serial situations. Videotapes are also invaluable in tracking development and documenting acquisition of skills that were either absent or just emerging at the time of a given taping.

The SLP who assesses bilingual children should be knowledgeable about the linguistic features of the languages the child uses and of their expected developmental sequences. Kayser[26] urges awareness of three principles of speech and language evaluation of bilingual children:

1. Both languages should be evaluated, even when the child only understands the home language.
2. If one of the languages is within normal limits, then a language disorder probably does not exist.
3. A concomitant disorder may exist, such as oral motor disorder, developmental apraxia of speech, phonological impairment, or developmental delay (p. 223).

In addition to thorough review of the case history, the SLP who conducts assessments with bilingual children should be alert to the presence of key clues that a possible language disorder might be present. Kayser's list of such clues that apply to toddlers includes the following:

- Inability to discriminate tones, phonemes, and morphemes
- Inability to associate sounds with objects or experiences
- Inappropriate verbal labels for common objects, actions, and persons
- Poor vocabulary
- Poor turn-taking
- Inappropriate comments
- Use of gestures rather than speech
- Apparent confusion (p. 224)

Novel situations also should be introduced during the serial assessment process. Wetherby and Prizant[27] provided suggestions that entice children to communicate during such encounters (see Appendix B, Table B-5, for an adapted list of communicative temptations). In a sense, the assessment process also can be used as a "trial intervention" strategy. The child's responses to natural and novel bids for communication on the part of the parent or of the examiner in connection with ongoing activities that capture the child's attention for the moment may yield information about the child's preferred communication modes. Videotaped samples of the child's responses to specific strategies could be used later as a part of the parent-education program. It is obvious that this procedure has a direct bearing on assessment of play activities because play is the tool used to elicit the child's behaviors. Just as the sequence of communication development is generally predictable, so too is the sequence of play development.[28,29]

Typical and Atypical Child Behaviors

Children with delayed or disordered communication often use a variety of other, sometimes inappropriate, behaviors to express their needs and feelings. Persistence of problematic behaviors over time is a cause for concern, because they can interfere with social and even cognitive development. Observation of the child in the home, daycare setting, or professional's waiting room can yield significant information about apparent motivation to use vocal, nonverbal, and verbal communication; the adults' reactions to the child's communicative attempts (or lack of attempts); and what forms of nonverbal behavior are typically used by the child.

If there are persistent problematic behaviors about which the family is concerned, a referral to a mental-health professional or a medical specialist may be indicated. Although there are no fixed guidelines for such referrals, Droter and Sturm[30] suggested referral to a mental health professional if (1) the child's aggressive behavior interferes with the capacity to negotiate developmental tasks to the level of his or her assessed mental age or cognitive development; (2) the child's behavior interferes with responsiveness to early intervention services; or (3) the child's parents indicate that they feel high levels of stress about the child's psychological or interpersonal functioning.

Sudden onset of extremely problematic behaviors in toddlers *may* suggest the possibility of childhood disintegrative disorder (one of the PDDs)[31] or even Landau-Kleffner syndrome, a rare neurological problem with similar symptoms, for which referral to a pediatric neurologist is appropriate.[21]

Predictors of Language Development

As McCatherine and colleagues[33] pointed out, there are:

four variables that appear to be closely related to language development and that independently predict language development irrespective of the presence or absence of other factors . . . . This small set of predictors includes three communication components that emerge during the prelinguistic period: (1) babbling, (2) development of pragmatic functions, and (3) vocabulary comprehension. The fourth predictor is the development of combinatorial and symbolic play skills (p. 58).

This set of four variables is expanded somewhat in terms of the pragmatic functions (see observations by Wetherby and Prizant in "Four Groups of Concern to the Speech-Language Pathologist" later in this chapter).

Calandrella and Wilcox[34] urge that at assessments of prelinguistic children with developmental delays special attention be directed at documenting nonverbal communication acts that include both (A) coordinated attention between the communication referent (e.g., an object) and the adult *and* (B) gestural indicating behavior and social interaction signals without coordinated attention to the adult. High rates of both behaviors were predictive of positive language development outcomes among prelinguistic children in follow-up testing at age 3 years.

By contrast, Wetherby[35] points to a series of predictors of persisting communication and language disorders that are identifiable in the prelinguistic child:

- Limited ability to share attention and affective states with eye gaze and facial expression
- Limited use of gaze shifts between people and objects
- Delay in following another person's point and eye gaze
- Low rate of communicating with gestures and/or vocalizations
- Limited range of communicative functions, particularly lacking in the joint attention function
- Limited repertoire of conventional gestures (giving, showing, reaching, pointing)
- Limited use of symbolic gestures (waving, nodding head, depictive gestures)
- Limited consonant inventory
- Immature syllable structure
- Delay in comprehension of words or sentences
- Delay in production of words or sentences
- Delay in spontaneous use or sequencing of action schemes in symbolic play
- Limited ability to imitate actions on objects

Traditional Assessment and Arena-Assessment Formats

Descriptions of multidisciplinary teams and their interactions are provided in Chapter 4. In their professional training programs, most practitioners in communicative disorders have been taught to assume significant, if not exclusive, responsibility for the communicative diagnostic or assessment process. The concept that individual SLP practitioners are legally and ethically responsible for their actions requires mastery of clinical skills in diagnosis, evaluation, and assessment. It is alarming to note that less than half of communicative-disorders program graduates have had exposure to the infant-toddler population. Over one-fourth of the respondents to a survey conducted by Dunn and colleagues[36] indicated that they "had no training with the birth-to-three population prior to graduation (not even units within a course); [only] 40% had an entire course" (p. 57). It is imperative that training programs provide students with opportunities to receive appropriate training with this age group.

Few training programs have implemented curriculum components that teach multidisciplinary or transdisciplinary team assessments, and even fewer provide training in arena assessment. Time constraints and competing priorities for curricular attention will probably continue to contribute to this dilemma. Fortunately, there is a considerable body of professional literature emerging on this subject, and increasing numbers of continuing-education programs are addressing these critical issues.

Although traditional clinical assessment methodology is essential, it appears that requirements of managed health care systems increasingly demand that practitioners also possess skills in team-assessment methodology, including arena assessment. Arena assessment is used when it is advantageous for one professional to handle the infant or young child while others look on. Planning of the assessment, including information desired by each participating professional, is completed either by the multidisciplinary professional team or by the parent(s) in conjunction with the professional team. A specialist in motor development is often designated to handle the child during the assessment so that muscle tone, reflex, and movement patterns can be judged. The entire multidisciplinary team, including the parents, participate in the process, exchanging information and providing each other with interpretations based on their individual areas of expertise. The process is different from either the solo evaluation or the traditional multidisciplinary assessment, both of which allow all participants direct access to the child.

Some emerging research is being directed at the arena-assessment issue and is also taking into consideration the increasing availability of electronic technology. Smith[37] reported on a developmental assessment model employed by the New York State Office of Mental Retardation and Developmental Disabilities that used a televideo network. Such assessment techniques have become common practice in some areas of medical practice. Perhaps some of the difficulties of providing appropriate services to children in rural or remote areas can be resolved in the future with refinement of technology and adaptation of procedures to the needs of very young children.

Play Assessment

Children's play is a rich source of information for professionals who study child development. Like physical growth, communication, and motor development, the development of play proceeds in a sequential manner along a reasonably pre-dictable continuum. Appendix A provides a synopsis of expectations of typically developing play associated with the child's advancing age. Through play, which by definition is *fun*, it is possible to observe how a child interacts with objects, the immediate environment, and play partners. Underlying abilities, such as joint attention, sustained attention, manner and form of manipulation of objects, bids for interaction in play activities, and other attributes, can be judged through skillful construction of opportunities to observe the child at play. Play is a window through which it is possible to have at least a rough estimate of a child's cognitive abilities (e.g., through observation of problem-solving attempts, satisfaction of curiosity), temperament (e.g., through observation of exploring objects and surroundings, responses to frustration or directed attention, endurance), receptive communication (e.g., through observation of responses to requests or directives), expressive communication (e.g., through observation of body language [facial expressions, gestures, eye gaze], vocal and verbal expressions), and socialization. The child's level of play schemes are also informative in connection with development of symbolic representations (e.g., use of a stick in place of a spoon in a kitchen play scheme). Demonstrated understanding of such representational symbols in play helps the SLP understand what is potentially available to the child in the area of verbal symbols.

Linder[38] provided an excellent format for using play as a means of communicative assessment within the framework of a more extensive multidisciplinary assessment. Resource references for using play as a foundation for assessment are provided in Appendix B, Tables B-1 and B-5.

▼ INTERPRETING TO THE FAMILY

Sufficient time must be scheduled to provide information to parents. Depending on the family, the structure of the assessment itself, the setting(s) in which the assessment is conducted, and the amount of information to be shared, the interpretation may be provided at a single visit or may require two or more visits to complete. Parents may express a preference about the type and timing of the interpretation, designation of who should be present to hear the results, and where it would be most convenient to convene. The option of collaborating with families in that manner may be readily available to practitioners who work for agencies that are publicly supported and tend to be more permissive in terms of how much staff time can be expended in such endeavors. Certainly, best practices would be served under such circumstances. However, in light of the managed care environment in which many practitioners work, time may be more constrained; therefore, it may be necessary to condense the available information or to share it through written reports, followed by telephone consultations or brief office visits with a limited agenda relating to interpreting results of the assessment.

Although logistical limitations may be imposed by administrative policy, SLPs must always keep in mind that they are talking to parents about their child: emotions are inevitably involved and must be dealt with in an appropriate way. The SLP must be alert to signs that anxiety-ridden parents receiving assessment results are confused by any vague or technical terminology being used or are misunderstanding the information being presented. Planning time for questions the parents may have *during* the presentation of assessment results, rather than at the end of the process, is advisable. When questions or comments are made by those receiving the news, professionals must truly listen and provide responses that are meaningful.[39,40]

It is difficult for most professionals to deliver bad news when the outcome of the assessment is likely to be upsetting to the family; it is also difficult for the family to receive bad news. Sensibility and sensitivity demand best efforts to be both truthful and compassionate in providing information and its interpretation to families. Emphasizing what the child *can do* and *is doing* is both truthful and sensitive; providing information about what the next developmental level is likely to be is constructive; providing guidance to the family as to what they can do to facilitate movement from the present level of functioning to the next level is empowering and inspiring of hope—a valued commodity among parents of children with any kind of developmental delay or disability.

The process of assessment seeks to answer the following questions that parents and professionals have about a given child:

- What is happening here?
- What are this child's capabilities and limitations?
- What approaches can be used to promote the child's development?

The process of diagnosis seeks to answer the following questions:

- What is the accepted label for this condition or behavior?
- Why is this happening to this child?
- What is the etiology?
- What is the future course of development likely to be on the basis of historic documentation of other instances of the same condition or disorder?
- What are the appropriate treatment, intervention, and management options?
- What are the prospects for a positive outcome?

To arrive at the answers to these questions, other questions must be addressed. To prepare parents for a focused discussion at the meeting at which results of the assessment, diagnosis, and evaluation are shared, it may be helpful to provide the family with a list of questions each procedure endeavors to answer, so that at the time the family receives the interpretation there is a common ground for understanding what the professional(s) hoped would emerge from the evaluation. The assessment seeks to answer the following questions about the child's communicative status:

- What level of communicative development is expected of a child this age with the same or a similar physical diagnosis?
- What level of communicative development does this particular child exhibit?
- If there is a significant discrepancy, can the causes be established?
- What would constitute functional communication for this child?
- What abilities and strengths does the child possess through which other communicative skills can be developed?
- What are the forms and functions of the child's present communicative attempts?
- Who are the preferred communicative partners?
- What are the child's preferred settings for interactions?
- What are the barriers and limitations affecting communication for which compensation may be required?
- What needs to be done to assist this child to establish functional communicative competence?
- What are the family's priorities with respect to the use of assistive communication strategies or devices if assistive communication is indicated?
- What are the options for providing any assistance the child or family may need to achieve the desired outcome?
- How will progress toward the chosen goals be evaluated?

▼ FOUR GROUPS OF CONCERN TO THE SPEECH-LANGUAGE PATHOLOGIST

As SLPs consider how to classify the population of infants and toddlers they evaluate, it is useful to consider the general categorical groupings to which a given child may be assigned based on the outcome of the assessment process. Broadly speaking there are four such groups. Children in the first group have a diagnosed, handicapping condition that is certain to contribute to atypical communicative development. The second group is comprised of children who are established risk, and for whom it is highly probable that impaired communicative development will occur. Children in the third group are risk suspect; that is, biological, medical, or environmental conditions place them at a higher-than-average risk for future problems in developing communicative competence. Finally, there is a group with no known risk factor whose members, nevertheless, develop atypical communication.

For convenience, the groups are referred to as follows:

Group I: confirmed condition (+)
Group II: established risk (risk +)
Group III: risk suspect (risk ?)
Group IV: no known risk (risk 0)

A taxonomy for classifying children into the four groups is presented in Table 8-2.

Infants in group I are usually identified at or shortly after birth and begin early on to receive services from a variety of professional disciplines, although there are exceptions that tend to cluster in the last two categories listed under group I in Table 8-2.

Babies in group II may be identified at or shortly after birth but more often become the focus of concern when speech fails to emerge at the expected time (i.e., around 14 to 18 months of age or adjusted age if the baby was born preterm). Group-II children often present clinically as being shy and exhibit meager social skills. However, some may present as aggressive children who are described as having behavior problems or suspected emotional problems. Their physical development and self-help skills may be age appropriate, but their lack of ability to communicate verbally contributes to inappropriate use of other means of expression.[41]

The same is true of children in group III. As Wetherby and Prizant[42] observed, [s]ignificantly delayed referral is more likely to occur when no risk factors (e.g., very low birthweight, perinatal complications) have been identified or when communication and language delays do not coexist with significant physical, sensory, or cognitive disabilities, any of which may lead to earlier identification and more definitive diagnosis of developmental problems (p. 291).

Several other professional groups have issued cautions to medical and allied health practitioners in this connection by way of their practice parameter statements.[43–45]

Concern for development of these children may emerge at or about 14 to 18 months of age (adjusted age if the infant was premature) and may initially be centered on delayed onset of speech. However, if a child uses even a few words, parental concern may not emerge until considerably later: Age 24 to 36 months is not an uncommon referral point for such children. This is important to recognize because a substantial number of children between 24 and 30 months who have delayed expressive language, but whose receptive language skills are apparently intact, continue to exhibit expressive problems at ages 3 and 4 years.[46–48]

The SLP should be aware, however, that about half of children with intact receptive language at age 3 "catch up" with age peers in expressive language skills by

TABLE 8-2
Suggested Taxonomy of Risk-Factor Groups Related to Communicative Impairment in Infants and Toddlers

Category	Examples of Specific Problems/Risks
Group 1: Diagnosed Conditions Associated With Atypical Communicative Development	
Sensory impairment	Hearing, vision, including retinopathy of prematurity, dual sensory impairment, and hyper- or hyporesponsivity to sensory stimuli
Physical conditions in which anatomical structures or neuromotor functions are impaired	Cerebral palsy, cleft palate, congenital craniofacial anomalies, intraventricular hemorrhage, bronchopulmonary dysplasia, laryngeal papillomatosis
Syndromes and genetic or chromosomal disorders associated with communicative disorders or mental retardation	Fragile X syndrome, Usher syndrome, Down syndrome, Cornelia de Lange syndrome, Cruzon syndrome, cri du chat syndrome, Prader-Willi syndrome
Prenatal exposure to teratogens	Fetal alcohol syndrome, cocaine, and other drug exposure
Diseases of newborns and infants in which known and unknown sequelae affect communicative development	Cytomegalovirus, human immunodeficiency virus, phenylketonuria, meningitis, rubella
Infant psychopathology (NOTE: Some problems can also be caused by genetic aberrations.)	Autism, pervasive developmental disorder, post-traumatic stress disorder
Problems of unknown etiology that are associated with impaired communicative development	Present with various, often multiple, disorders involving state regulation, neuromotor or sensory deficits, pervasive developmental delay, failure to thrive
Group II: Established Risk: Biological, Medical, Environmental Risk Factors Associated With Atypical Communicative Development	
Confirmed presence of family history for specific disorders	Learning disability, progressive hearing loss, language disability
Prenatal exposure to toxic substances without diagnosed sequelae at birth or during postpartum course	Cocaine, alcohol, prescription drugs (e.g., anticonvulsants)
Postpartum exposure to toxic substances	Antibiotic ototoxins, lead, neurotoxins
Prematurity and low birth weight, intrauterine growth retardation	<1599 g <Tenth percentile in head circumference <37 weeks gestation Significant increase in risk if mother has little education and family is in a low SES group
Postmaturity	>40 weeks gestation (NOTE: Placental deterioration can be a factor in problems of postmaturity.)
Fetal distress or birth complications with or without diagnosed handicap at time of hospital discharge	Significantly prolonged labor, fetal distress, injuries from instruments Meconium aspiration, significant hypoxia or anoxia
Diseases and conditions	Rh incompatibility Apgar score lower than 7 at 5 min

Continued

TABLE 8-2
Suggested Taxonomy of Risk-Factor Groups Related to
Communicative Impairment in Infants and Toddlers—Cont'd

Category	Examples of Specific Problems/Risks
Atypical neuromotor or neurobehavioral function in infancy	Feeding or swallowing problems, hypersensitivity, inconsolability, hyposensitivity, floppiness, difficulty with state regulation, failure to thrive
Environmental	Very young mother in low socioeconomic status group with little or no formal education Strong family history of abuse or neglect Combination of such factors
Multifactorial	Early signs of possible developmental delay, attention deficit disorder, or learning disability

Group III: Risk Suspect: Conditions That Suggest a Significant Risk of Atypical
Communicative Development
(Cumulative factors increase probability of atypical communicative development.)

Biological	Any inherent condition or combination of conditions that can interfere with normal neuromotor, physical, or sensory growth and development Soft neurological signs
Medical	Any acquired disease, injury, condition, or combination thereof having the potential to interfere with normal neuromotor or physical growth and development or sensory integrity
Environmental	Any condition or combination of conditions having the potential to interfere with normal cognitive, social, psychoemotional, communicative, or other developmental process

Group IV: No Known Risk Factors in the Presence of Communicative Delay or Disorder
(Children in group IV can be reassigned to another group as maturation and discovery of applicable data lead to identification of previously unrecognized causative factors.)

the time of school entry. Parsing out which language-delayed children should receive treatment to optimize chances of normal language skills on school entry age is a challenge. Wetherby and Prizant[42] (p. 294) summarized the most pertinent indicators for persisting language problems in young children as follows:

- Deficits in the ability to share attention and affective states with eye gaze and facial expression
- A low rate of communicating with gestures and/or vocalizations
- A limited range of communicative functions, particularly lacking in the joint attention function
- A reliance on gestures and a limited use of vocalizations to communicate

- A limited consonant inventory and a less complex syllabic structure in vocal communication
- A delay in both language comprehension and production
- A delay in the spontaneous use of action schemes in symbolic play and the imitation of action schemes

These characteristics can be identified in children under the age of 18 months.

Concern for children in group IV may not develop until even later because some limited functional verbalization is almost always present early in life. Children who are initially considered to be group IV often escape notice until they reach the age of school entry, by which time standardized testing can be applied more reliably.

An interesting observation about children in group IV is that a significant number of them are observed to be "toe walkers." For reasons not yet clear, idiopathic toe walking (i.e., a diagnosis of exclusion in which diagnoses of spastic cerebral palsy, spinal dysraphism or injury, myopathy, neuropathy, autism, and pervasive developmental disorder [PDD] have been ruled out) seems to be a diagnostic sign of developmental language disorder (DLD). Accardo[49] and Schulman and colleagues[50] urged pediatricians to be aware of that phenomenon. Accardo stated, "[t]oe walking is a finding whose presence or history should strongly incline the clinician toward a neurologically based DLD" (p. 510). Schulman and colleagues,[50] in their study of 799 children referred to an orthopedic clinic and seen by a multidisciplinary developmental evaluation team when toe walking was verified, observed that "[t]he [19] children in our study demonstrated delays in multiple developmental areas. Significant language delays were the most prevalent, occurring in more than 75% of the cases" (p. 545). They further commented that "an increase in the severity of language impairment was associated with an increase in the frequency of toe walking" (p. 545).

As noted throughout this book, value should be invested in the family's role in helping to identify children who are in need of communicative assessment. When parents are concerned about any aspect of their child's development, professionals should pay attention. Professional training programs usually include a study of the phenomenon of "parental denial" that can occur in the presence of identified problems, and instruction is provided on methods of dealing with it. Until recently, however, little attention was focused on the phenomenon of "professional denial," although parents have complained through the years about knowing something was wrong with their child and not being able to convince professionals to acknowledge the validity of their concern. Assurances by many professionals that the child would "outgrow" the problem were sometimes accurate but often represented a limited understanding of facts and resulted in delayed provision of appropriate care. When professional denial occurs, many months and sometimes years are lost to what might be appropriate preventive treatment or intervention during the optimal neurophysiological developmental period.

▼ ASSESSMENTS AND COMMUNICATIVE DIAGNOSES

Very young children who experienced professionals and parents place in one of the four risk groups defined above should have the benefit of a communicative assessment or full communication diagnosis. Determining which of the two processes is appropriate at any point in time depends on individual circumstances, including the age and developmental status of the child for whom services are to be provided. Assessment is an ongoing process through which the child's present level of functioning is documented and strategies to enhance development and attainment of the next level of development are recommended. Many practitioners view the assessment process as part of developmental intervention activities. By contrast, as noted in Chapter 2 (see "Screening, Evaluation, Diagnosis, and Assessment"), the process of diagnosis has different goals and can be concluded with a referral to other personnel for habilitation or intervention services. Assessment of function is always a part of a diagnostic evaluation, but diagnosis is not necessarily a part of the assessment process. The two processes are intimately related but should not be considered interchangeable, although planning for both processes requires making decisions about what will be included in the process when it takes place.

As professionals consider the categories into which particular traits assign the child to diagnostic labels or functional descriptors, it is imperative that the implications of such labels and descriptors be considered.

Planning the Assessment

It may be useful to adopt a formal protocol for planning the process to be used. Adoption of such a planning protocol, which guides the sequence of activities and probably identifies personnel responsible for each step of the process, organizes the process for all participants and builds in a degree of predictability. It can also assist in developing projected timelines for the family and team of professionals involved. Table 8-3 illustrates what such a planning protocol can look like. The sequences can be modified to meet the needs of designated agencies or teams.

Communication Assessment Tools

Standardized Tests

Extreme caution should be exercised in using standardized tests with infants and toddlers. Careful consideration should be given to the norming population on which standardized scores are based: Potential exclusion from that group of children with the same diagnosed conditions as that of the child to be tested must make scores invalid. Extremely small samples or extremely varied conditions among children included in the normative group may make interpretation of individual scores extremely difficult. Very young children may not be able to comply with the protocol required in the prescribed testing procedures. Broad variations in developmental patterns among individual children can compromise reliability of test scores. Having said that, however, it must be recognized that in some states Part C service-eligibility regulations call for documentation of specific, quantifiable, deviations from the norm of standardized test scores. Hence, in some states, standardized testing is required to qualify children and families for Part C early intervention services. Practitioners must be aware of such regulatory requirements.

TABLE 8-3
Suggested Sequence for Planning the Assessment

Receive
  Presenting concern or complaint
    Presented by whom (e.g., parent, other family member, professional[s], team)?
    What are the specifics of the concern or complaint?
Consider
  Validity of communicative concerns expressed in terms of risk groups shown in
    Table 8-2 or other taxonomy
Evaluate
  Expressed or apparent need or rationale for service(s)
    Prevention (e.g., secondary, tertiary)?
    Scheduled monitoring (of developmental status, specific condition)?
    Evaluation? Assessment? Diagnosis?
    Statutory or regulatory compliance issues?
    Parent information, education, training?
    Habilitation?
    Rehabilitation?
Identify
  Protocol(s) to be employed and disciplines that need to participate
    Option 1: evaluation and assessment
      Neonatal intensive care unit assessment(s)
      Full developmental assessment
      Communicative assessment
    Option 2: diagnosis
      Comprehensive
      Communicative
Select
  Methods, tools, approaches to be used in developing the following:
    Case history
    Records review
    Observation of child and family
    Examination protocols: initial, serial
    Monodisciplinary, multidisciplinary settings
      Center
      Home
      Other site
      Combination of sites
    Approaches
      Multidisciplinary
      Transdisciplinary
      Interdisciplinary
      Arena format (standard or tele-electronic?)
      Consultation(s) needed
      Serial visit schedule (in consultation with family)
    Instruments, tools, procedures to be used
Conduct
  Assessment, evaluation, diagnostic examination(s)
Record
  Data generated by process used
Document
  Outcomes and impressions
  Evaluation and assessment of status
  Diagnosis

Continued

TABLE 8-3
Suggested Sequence for Planning the Assessment—Cont'd

Document—Cont'd
    Identified skills
    Strengths
    Needs
    Other findings
Prognosis (optional)
    For what?
        Development of functional communication?
        Development of oral communication skills?
        Development of age-appropriate oral communication?
        Other? (specify)
Determine
    What are the keys to a successful communicative and developmental outcome?
        Etiology and prognosis?
        Modifying identified perpetuating factors?
        Parent information, education, training, or any combination of these?
        Family involvement?
        Specific intervention, treatment, and management methods (e.g., assistive or
            augmentative communication)?
        Other means (e.g., referral for consideration of medical, surgical, or other
            management)?
Recommend
    Treatment, management, and intervention plan
        Child-centered, traditional approach?
        Child-centered, family-focused approach? (Individual Family Services Plan)
        Other approach(es)? Special circumstances?
    Referral(s)
        For what?
        To whom?
Implement
    Intervention: treatment, management, or intervention plan
        Make appropriate referrals
        Recommend periodic reevaluations if needed
        Implement active treatment, management, education
            Child
            Parents and family
            Other caregivers
        Monitoring and follow-up as recommended
Evaluate
    Outcomes
        Status
        Progress made since last visit or anticipated at next visit
        Need for modification of treatment or intervention plan

Judgment-Based Assessment

Judgment-based assessment (JBA) is a term used to describe the professional's authority, based on knowledge, training, experience, and status as a "qualified provider" under Part C, to determine a child's developmental status, strengths, and need for early intervention services. In some states, JBA is written into the assessment guidelines, having the effect of statutory authority invested in designated professionals to determine eligibility of infants and toddlers for Part C early-intervention services.

Practitioners who apply JBA procedures use clinical-observation skills; devise situations in which the child's best "performance" can be expected or elicited; and integrate information from a wide range of sources to formulate an informed professional determination of the child's developmental status, observed strengths and needs, and recommendations for appropriate interventions. In some states, a combination of JBA and standardized testing is either required or suggested.

Initial concerns about a child's suspected atypical development are almost always based on JBA in the absence of conditions or diseases present that are known to be associated with developmental disorders. As Morisset[51] observed, "[e]ven though the range of normal variation in language acquisition is wide, there are robust indicators of potential difficulty, and these should not be ignored" (p. vii). The classic indicators are outlined by many researchers, including Wetherby, Rossetti, and Prizant; they are generally agreed to be as follows: lack of response and orientation to sound, poor social responsivity, and lack of vocal play during infancy. They also include lack of development of vocal inflection patterns of the language spoken in the home, absence of or delayed development of consistent sound combinations that label familiar objects, and lack of conventional gestures by 12 months; scant use of spoken words, little or no comprehension of adult requests, and lack of development of two-word combinations by age 24 months.

Decisions that any one of those difficulties is present rest on JBA. Confirmation by formal testing may or may not be required under regulatory guidelines in the family's state of residence.

Multiple Strategies

Multiple strategies are required to develop an accurate picture of a child's communication system. Reliance on any one means or tool of assessment is to be avoided. The SLP employs both formally developed tools and JBA. Anecdotal reports can be as valuable to the assessment process as "hard data" (e.g., test results and physical measurements). The practitioner must be equally aware of available technology and equipment and of the ever-increasing number of tools and procedures that are being made available in contributions to the professional literature by commercial enterprise.

A number of formal diagnostic and assessment tools or instruments are available to practitioners. Some are standardized, some are criterion referenced (often to demonstrated attainment of specific skills or to generally accepted age norms for such attainment). Other tools are procedural strategies through which the child's behaviors can be analyzed with some degree of uniformity across populations. There are also questionnaires to be completed by parents or caregivers that are designed to elicit specific information about the child's developmental status, behavior, or specifics of health and treatments of record. Other tools deal with coping strategies used by parents, such as attitudinal scales by which it is possible to ascertain how designated individuals respond to the child or the disability or that identify family priorities with respect to enhancing parent's abilities to optimize their child's development.

Commercially available instruments vary widely in terms of (1) breadth of communication skills sampled; (2) depth of sampling; (3) methods of sampling used; (4) means of recording findings; (5) intended ages or conditions for which the instrument is applicable; and (6) criteria against which behaviors are compared. It is wise to be cautious in selection and application of instruments. This is doubly true when the child being assessed is known to possess sensory, cognitive, or motor impairments.

Qualitative and Multidimensional Scoring Systems

In some instances, consideration should be given to using a qualitative scoring system to document clinical observations. The child's mastery of a particular skill can be described as being present or absent, but it also may be valuable to describe the manner in which the child responds to specific stimuli. In this regard, examiners who are familiar with Porch's 16-point scoring system[52] or similar multidimensional systems may find them useful in conducting JBAs. Use of such systems is especially recommended in dealing with children who exhibit poor motor coordination.

Although such scoring systems do not yield standard, average, or mean scores, they are meaningful systems of describing skills or behaviors. Such systems, when used by groups of trained observers, also enable cross validation of data for purposes of research and clinical application.

The Professional's Toolbox

Just as carpenters and plumbers need appropriate tools to fit a particular need, so does the SLP. To extend the analogy, master carpenters select among an array of hammers, saws, planes, and other tools the ones that will do a job most efficiently. In the same way, master plumbers rely on a variety of wrenches (e.g., monkey, crescent, ratchet, torque), knowing that different circumstances require different tools. Likewise, the SLP and other professionals who work with the infant-toddler-family population recognize the need for an array of tools that lend themselves to the requirements of specific situations.

A basic "toolbox" for the communicative disorders specialist may include the items listed in Table 8-4. Each practitioner discovers preferred instruments that meet the needs of a particular situation, practice setting, or both, as new products and protocols are developed. The list provided in Table 8-4 reflects the author's selection of basic tools appropriate to a practice based in a university training program and its affiliated clinic. An expanded list of assessment tools is provided in Appendix B, Table B-1.

▼ REPORTING RESULTS

Written reports are generally required and can be presented to the family at the time the results are interpreted to them by the professional team, its representative, or the individual practitioner. The format of written reports is often dictated by the agency, protocols of the practice group or practitioner, requirements of a funding agent, or other entity. Some written reports are lengthy (this is usually the case in clinical training programs); some are very brief (sometimes even to the point of being formatted as checklists or fill-in-the-blank forms); and others fall somewhere

TABLE 8-4
Selected Infant and Toddler Communication Assessment Tools

Instrument	Features	Recommended Ages
Assessing Prelinguistic and Linguistic Behaviors[53]	Observation and elicited interactions are used to assess cognitive antecedents to language, communicative intent, production and comprehension of language	Birth to 2 yr
Assessment of Infants and Toddlers in Naturalistic Contexts[54]	Descriptive, nonstandardized language assessment protocol that may be used in the home or at daycare sites	Children functioning as infants-toddlers developmentally
Assessment of Mother-Infant Interaction[55]	Observer rates mother-child interactions that are important to communicative development	Birth to toddler
Assessment, Evaluation, and Programming System (AEPS)[56]	Designed as an interdisciplinary tool; the "Social-Communication" section can be used separately by SLPs	Birth to 3 yr
Communication and Symbolic Behavior Scales[57]	A normed measure of communicative means, reciprocity, and social and affective signaling based on play activities and interactions with objects	8 mo–2 yr
Communicative Development Inventory for Infants[58]	Inventory relies on parent reports of child's knowledge and use of pragmatic skills and early language	10–36 mo
Communicative Development Inventory for Toddlers[59]	Inventory relies on parent reports of child's understanding and use of early language components; recommended for children who have begun to use single words or connected speech	10 mo–3 yr
Cue Questions[59]	Parent questionnaire that gathers information on communicative means and functions of children with severe developmental delays or multiple handicaps and who function at levels expected of infants and toddlers; checklist ranges from preverbal and nonverbal levels to phrase and sentence level (See replica of form in Appendix B)	Any age, but nicely adapted to situations in which time constraints are present

Continued

TABLE 8-4
Selected Infant and Toddler Communication Assessment Tools—Cont'd

Instrument	Features	Recommended Ages
Integrated Developmental Experiences Assessment (IDEAS)[60]	A functional-language assessment based on observation of cognitive, social, and communicative behaviors in naturalistic settings; the focus is on integration of junctions	Birth to 36 mo
The Language Development Survey[61]	A parent questionnaire that documents language usage of 2 year olds; can be administered as a paper and pencil task or by interview if parent/caregiver does not read	2 yr only
Preschool Language Scale-3[62]	Standardized tool that evaluates auditory comprehension, articulation, grammatical form and structure, and basic concepts of toddlers; requires child's ability to focus attention on picture prompts and oral directions.	Toddlers
The Rossetti Infant-Toddler Language Development Scale[63]	Single-volume tool that contains a parent questionnaire and protocol for complete language assessment. Criterion referenced; observation, parent report, and elicitation of behaviors in play settings used to generate data; focus is broad and includes attention to attachment-interaction, pragmatics, gesture, play, preverbal communication, language expression and comprehension	Birth to 3 yr
Transdisciplinary Play-Based Assessment[64]	Intended for use by transdisciplinary early intervention teams; section on language assessment can be used independently by SLPs if desired	Developmental levels of 6 mo–6 yr

between those extremes. Reporting results to parents following the assessment or diagnostic process is discussed under "Interpreting to the Family" earlier in this chapter. Written reports of professionals are generally considered to be eligible for subpoena in lawsuits as legal documents relating to the child's status.

Individual Family Services Plan

The individual family services plan (IFSP) is a unique requirement of Part C. It is viewed as both a process and a document that serves as a guide for intervention services selected by the family for their child or for the family itself as a means to enhance their ability to maximize the child's development. The IFSP is flexible, subject to change as the parents desire, and developed by the family in conjunction with members of the multidisciplinary team or the designated family services coordinator. By law, the IFSP must contain the following[65,66]:

- A statement of the child's present health status
- A statement of the child's developmental levels: physical (including sensory), cognitive, motor (gross and fine), communicative (speech and language), and social and emotional
- The service coordinator's name
- Expected outcomes (functional goals) for the child and family
- A listing of services to be provided
- Starting date and expected duration of the services and the person or agency responsible for providing the services
- Identification of the environment in which the services are to be provided (The child's "natural environments" [e.g., home, daycare center] are preferred and must be used to the extent possible.)
- A transition plan in anticipation of any major changes as the child moves from service to service or approaches the age of 36 months, at which time Part C services are terminated

In some instances, the IFSP can itself be regarded as the assessment report. Most agencies and practitioners, however, feel obligated by standards of practice to generate more specific written reports of assessment or diagnostic findings.

The family service coordinator is required to document how the IFSP services are to be financed. Payment through Part C funds in participating states is available only as a last resort; all other possible sources of payment must be tapped and exhausted before Part C funding can be requested. Some Part C services must be provided free of charge to eligible infants, toddlers, and their families. These include screening and evaluation, multidisciplinary assessment, medical services and equipment that are required to complete the multidisciplinary assessment, development of the IFSP, service coordination (case management), and transition planning.

Once an IFSP has been developed, the lead agency in the participating state is ultimately responsible for seeing that the designated services are provided through the family-focused, community-based system. Families can change the services that they request from time to time and can decline to participate in services for which they and the child are eligible. Any variation from the original IFSP requires a modification of that document. Families are entitled to initiate due-process proceedings when conflicts about desired services cannot be resolved with service providers. Eligibility criteria, policies relating to confidentiality and due process, and other components of a state's Part C implementation plan vary widely among participating states. Diagnostic and assessment processes can be affected by the rules and regulations pertaining to those aspects of the Part C system. Information about implementation is available from the state's lead agency. Lead agencies are listed in Appendix C, Table C-1.

Documentation must be made available by agencies and practitioners to designated monitors of the Part C system. Thus assessment and diagnostic reports are essential records of the agencies and practitioners serving the Part C population.

Other Report Formats

Reports provided to other professionals can take the form of a personal letter or memo summarizing findings to which a more detailed report may be appended. Physicians and other professionals often prefer receiving one- (or at most two-) page summaries of findings with a note that a more detailed report is available on request. In private practices and in managed health care environments, where time is a crucial element of the economic picture, economy of writing (and reading) time is at a premium. SLPs should cultivate skills in preparing information-dense but concise reports. However, there also must be a means of capturing the "fine-grained" information generated during the assessment or diagnostic process that leads to formulation of conclusions about a given child's communication system. Guidelines for making a referral for specialized medical evaluation are suggested in Chapter 7.

▼ Summary

Certain philosophical and procedural adaptations are required when different service-delivery models are used. Practitioners who serve the youngest segment of the pediatric population and their families need to keep abreast of rapidly developing legislative mandates, guidelines of practice, and technical advances through

TABLE 8-5
Quick Review of Items Essential to Communicative Assessment and Diagnosis

Review of records
  Medical and surgical
  Developmental
    Health status
    Physical and sensory development
    Cognitive development
    Motor development (i.e., gross and fine)
    Social-behavioral development (i.e., attachment, temperament, adjustment, coping behaviors)
    Communicative development (i.e., interactions, turn-taking, means, intent, preverbal, receptive, expressive, nonverbal, verbal)

TABLE 8-5
Quick Review of Items Essential to Communicative Assessment and Diagnosis—Cont'd

Pertinent history by interview
  Family (i.e., medical, social, and educational)
  Prenatal (child and mother)
  Postnatal
  Developmental
    Attainment of milestones
    Variations in development
    Problems and delays encountered
Presumed cause of present concern
  By family
  By professionals
Observation
  Child, parent, and family interactive styles
  In familiar and unfamiliar settings
  Videotaped record, if possible
Team participation*
  Family member(s)
  Speech-language pathologist
  Audiologist
  Psychologist
  Physician(s) (e.g., pediatrician, neurologist, ophthalmologist, orthopedist, radiologist,
    otorhinolaryngologist, gastroenterologist, plastic surgeon, geneticist, cardiologist,
    other specialist)
  Physical therapist
  Occupational therapist
  Nurse
  Social worker
  Early childhood educator, early interventionist, early childhood special educator, child
    development specialist
  Other(s)
Examination, assessment, and evaluation
  Evaluation of sensory integrity (especially hearing, taction, vision, balance, tolerance
    for sensory stimuli)
  Evaluation of anatomical structures required for communication, including the peripheral
    oral mechanism and related physical structures
  Evaluation of physiological function required for communication
  Documentation of known conditions and syndromes that are or may be associated
    with atypical communicative development
  Assessment of feeding and swallowing functions, if needed
  Identification of communicative means, modes, functions, and intent
  Assessment of communication status†
    Presymbolic
    Nonverbal symbolic
    Verbal
The communication examination and assessment also includes evaluation of the following:
  Interaction between child and primary caregiver(s) and interactive styles of family unit
  Cultural milieu in regard to communicative development
  Motivation for communicative effort
  Opportunities presented for communication within daily routines
  Play behaviors (i.e., cognitive and motor abilities, social interactions, coping skills, and
    communication skills exhibited)

Continued

> ## TABLE 8-5
> ## Quick Review of Items Essential to Communicative Assessment and Diagnosis—Cont'd
>
> Decisions to be made
>   What to cover in examination(s)
>   When examination(s) will be conducted
>   Where examination(s) will be conducted
>   How examination(s) will be conducted
>   What special methods and tools are needed
>   Laboratory tests
>   Developmental inventories
>   Specific test materials, instruments, equipment
>   Special handling (e.g., therapeutic positioning)
>   Videotaping of all or portions of the examination (for baseline reference and later
>   comparison? for verification of findings? to free up examiners from documentation
>   chores during the examination? for viewing by team members not available at
>   scheduled examination appointment?)
>   To what extent will judgment-based assessment be accepted as part of the findings?
>   In what format will documentation and reports be developed and disseminated?
>   What permissions and informed consent documents are required, and whose responsibility
>   are they?

*Part C regulations define the multidisciplinary team as having at least two professional members. A minimal team considered appropriate to communication examination comprises parent(s), the speech-language pathologist, and the audiologist.
†See Appendix A for helpful reference data.

continuing professional education. The material presented in this chapter should confirm the reader's perception that mastery of specific technical skills, along with a healthy dose of common sense, go into the processes of assessment and diagnosis with very young children and their families, and that work with infants and toddlers is not simply a downward extension of skills applied with older preschool children.

Table 8-5 provides the reader with a condensed review of the necessary elements of a communication assessment.

▼ REFERENCES

1. Lewis ML, Fox N: Issues in infant assessment. In CC Brown, editor: *Childhood prenatal risk: pediatric round table #9*, Skillman, NJ, 1983, Johnson & Johnson Products, p 78.
2. Menyuk P, Liebergott JW, Schultz MC: *Early development in full-term and premature infants*, Hillsdale, NJ, 1995, Erlbaum, p 193.
3. Keefe KA, Feldman HM, Holland AL: Lexical learning and language abilities in preschoolers with perinatal brain damage, *J Speech Hear Disord* 54:395, 1989.
4. Sherman T, Shulman BB: Low birthweight and developmental delays: research issues in communication sciences and disorders, *Contemp Issues Commun Sci Disord* 24:79, 1997.
5. Glascoe FP, Altemeier WK, MacLean WE: The importance of parents' concerns about their child's development, *Am J Dis Child* 143:855, 1989.
6. Glascoe FP: Parents' concerns about children's development: prescreening technique or screening test? *Pediatrics* 99:522, 1997.

7. Wetherby A, Prizant B: *CSBS developmental profile,* Vero Beach, Fla, The Speech Bin, n.d.
8. Frankenburg WK, Dodds JB: *Denver developmental screening II,* Denver, 1990, Ladoca Project and Publishing Foundation.
9. Bricker D: *Assessment, evaluation, and programming system (AEPS) for infants and children, vol 1, AEPS measurement for birth to three years,* Baltimore, 1993, Paul H. Brookes.
10. Provence S, Apfel NH: *Infant-toddler and family instrument,* Baltimore, 2001, Brookes Publishing.
11. Fenson L, et al: *MacArthur communicative development inventories for infants and toddlers,* San Diego, 1991, Singular.
12. Rescorla L: The language development survey: a screening tool for delayed language in toddlers, *J Speech Hear Disord* 54:598–599, 1989.
13. Rossetti LM: *The Rossetti infant-toddler language scale: a measure of communication and interaction,* East Moline, Ill, 1990, LinguiSystems.
14. Schuler AL, et al: Assessment of communicative means and functions through interview: assessing the communicative capabilities of individuals with limited language, *Semin Speech Lang* 10:51–56, 1989.
15. Bzoch KR, League R: Receptive expressive emergent language scale, ed 2, Austin, Tex, 1991, PRO-ED.
16. Crais E: Communication report form. In Bailey DB, Jr, Wolery M, editors: *Assessing infants and preschoolers with handicaps.* ed 2, New York, 1996, Merrill, pp 366–367.
17. Lewis B, et al: Family pedigrees of children with suspected developmental apraxia of speech. Paper presented at the American Speech-Language-Hearing Association, New Orleans, Nov 2001.
18. Lohman P, Manning RK, Dean CR: Current trends in developmental apraxia of speech. Poster session presented at the American Speech-Language-Hearing Association, New Orleans, La, Nov 2001.
19. Jakielski KJ: Clinical management of developmental apraxia of speech. Seminar presented at the convention of the Louisiana Speech-Language-Hearing Association, Baton Rouge, La, Nov 5, 2000.
20. Brunetti V, et al: Chronic hoarseness misdiagnosed in children. Paper presented at the American Broncho-Esophageal Association Annual Meeting, Palm Springs, Calif, May 14, 2002.
21. Mitchell PR: Prelinguistic vocal development: a clinical primer, *Contemp Issues Commun Sci Disord* 24:87, 1997.
22. Wetherby AM: Alton Ochsner Clinic Annual Continuing Medical Education Program: Infants and Toddlers with Special Needs, New Orleans, May 1999.
23. Bell RQ: Minor physical anomalies: relation to later achievement. In Paul NW, editor: *Research in infant assessment,* White Plains, NY, 1989, March of Dimes Birth Defects Foundation, p 25.
24. Superneau DW: Subtle signs of undiagnosed genetic disorders ("The Dysmorphology Detective"). Paper presented at Conference on the Child with Special Needs, New Orleans, April 1997.
25. LeVan RR: Clinical sampling in the assessment of young children with handicaps: shopping for skills, *Top Early Child Special Educ* 10:65, 1990.
26. Kayser HR: Bilingual language development and language disorders. In Battle DE: *Communication disorders in multicultural populations,* ed 3,. Boston, 2002, Butterworth-Heinemann, pp 205–232.
27. Wetherby AM, Prizant BM: *Communication and symbolic behavior scale* [CSBS]-Normed edition, Chicago, 1993, Applied Symbolix.
28. Fewell R: *Play assessment scale,* Miami, 1991, University of Miami.
29. Fewell R: *Assessing the child with special needs using play observations: evaluating communication, cognition, and motor behavior.* Paper presented at the Conference on the Child with Special Needs, New Orleans, April 1997.
30. Droter D, Sturm L: Mental health intervention with infants and young children with behavioral and developmental problems, *Infant Young Child* 3:1, 1991.
31. American Psychiatric Association: *Diagnostic and statistical manual,* ed 4, Washington, DC, 1994, Author.

32. National Institute of Neurological Diseases and Stroke: *Fact sheet: Landau-Kleffner syndrome.* Available at http://www.ninds.nih.gov/health_and_medical/disorders/landaukleffnersyndrome_doc.htm.
33. McCatherine RB, Warren SF, Yoder PJ: Prelinguistic predictors of later language development. In Cole KN, Dale PS, Thal DJ: *Assessment of communication and language, vol 6, Communication and language intervention series,* Baltimore, 1996. Paul H. Brookes, p 57.
34. Calendrella AM, Wilcox MJ: Predicting language outcomes for young prelinguistic children with developmental delay, *JSLHR* 43(6):1061–1071, 2000.
35. Wetherby AM: First words project: improving early identification of communication disorders. Seminar presented at the convention of the Louisiana Speech-Language-Hearing Association, Baton Rouge, La, Nov 6, 2000.
36. Dunn SL, van Kleeck A, Rossetti LM: Current roles and continuing needs of speech-language pathologists working in neonatal intensive care units, *Am J Speech-Lang Pathol* 2:52, 1993.
37. Smith DL: Teleassessment: a model for team developmental assessment of high-risk infants using a televideo network, *Infant Young Child* 9:58, 1997.
38. Linder TW: *Transdisciplinary play based assessment,* Baltimore, 1993, Paul H. Brookes.
39. Kovarsky D, Kurtzner-White E: Delivering and formulating diagnostic news. Miniseminar presented at the American Speech-Language-Hearing Association Conference, New Orleans, Nov 17, 2001.
40. Mastergeorge AM: *Discourse in diagnostic news delivery: What is said, what is not said, and what is mis(understood),* Miniseminar presented at the American Speech-Language-Hearing Association conference, New Orleans, La, Nov 17, 2001.
41. Prizant BM, Meyer EC: Socioemotional aspects of language and social communication disorders in young children, *Am J Speech-Lang Pathol* 2:56, 1993.
42. Wetherby AM, Prizant BM: Toward earlier identification of communication and language problems in infants and young children. In Meisels SJ, Fenichel E, editors: *New visions for the developmental assessment of infants and young children,* Washington, DC, 1996, Zero to Three/National Center for Infants, Toddlers, and Families, p 289.
43. American Academy of Pediatrics: Policy statement: Developmental surveillance and screening of infants and young children (RE0062), *Pediatrics* 108(1):192–196, 2001.
44. American Academy of Neurology: *Practice parameter: screening and diagnosis of autistic spectrum disorders* (a multi-society consensus statement, 02/25/00). Summary statement prepared by PA Filipek, corresponding author and project chair (E-mail: filipek@uci.edu).
45. Interdisciplinary Council on Development and Learning Disorders: *ICDL clinical practice guidelines,* Bethesda, Md, 2000, Author. [Free download at http://icdl.com/ICDLguidelines]
46. Rescorla L, Schwartz E: Outcome of specific language delay (SELD). Paper presented at the meeting of the International Conference on Infant Studies, Washington, DC, April 1988.
47. Fischel J, Whithurst G, DeBaryshe B: Language growth in children with expressive language delay, *Pediatrics* 83:218, 1989.
48. Rescorla L, Roberts J, Dahlsgaard K: Late talkers at 2: outcome at age 3, *J Speech Hear Res* 40:556, 1997.
49. Accardo P: On one's toes about developmental language disorders, *J Pediatr* 130:509, 1997.
50. Schulman LH, et al: Developmental implications of idiopathic toe walking, *J Pediatr* 130:541, 1997.
51. Morisset CE: Perspective, *Infants Young Child* 9(4):vi, 1997.
52. Porch BE: *Porch index of communicative ability in children,* Palo Alto, Calif, 1979, Consulting Psychologists Press.
53. Olswang L, et al: *Assessing linguistic behaviors,* Seattle, 1987, University of Washington Press.
54. Norris JA: Assessment of infants and toddlers in naturalistic contexts. In Secord WA, Damico JS, editors: *Best practices in school speech-language pathology: descriptive/nonstandard language assessment,* San Antonio, Tex, 1992, The Psychological Corporation.

55. Klein MD, Briggs MH: *Observation of communicative interaction*, Los Angeles, 1987, Mother-Infant Communication Project, University of California at Los Angeles.
56. Bricker D: *Assessment, evaluation, and programming system (AEPS) for infants and children*, Baltimore, 1993, Brookes Publishing.
57. Wetherby A, Prizant BM: *Communication and symbolic behavior scales*, Baltimore, Md, 1993, Brookes Publishing.
58. Fenson L, et al: *MacArthur communicative development inventories for infants and toddlers*, San Diego, Calif, 1991, Singular.
59. Schuler AL, et al: Assessment of communicative means and functions through interview: assessing the communicative capabilities of individuals with limited language, *Semin Speech Lang* 10:51–56, 1989.
60. Norris JA: Assessment of infants and toddlers in naturalistic contexts. In Secord WA, Damico JS, editors: *Best practices in school speech-language pathology: descriptive/nonstandard language assessment*, San Antonio, 1992, The Psychological Corporation.
61. Rescorla L: The language development survey: a screening tool for delayed language in toddlers, *J Speech Hear Disord* 54:598–599, 1989.
62. Zimmerman IL, Steiner VG, Pond P: *Preschool language scale*, ed 3, San Antonio, 1992, The Psychological Corporation.
63. Rossetti LM: *The Rossetti infant-toddler language scale: a measure of communication and interaction*, East Moline, Ill, 1990, LinguiSystems.
64. Dickson K, Linder TW, Hudson P: Observation of communication and language development. In Linder TW: *Transdisciplinary play-based assessment*, Baltimore, 1993, Paul H. Brookes.
65. Public Law 102-119. Amendments to the Individuals with Disabilities Education Act [IDEA] of 1991.
66. US Department of Education: Assistance to states for the education of children with disabilities and early intervention program for infants and toddlers with disabilities. 34CFR Part 303: Early intervention program for infants and toddlers with disabilities, *The Federal Register*, 64(48):12505–12554, 1999. [Full text of final regulations for IDEA available at http://www.icase.org/idea/regulations/12415.htm]

CHAPTER 9

OPTIMIZING COMMUNICATION DEVELOPMENT

Treatment, Management, Intervention

Frances P. Billeaud

▼ INDIVIDUALIZED CARE

Once it has been determined that a child needs developmental assistance, it is imperative that the assistance be appropriate to that child's needs. Brazelton[1] pointed out that oversimplified, nonindividualized intervention programs can do more harm than good. The individualization of intervention programs and attempts to help the young child acquire the power of functional communication are critical to creating optimal results. Individualized plans accentuate what the child *can already do* and what the parent-professional team can do to build on existing abilities. A positive and productive starting point is to identify the parents' priorities for the child. The professional's knowledge and technical expertise can then be used to assist in guiding family efforts to enhance the child's development. Goals can be modified over time, but the initial objectives that help the child progress from present status to the next developmental level provide a positive framework with a sense of purpose for all involved in the child's care.

▼ IS IT TREATMENT, MANAGEMENT, OR INTERVENTION?

The terms *treatment, management,* and *intervention* have distinct meanings to practitioners in different work settings. For many, *treatment* implies a medical or allied-health approach to ameliorating or eliminating a diagnosed problem. *Management,* on the other hand, can subsume treatment but includes other processes through which a positive outcome is achieved. Management can include parent education, genetic counseling, and other measures not involving medication, direct therapeutic strategies, or surgical intervention. Treatment is often thought of as what is done to or for the individual possessing the diagnosed problem, whereas management usually involves parents, other caregivers, and possibly program personnel. *Intervention* is designed to produce a favorable result for an identified problem. In the context of working with infants, toddlers, and their families, intervention has come to mean anything done that has a positive effect on enhancing the child's development. By contrast, intervention, as it is used in the field of mental health or substance abuse, implies a confrontation of the individual with the problem by loved ones, coworkers, or both to force the individual to face the seriousness of a situation and to initiate treatment. Because these terms are used in various ways by practitioners in different work settings, different disciplines, and the public, it is wise to ensure that professionals and family members understand what is meant

TABLE 9-1
Treatment, Management, and Intervention Targets for Infants and Toddlers at Risk for Communicative Disorders

Child Centered	Family Focused	Environment Focused
For children with conditions that affect growth, structures, or functional integrity needed for communicative purposes	Parent training in techniques and methods specific to their child's physical and developmental needs	Modifications (e.g., special equipment, furnishings, room arrangements, schedules) to enhance the child's development in various settings:
Single-discipline or multidisciplinary management by the following:	Parent information and education about the following:	Hospital
Medical practitioners in various specialties	Decision making	Home
Surgical practitioners in various specialties	Advocacy	Center
Occupational therapist	Child development	Child care site
Physical therapist	Their child's condition or diagnosis	Preschool
Nutritionist	Financial resources	Clinic
Audiologist	Legal rights of child and family	
Speech-language pathologist	Available management options	
Psychologist	Gaps in the service-delivery system	
Early childhood educator	Family empowerment (identifying, selecting, and using services)	
Specialists in prosthetic appliances and augmentative devices	Self-advocacy	
Case manager or service coordinator	Service coordination	
	Family support for individual family members and the family unit as a whole	
	Social services	

when specific terms are used. The power of such terms to affect cooperation and involvement should never be underestimated.

Whatever the mechanism (management, treatment, or intervention) used, the same goal is operative: all efforts are directed by those involved to optimize the child's development. The speech-language pathologist's (SLP's) role in treating, managing, or intervening with the target population is multifaceted. Circumstances surrounding the child's care can be complicated or relatively straightforward. The activities in which the SLP engages are affected by philosophies of care, timing of treatment or intervention, the contributions of other professionals and caregivers to the processes, the child's condition and need for specific types of intervention, and other factors. Table 9-1 provides an overview of the many elements that must be considered.

▼ Strategies of the Speech-Language Pathologist with the Pediatric Population

Services provided by the SLP can include one or a combination of the following:

- Screening, referral, and follow-up
- Consultation
- Parent education
- Parent training
- Direct treatment and management of the delay or disorder
- Prevention
- Application of Part C intervention mandates

Screening, Referral, and Follow-Up

Parents or others may bring their concerns about the child's communicative development to the SLP through their own initiative or as a result of a referral from another parent or a professional. When the concern is reviewed by the SLP, it becomes apparent whether an immediate referral to another professional discipline or program is warranted or whether the SLP should personally see the child to evaluate reported behaviors that may validate the need for concern or reassure the family that development is proceeding along a typical course. On the basis of these findings, the SLP can suggest a follow-up phone call or visit at some future date for the purpose of tracking the child's development.

Medical and surgical treatment may be warranted for some youngsters with delays or disorders in communicative development. Perhaps the most obvious problems for which surgical treatment would be appropriate are cleft lip, cleft palate, and other craniofacial anomalies. Surgical treatment can also be appropriate for certain laryngeal structural anomalies, granulomas, papillomatosis, and laryngeal trauma. Tracheotomies are required for a variety of problems. Pressure-equalization tubes are the treatment of choice for some chronic middle-ear infections. The role of the SLP in such instances can include referral to the medical practitioner on the basis of the quality of the child's vocalizations, parent reports of repeated earaches (especially if they have gone untreated), or physical characteristics that can be suggestive of a recognizable syndrome or that are associated with atypical motoric functioning of the oral mechanism.

The cost of referral service varies from one work setting to the next. Because the SLP's time is a commodity in the health care marketplace, a nominal fee may be charged. The service is one of the designated "free" services under Part C legislation, however, and many agencies absorb its cost as a function of public awareness and prevention activities.

Consultation

Consultation services are often provided in connection with care options considered or offered by other professionals (e.g., physicians, early interventionists, physical and occupational therapists). Such services are often part of the process for developing the individualized care plan. Consultation can be conducted as part of the discharge plan when an infant or young child is being released from a stay in the hospital, as part of an overall health care plan for a child with specific medical or surgical needs, or as part of the individual family services plan (IFSP) process when the multidisciplinary evaluation has been completed. When the service is provided as part of the development of the IFSP, it is free of charge to the family, and the agency can bill the Part C system directly for the allowable costs. When it is done as part of the planning process with peer professionals, the work setting generally dictates how the costs of providing the professionals' time are covered.

Coleman and colleagues[2] provided a perspective on the professional's role in serving as a consultant to parents. They observed that this form of consultation generally takes the form of (1) determining the nature of the problem at hand; (2) devising a plan to observe and record instances of the child's behavior that the family wishes to modify; and (3) helping the family to develop a plan of action to change the behavior to a desired outcome. The success of the process hinges on the family's active participation in developing the plan that is to be implemented. They stated,

"Consultees are asked to contribute information on strategies that they have tried and on the level of success or failure of a particular strategy. . . . Most important, consultees assist in developing a plan of implementation that best suits their particular situation (p. 194).

They concluded that parents' stated needs for information and support are both met in the consultation process, which "readily provides in a less intrusive format" than does the traditional interview model (p. 198).

Formal and informal opportunities to provide in-service training and staff-development training are also forms of consultative services. If the medical staff is unfamiliar with the range of assistance the SLP can provide, a written communication or face-to-face meeting may be warranted. Seeking opportunities to address groups of specialists at their professional meetings is one way of conveying information about the SLP's technical competencies and desire to enhance the provision of comprehensive patient care. Providing copies (or abstracts) of pertinent articles from professional journals (both theirs and SLP journals) or reviews of pertinent new books, along with a short personal note to the appropriate medical staff members, is another way of "breaking the ice" with pediatric care providers; it is also a legitimate form of consultation.

Children who are under medical care for acute or chronic conditions can also benefit from what the SLP has to offer. Hospital pediatric care plans often reflect a concern for the child's lack of normal social stimulation and separation from family routines that are necessitated by periods of hospitalization. Staff communication with the child and with the family is a primary concern. The SLP can be of assistance in consulting with the medical and nursing staff about how to make the child's communicative stimulation as normal as possible under the circumstances. When children are under specific treatment protocols that require special equipment or pharmacological management, the SLP can provide counseling to families concerning how to establish, strengthen, or optimize communication under such unusual circumstances. The SLP can also design temporary assistive communication strategies (e.g., basic communication boards for toddlers) and train the family and staff in their use.

Because development of communication skills occurs simultaneously with other aspects of child development, specialists can learn from one another. Sharing information about standard protocols of treatment, criteria for selecting or administering specific kinds of care, pertinent research findings, and how each member of the developmental team can assist the others in attaining their respective goals is an invaluable activity of the team. That type of consultation promotes a deeper understanding of the contributions of each discipline to optimal outcomes, enhances the skills of all team members, and improves the ability of members of the team to make appropriate referrals and provide more comprehensive information to families with whom they work.

Parent Education

Parent education services involve the provision of information about the expected course of child development. Typical sequences of development, acceptable variations, anticipated difficulties in the presence of stressful events, and finding the right kind of help when the parent has questions or needs guidance can be subjects covered in parent-education programs. Such services can be provided in the context of a scheduled workshop or series of workshops or can involve use of a longer sequence of meetings (or even a formal academic course). A number of excellent commercial programs are available for implementing parent education programs that the SLP may wish to review. Merely providing parents with information on child development and engaging them in problem solving has produced positive developmental outcomes in some cases.[3–6]

Generally speaking, few parents have had any formal coursework in child development; even fewer have had exposure to information about syndromes, diseases, anomalies, or other conditions their children may have. Information about expected variations in acquisition of communication skills, available treatment options, how to locate credentialed professionals, traditional and experimental or controversial approaches, legal entitlements and responsibilities, and how to locate parent-support groups or organizations that provide specific information about a given condition are examples of topics that could be covered in a more targeted parent-education program for families whose children are known to have (or to be at high risk for) developmental problems. Because the SLP has a broad understanding of available resources (e.g., printed materials, organizations, videotapes, and other educational materials), he or she may serve as a specialist in accessing the information parents need.

The costs of parent-education programs, including the time of professionals involved, an assigned share of operation costs of the facility, and materials and supplies, are sometimes contributed by an agency as part of their dedication to public awareness, information, and prevention. When that is not the case, families or a third-party payer (e.g., social-service agency, sponsoring organization that underwrites the service) may be charged an enrollment or tuition fee. A point to remember is that there *is* a cost to providing such programs.

Parent Training

Parent training is distinguishable from parent education in that it is directed toward parental acquisition of information and specific skills and strategies used in treatment regimens or management procedures delineated in the care plan for their child. For example, families of babies who are tube fed are trained by nursing professionals in appropriate procedures to complete the feedings. Such training includes such strategies as sterilization of the tube area and implements used in the feeding, prevention of common misapplications that result in stomach cramps, and management of bowel problems that can be associated with tube feedings. Children who are tube fed are often provided with non-nutritive sucking devices, so that normal motor coordination for the functions underlying speech develop in spite of the fact that food is not ingested orally. Parents of youngsters with tracheostomies, apnea monitors, supplementary oxygen, and other devices require training to anticipate emergencies and respond to them, to understand how their child's developmental patterns may be affected by the devices, and to implement compensatory strategies when appropriate.

The SLP with appropriate training and experience in specialized care strategies can be involved in providing parent training on feeding and swallowing; communication development in tracheostomized infants and toddlers; pre- and postsurgical counseling for families whose children have craniofacial disorders; and specific strategies to promote communication development for children with diagnosed diseases, conditions, and syndromes. Collaboration with other health professionals in parent-training efforts is often necessary when the nature of the child's problem is complex. Physical and occupational therapists can assist the SLP in advising parents about positioning of the child to optimize communicative efforts. Along with nurses and medical practitioners, they can help "read" infant signals that assist adults to interpret the baby's physical condition, state of alertness, and stress levels.

Of particular value to families of infants and young toddlers is training in specific techniques relating to (1) appropriate communicative stimulation and its timing; (2) techniques to calm a child (e.g., swaddling, positioning, and handling to accommodate for hypersensitivity); and (3) optimizing attentiveness and interaction.

Direct billing for parent training is generally appropriate, but the manner in which billing procedures are handled can vary from one employment setting to the next. Some third-party payers require a physician order for such training; others may accept parent training as a standard protocol under certain conditions.

Direct Treatment and Management of Communicative Delays or Disorders

The SLP can be involved in direct treatment strategies necessitated by issues of the child's health and survival. Chapter 5 explores a number of such instances and elaborates on the SLP's role in developing, implementing, and monitoring the feeding and swallowing treatment plans for infants in the neonatal intensive care unit. Of particular importance in this discussion are issues concerning the scope of practice appropriate to specific professional disciplines, licensure stipulations (i.e., who is licensed by the state to do what), what constitutes best practices for the situation at hand, costs associated with specialized care, conservation of resources through staff collaboration, and competencies of individual staff members.

Many children with developmental delays or disorders can benefit from child-centered, family-focused management approaches that employ a range of activities and do not require a traditional clinical treatment regimen. There are instances, however, when direct management or treatment of the child's communication problem is required. Examples of this situation include instances in which the child is in need of amplification, augmentative communication training, management of developing oral communication in the presence of a tracheostomy, or when implementation of compensatory strategies are necessary. Sometimes parents request direct treatment in the traditional model even when their children do not have such unusual problems. Families may prefer the privacy of the traditional clinical model.

After reviewing the array of treatments available, some parents conclude that a direct one-on-one therapeutic intervention protocol is optimal for their child. An example of this is the applied behavioral analysis (ABA) approach (e.g., the Lovaas program or one of its modifications) for management of behaviors, including communicative behaviors associated with pervasive developmental delay and autism.

In most cases, application of direct treatment strategies does not necessarily eliminate access to additional forms of management. In many cases, direct treatment programs are administered in addition to or in conjunction with other management programs in which the child is enrolled.

Prevention

Prevention is an emerging and important role for the SLP. Families of children diagnosed with inherited conditions may wish to know the probability of bearing another child with the same disorder. In the case of primary prevention, when there is hesitancy about accepting a recommendation for genetic counseling, the SLP may assist other health care providers by listening to the concerns of the parents, providing appropriate information to them in layperson's terms, and allaying fears about the procedure of obtaining the necessary samples and subsequent medical counseling.

Placement of the discussion of prevention toward the end of the list of services the SLP provides or collaborates on with other professionals may seem strange. However, it is often the occurrence of one child's developmental problems that initiates parental interest in issues of preventing the recurrence of such problems in the future. The current explosion of knowledge about genetic problems, however, does not extend to other causes of communication disorders, and it is the SLP's knowledge of available resources in the professional literature that is often sought by families. Language-learning disabilities, familial stuttering, and other communication difficulties experienced by very young children are examples of problems for which information on prevention might be sought.

Secondary prevention, in which the focus is on avoiding exacerbation of an existing problem, is certainly a strategy used by the SLP (e.g., in instances of early onset of dysfluencies). Strategies are routinely recommended to parents to reduce the probability that the dysfluencies will progress to true stuttering. Other examples include recommendations that toddlers who are only children be provided opportunities to play with age peers to increase their need or desire to communicate and that parents reduce the level of language used with their children who are experiencing delayed language development. The latter, of course, is intended to provide appropriate speech models the children find easier to emulate.

Tertiary prevention is the application of therapeutic strategies to eliminate or modify an existing disorder and has been discussed in Chapter 2 (see "The Concept of Prevention").

Application of Part C Intervention Mandates

Throughout this section, *Part C* is used to refer to strategies the SLP and others employ in their implementation of early intervention as mandated by federal statute and companion legislation in participating states. Under the Part C system, services must be provided in accordance with the IFSP. Thus the SLP, as a member of the early intervention team, can provide a wide range of the services in one or more designated settings.

Home-based services are considered optimal for early intervention, because young children and their families have daily routines in which developmental stimulation can be implemented without setting aside "special" times or excluding other members of the family. The ability of individual family members to participate directly in intervention activities is a natural function of family interaction. Communication development typically occurs during the child's experiences in the natural environment of the home and with familiar people in that environment. Thus meal times, bath time, routines of dressing and grooming, and other day-to-day experiences can be the "vehicle" for communicative development.

Many children spend a significant amount of time in child care settings, either homes in which a few children are cared for while parents work or larger centers licensed to care for many children across a range of ages. Such settings are also considered to be "naturalistic settings" under the law. Hence, many SLPs provide direct services, indirect services, or both, to children in these environments. It is important to keep in mind that most states require that directors of such centers possess credentials that reflect their knowledge of child development, but it is also true that the minimum requirements for child care workers employed in the centers are generally proof of having reached a minimum age (often 18 years), a health certificate verifying that the worker is free of communicable diseases, and basic understanding of universal precautions and the requirements for reporting child abuse and neglect. Strategies described above in the sections on parent education and parent training can be adapted by the SLP in working collaboratively with employees of child care agencies. Consultation services, demonstration of specific strategies, and assistance in devising efficient records that relate to the child's behaviors involving communication development can be appropriate means of extending care to the child through daily activities and the caregivers.

Some Head Start centers and school districts have established programs for infants and toddlers with special needs. If Part C services are offered through those entities, employers are required to adhere to hiring "qualified providers" as defined under the statutes. Early interventionists and teachers who work in those settings are likely to have had more exposure to formal educational programs relating to early childhood development and to be required to participate in ongoing professional development programs. It is wise to bear in mind, however, that personnel shortages often necessitate the hiring of uncertified individuals. (Unfortunately, in some states the proportion of uncertified to certified personnel approaches 50%.) SLPs working in those settings should be sensitive to the needs of employees who work with at-risk infants and toddlers and tailor their strategies to use staff strengths and be responsive to areas in which the need for more information, education, and training is identified.

There are many dedicated, effective, and caring individuals who work in daycare settings and early-intervention programs throughout the country. Collaboration with these staff members extends the care given to children enrolled in such settings by encouraging and directing the efforts of the staff as they engage children in their daily activities.

Special Features and Requirements of Part C Early Intervention

Compliance with several requirements of Part C legislation should be noted by the SLP:

1. The IFSP must be reviewed and updated at least every 6 months and before that if conditions warrant or a parent requests the review or a change in its provisions.
2. When the child approaches the age of 3 years, transition planning is required. A change in the setting in which services are provided, personnel providing the services, and programs under which the child is (or is not) eligible to continue services must be identified. A plan of action to accomplish the transition from Part C services must be completed with the parent's participation.
3. Parents can choose at any time to participate or withdraw themselves, their child, or both, from services recommended or actually undertaken. They can select those services they believe will help them optimize their child's development, even if the professional recommends another approach or priority.
4. Access by professionals to payment for services rendered is dictated by the state's Part C system. Some court cases have prohibited states from accessing the family's private insurance if payments from those funds jeopardize the family's ability to maintain that coverage or burden the family in other ways with respect to their future access to that coverage.

National Effort to Make a Difference for Infants and Toddlers With Special Needs

Despite occasional difficulties in meeting timelines, navigating Part C rules and regulations, and keeping abreast of the ongoing process of legislative reauthorization with its attendant procedural modifications, Part C has established national recognition of the importance of early intervention for children with special needs. Through substantial funding to participating states, it provides the means by which families that would otherwise be unable to access services for their at-risk infants and toddlers can access such care. Through judicial rulings, the Part C rights of families of very young children with developmental delays and disabilities have been affirmed. No other country in the world can boast such a record on behalf of their youngest and most vulnerable citizens.

▼ BEST PRACTICES UNDER ALL SERVICE-DELIVERY MODELS

Regardless of the specific service-delivery model or the set of strategies used by the SLP, individualization of intervention plans and attempts to help the young child acquire the power of functional communication are common features of effective treatment, management, and intervention. To those ends, best practices call for employment of qualified, credentialed personnel; application of appropriate strategies and techniques; collaboration among agencies and personnel for the benefit of the child; involvement of the family in planning and implementing care; adherence to standards of care and ethical practices; and personal dedication to the goal of helping the child achieve optimal communicative function.

▼ PRACTICAL PROBLEM-SOLVING APPROACHES FOR INFANTS AND TODDLERS WITH DELAYED OR IMPAIRED COMMUNICATION

"I understand all that, but what do I *do*?" When that question comes up, as it inevitably does with students, there is only one correct answer: identify the needs and solve the problem of how they can be met most efficiently. It has been the author's experience that this is not the answer students hope to get. Experienced practitioners, however, know that it is the only way to get things done. They also know that the fund of knowledge from which to draw in designing what to do comes from accumulated experience over time, with each experience contributing another bit of critical information to one's personal database. To say that one "does by doing" is an oversimplification, because it is the *integration* of information and experiences that leads the practitioner to make decisions that are likely to produce an effective treatment, management, or intervention plan.

Personnel employed in health care settings may be required to use standardized, agency-approved plan formats. These can take the form of notes in the medical chart, discharge plans, or other documents maintained in accordance with agency accreditation bodies. Copies of such procedural requirements may be available for individual practitioners who wish to compare what is done in other settings with their own. Some practitioners are required by their employers to use computerized forms for generating intervention plans. Sometimes the motivation for adopting such formats is to optimize the professional's planning time; sometimes it is to have data sets that are readily available for record keeping and monitoring purposes; sometimes it is done on the basis of personal preference. How much plan individualization is truly achievable is beyond the scope of this discussion.

Crais and Roberts[7] and Wetherby[8] have devised exemplary and complementary, but quite different, problem-solving formats by which the SLP can be guided in making critical therapeutic decisions. Crais and Roberts' "decision tree" approach helps the practitioner formulate what is known about a given child's communicative skills and follow binary choices regarding "next steps" in planning how to deal with the problem or problems. The tree is arranged to address the needs of prelinguistic children, with subsequent sections focusing on the needs of children with increasingly sophisticated communication skill levels. It is easy to use and helpful in explaining procedural decisions to parents.

Wetherby's approach is based on the research that led to development of the Communication and Symbolic Behaviors Scale (CSBS).[9] After completing an assessment of the child's communicative abilities and needs, she recommends completing a profile that pinpoints strengths, weaknesses, and recommendations with reference to the child's communicative functions, communicative means (i.e., gestural, vocal, and verbal), reciprocity, social-affective signaling, and symbolic behavior. The method is adaptable to any means of assessing the child's communicative abilities, although the examiner may have to recast the resulting data into the definitional categories used with the CSBS. A statement of the differential diagnosis, if available, is also recorded.

Once that process is completed, the next step in Wetherby's approach is to prioritize intervention goals for children with emerging language. Goals are set for both the child and for the communication partner. A portion of a sample plan for an infant with limited skills, for example, may include the following (p. 11)[8]:

Goal for learner: Expand use of social-affective signals
Goal for partner: Foster facilitative interaction style
Strategies: Follow child's lead by imitating child's behavior and attuning to child's display of affect. Use proximity in positioning and presentation of materials to enhance social referencing.

Use of this problem-solving approach to develop individualized plans allows the practitioner a great deal of latitude in providing clearly worded functional goals preserving considerable variety in the means by which the goals can be implemented. The goals can be selected jointly by the family and the SLP. Attaining the goal can include strategies that involve parent education regarding the expected types of responses the child may exhibit, parent training involving demonstration of specific techniques that could be used during different caregiving and play routines, and easy ways to document what was tried and the results, so that the professional can monitor progress from visit to visit.

Excerpts from a plan for a toddler with more advanced emerging communication may include the following (p. 11)[8]:

Goal for learner: Enhance symbolic level from presymbolic communication to referential language, from nonlinguistic comprehension strategies to linguistic comprehension, from exploratory actions on objects to functional object use and single and multiple action schemes toward self and others, and from exploratory actions to combinatorial actions to construct a simple product
Goal for partner: Adjust language input to match and be slightly above child's language level and provide 'scaffolding' to foster learning

Strategies: Provide opportunities to engage child in appropriate use of objects and to model play at appropriate level for child during a variety of symbolic and constructive play experiences. Provide developmentally appropriate activities and use areas of relative strength to enhance areas of weakness (e.g., types of play, communicative functions); when play demands are more difficult for child, minimize communicative demands, but model and prompt developmentally appropriate behaviors.

Note that the format remains the same for developing the plan and that the plan is not cast in terms of traditionally worded behavioral objectives (e.g., given a situation in which a vocalized "request" is expected, the child will demonstrate the ability to spontaneously initiate inflected vocalization a minimum of 15 times over 20 consecutive opportunities). Wetherby's emphasis is on functional communicative skills rather than on task-specific criteria. This change in emphasis is in keeping with practices with which managed care providers (insurers) are familiar: functional goal attainment. By definition, *functional goals* relate to skills that can be applied across a variety of situations as opposed to discrete applications to designated situations. Readers who are interested in more information about functional treatment outcomes can obtain a packet of materials on the topic from the American Speech-Language-Hearing Association.[10]

▼ FITTING SPECIFICS INTO THE TREATMENT AND INTERVENTION FRAMEWORK

Facilitating Communicative Development in Infancy

The focus of services during the early months is to promote the family's ability to (1) understand and encourage interactions between the infant and caregivers; (2) facilitate the child's physical development to support preverbal vocalization and other forms of communication; (3) provide opportunities for cognitive development; (4) support any special care that is necessitated by the child's condition; and (5) monitor and report changes in the child's physical and behavioral status. Ongoing assessment of the child's communicative development is also an important contribution of the SLP to these efforts.

As practitioners work with families in their homes or center-based programs, with child care workers in daycare centers, and with other communicative partners of the child, it is imperative that cultural issues be considered. Customs, preferred languages, and attitudes about expected interactions among adults and children can be different from those that seem natural to an SLP with a different cultural background.

Ongoing assessment of language development in children whose communicative partners speak more than one language must take that fact into account. As Kayser[11] points out, "[l]anguage mixing, using the features of both languages, occurs up to [age] 3.5 years in the simultaneous bilingual [child]. The caregiver's use of the two languages, frequency of language mixing, and type of language switching are important variables in the use of language mixing" (p. 210). Kayser also notes that in the typically developing child, early exposure to two languages does not retard the onset of speech nor development of vocabulary if one considers words used from both languages. It is assessment of comprehension in both languages that determines the presence or absence of a language disorder (pp. 211–212). When working with children who are found to have delays or disorders of language development, adaptations of the suggestions presented in "Facilitating Interactions Between the Infant and Caregivers," below, may be required, although most are acceptable to families who are members of most cultures.

Facilitating Interactions Between the Infant and Caregivers

The SLP must have access to the child's caregivers to be able to provide information to those with whom the infant interacts. In some families, the only caregiver is the mother; in others, both parents are caregivers; in others, caregiving is provided by personnel at a child care center. Older siblings, members of the extended family, in-home sitters, or home-health professionals also may interact with the baby on a regular basis. With the help of the family, it can be determined who needs the information and how it can be provided to them most effectively.

The next step is to decide what information it is necessary to provide. This varies from situation to situation and is largely dependent on how much information the caregivers already have about infant development and physical, cognitive, social, and communicative expectations. Subjects selected for discussion can include the following:

- The baby's state-regulation abilities and the "rhythms" or cycles associated with daily activities involving the baby and family
- How to "read" the baby's signals (e.g., evidence of stress, readiness to interact)
- The importance of talking to the baby, especially if the infant's condition is predictive of limited ability, to provide the same quality of response or reward to the adult's efforts to interact
- The concept of dyads (partnerships) in interactions and providing opportunities for turn-taking by the baby
- Management of social routines, that is, creating brief opportunities for interaction during caregiving activities without creating overstimulation, fatigue, or aversive reactions
- The importance of sharing information about communication with other family members and caregivers

The underpinnings of receptive language development are obviously operative from the earliest exposure to interaction with caregivers. The SLP may wish to stress that even very young infants with adequate hearing and cognitive ability can discern the difference between similar phonemes and intonation patterns used by caregivers. Informative videotape recordings or printed handouts can be used as part of the family training and education effort. Such materials can be developed for a particular set of circumstances, or commercially available products can be used.

Facilitating Physical Development to Promote Readiness for Communication

The transactional linkage between physical development and communicative development is not always evident to caregivers. It may, therefore, be necessary to provide information about the important relationship between a child's physical health and maturation and ongoing communicative development. Topics that the SLP may wish to cover in this connection include the following:

- Feeding as a pleasurable experience, especially with reference to oral-motor stimulation. For children who are tube-fed, nonnutritive sucking can be used to simulate this pleasurable experience.
- Handling and positioning the baby to enhance physical development. If the infant is physically handicapped, the information given to parents should be chosen in consultation with the infant's physician or physical or occupational therapist. Babies who are prenatally exposed to drugs need specific handling techniques to assist in behavioral organization. If the family was given instructions regarding physical handling at the time of hospital discharge, reconfirming their importance can be helpful.
- Respiratory considerations that also can require special handling, positioning, or supportive technology. Consultation with other members of the child's multidisciplinary team may be required to address this issue appropriately. Babies with a combined history of bronchopulmonary dysplasia and intraventricular hemorrhage are at significant risk for development of communicative disorders.
- Care of the ears and information about the importance of seeking prompt care for ear infections. This topic probably should be included in all early parent-education and parent-training plans because special-needs babies as a group have a significantly higher risk of developing frequent ear infections. Caregivers of infants with craniofacial anomalies should be especially alert for such problems, and they may require instruction on how to position the child during feedings to avoid leakage of fluids into the nasal chamber or eustachian tubes. Propping bottles should be discouraged for all infants, not only because of potential ear infections but also because it deprives the infant of important tactile stimulation, mutual gaze with the adult during feedings, and early turn-taking interactions that promote communicative development.
- Visual impairment and adaptations for stimulation. Babies with known visual impairment often lack the richness of environmental stimulation available to other children during infancy. Compensation for the reduced visual stimulation should begin early. The infant can benefit from enhanced auditory and tactile stimulation. Care should be given in selecting objects for exploration on the basis of variations in size and texture. (Hint: Surface patterns can be raised by outlining them with nontoxic "puff paint" so that they can be felt.) Scent, weight, temperature, movement patterns, and auditory properties of play materials also can be varied. The baby should be stimulated to use residual vision, even if it is severely limited. Sensory interactions between the infant and caregiver can include placing the baby's hand on the side of the partner's nose or on the lips or larynx as speech is produced, so that the baby can feel vibrations and movement associated with speech.

Facilitating Cognitive Development

Many caregivers are content to allow a quiet, compliant child to be left undisturbed. There may be little understanding of the importance of exposing the child to a range of experiences to promote cognitive development. Classic studies of children in orphanages in the United States during the 1930s and studies done in Romania in the late 1980s and early 1990s testify to the ravages that "benign neglect" have on infant development. It is particularly critical that infants at risk for mental retardation receive regular stimulation from other people. During caregiving routines and periods of purely social interaction, it is relatively easy to establish stimulating experiences that enhance cognitive development. The SLP may wish to provide information to caregivers about ways to provide the following:

- Appropriate tactile stimulation—through handling, positioning, touch, and pressure. This is especially important with children who have or are at risk for cerebral palsy and for those who have had prenatal drug exposure.
- Appropriate visual stimulation—by varying the baby's opportunities to view shapes, colors, light, shadows, and movement. It may be appropriate to provide information to caregivers about the importance of visual acuity to cognitive, social, and communicative development. Consultation with the physician or vision specialist is appropriate before providing any information of this nature if the infant is known to be visually impaired.
- Appropriate auditory stimulation—by providing opportunities for the child to hear a variety of sounds throughout the day and by avoiding exposure to excessively loud noises, including amplified music. Even from the earliest weeks, the infant is able to separate the human voice and many of its variations from other sounds in the environment. It is from consistent exposure to the sounds of speech that the child begins to build an awareness that strings of sounds are means of communication and to discern the fundamental phonemes of the language of the home. Early in life, emotional content is perceived by the child as it is conveyed by intonation, loudness, and stress patterns used by the adult. In fact, intonational patterns emerge quite early in the child's own vocalization patterns. Surprisingly, the importance of giving the infant opportunities to hear the human voice is not universally known. Children who spend long hours away from the mother in child care settings can benefit from having the mother's tape-recorded voice available at times of stress or to soothe them to sleep. Family members or others charged with providing care to an especially fussy baby or one who is difficult to console also may find that a tape recording of the mother reading a story, singing, talking on the phone, or uttering comforting phrases has a calming effect. The SLP may wish to consult the infant mental-health literature for specific information about the importance of the tone of voice used by caregivers who influence the child's development of a sense of emotional security.
- Appropriate motor stimulation—which is associated with cognitive development. Babies with atypical physical development benefit from information prepared by physical and occupational therapists with respect to motor stimulation. Some children profit from application of neurodevelopmental and sensory integration techniques. Collaboration with motor development specialists is productive.
- Opportunities to experience different environments—both indoors (different rooms of the house) and outdoors where sights; sounds; lights and shadows; and features of the sky, wind, and earth change with the time of day and season of the year is healthy. An exception to encouraging environmental variety, of course, applies when the child's health is at significant risk. If that exception does

not apply, it is probable that confining children to a limited environment because of atypical physical features or the caregiver's anticipation of personal stress is unwarranted.

The sense of security that is so important in infancy and that allows the child to enjoy a variety of experiences from an early age derives, at least in part, from the baby's relationship with primary caregivers.[11-13] Sparks[12] discussed this in terms of "goodness of fit" between the baby and (initially) the mother. Zeanah and colleagues[13] referred to the phenomenon as *infant attachment*. The baby's sense of security is also related to development of a sense of the rhythms of the total environment, which some practitioners refer to as the child's *ecosystem*. Infants who exhibit significant and persistent difficulty in adjustment are likely to have difficulties with cognitive, social, and communication skill development. When such problems are noted by the SLP, collaboration with the child's physician or mental-health specialist is in order.

Severe difficulty in psychobehavioral adjustment is a characteristic of many children who were exposed prenatally to cocaine and other drugs. It is also characteristic of children with certain psychopathologies, such as autism. Sometimes medical or nutritional problems are implicated. For those reasons, persistent problems with adjustment should be investigated in a timely manner and with the utmost care by appropriately selected specialists.

Supporting Special Care Necessitated by the Child's Condition

Children with a wide variety of handicapping conditions require special care, a portion of which is related directly to promoting communicative development.[14] Obvious examples are children with cleft lip and palate, congenital hearing impairment, or "floppy" muscle tone; babies who exhibit hypersensitivity to sensory stimuli; infants who are excessively irritable or difficult to console; very low birth weight babies; and babies with diagnosed syndromes. It is essential that the SLP be sensitive to the fact that the family undergoes a tremendous amount of stress when they learn their child has special problems. Their receptivity to and desire for information pertinent to the baby's condition varies significantly within and across families. Even the *same* family member may relate to the professional on different levels at different times, depending on the stresses and concerns that affect the adult at a given moment and on that person's means of coping with them.

The SLP who is involved with the treatment and management of children with significant impairments may need to assist the family with incorporating communicative interventions with care prescribed by other members of the multidisciplinary team. Attempts to do this should always be accompanied by an appreciation for the family's priorities and their readiness to interact both on a personal level with the SLP and on a subjective and emotional level with the management plan per se.

Providing the family with information about available resources can be helpful (see Appendix C, Table C-3, and Appendix D). Assisting them in understanding technical terms that other professionals may use and fail to explain also can be a way of assisting. Any family, but especially those dealing with the stresses of decision making for a child with extensive special needs, is only able to absorb so much information at one time. Being considerate by giving information that is a priority at the moment and reserving the rest for a later meeting helps families retain important data and reassures them that additional information will be made available when they indicate that they are ready for it.

Depending on the condition(s) the child possesses, the SLP may need to be prepared to provide information in the following areas:

- Respiration and respiratory functions for speech
- Special feeding considerations
- Positioning and handling the baby for optimal interactions
- Physical therapy and occupational therapy
- Presurgical and postsurgical care
- Communication considerations during recovery
- Overt physical and cognitive limitations
- Expectations for atypically developing children

Monitoring Changes in Physical and Behavioral Status

Because communicative development is so intimately interwoven with all facets of a child's development, it is essential that the other aspects of maturation be monitored and that the SLP have knowledge of what is happening with the whole child. To this end, the SLP may ask the family to engage in specific activities that provide a summary of pertinent information that can be incorporated into the management-planning process. Some information is available from formal reports of other professionals who see the child. However, the time lag between requests for reports and their receipt can slow down the process of efficient monitoring and interfere with planning efforts. For that reason, certain information can be monitored and recorded by the family on an ongoing basis using checklists or other simple forms to report observed changes in the following:

- Physical growth—by recording the baby's weight at specified intervals or at the time of regular health care visits
- Maturation—by recording attainment of specified milestones (e.g., sitting independently, responding to his or her name, crawling, pulling to stand, cruising)
- Behavioral characteristics—by recording new behaviors that are significant in communicative development as they emerge (e.g., cooing, babbling, emergence of first word)
- Plateaus or reversals in development—by recording, in anecdotal form, any apparent lack of progress that can signal a need for attention from the SLP or other members of the multidisciplinary professional team or a need to revise the intervention and treatment plan. The SLP should alert the parents to expected plateaus (e.g., reduction in vocalization during rapid acquisition of major physical milestones). *Reversals in development, however, can be of great significance and should be noted.*

The system of collecting information should be simple and clearly specified. Parental preferences should be honored. The SLP or multidisciplinary team may wish to provide the materials for record keeping (e.g., charts, checklists, forms, notebook, or journal). Some multidisciplinary teams have developed booklets that can be tucked into the mother's purse or diaper bag and be readily available for visits to the doctor's office, as well as being accessible to team members in their offices or on home visits.

The tasks requested of parents in connection with record keeping should be reasonable in terms of time requirements and simplicity (excessively detailed information requires time and effort to generate). New parents seldom have either extra time or abundant energy. When the child is at risk or has a diagnosed condition, the conditions may be doubly stressful and reduce the probability that record keeping will be done. The parents' reading level and familiarity with English are also considerations. Written materials may need to be made available in the home language of the child's family. Acknowledgment of parental efforts to collect requested data should be provided by members of the professional team. The family needs to know that they are regarded as important participants in their child's program of care and that information they supply is valuable in planning and evaluating the effectiveness of that program.

Treatment, Management, and Intervention With Toddlers

At 12 to 14 months of age, children are classified as toddlers whether or not they are physically capable of walking. The designation presumes exposure to an array of life experiences and a certain degree of developmental maturation. Children with severe disabilities are less likely to have attained the milestones achieved by their typically developing peers in either physical or communication domains. Even among children who exhibit no overt disability, some fail to develop satisfactory receptive communication, expressive communication, or both. Most, however, have developed at least a meager understanding of the efforts made to communicate with them and have at least some form of expression, whether it be eye gaze to indicate a choice, pointing and grunting to make a request, gesturing, inflected vocalizations, or true efforts to use words. A determination of whether a child's expressive communication is merely delayed or is probably disordered is possible even before the second birthday (see Chapter 8). That determination assists in guiding the specific techniques applied in the treatment and management plan for an individual child.

Adult Instruction

Because parents and other adult caregivers are intimately involved in meeting the needs of atypically developing infants and toddlers, it is important that the SLP understand not only child development, assessment, and treatment protocols but also have a working knowledge of the principles of adult education. Effectiveness of any treatment or management plan to achieve communication goals for the child depends to a large extent on how effectively the SLP succeeds in collaborating with adults who interact regularly with the child. This involves both imparting needed information to them and assisting them with development of specific skills.

Adult instruction includes some or all of the following:

- Provision of written materials about the child's diagnosed condition, developmental expectations, and other pertinent matters
- Provision of information about the developmental stage at which their child presently functions

- Demonstration of specific techniques
- Discussion of the use of play and family routines as vehicles for communicative development
- Observation of the efforts of parents and caregivers in implementing recommended practices or techniques
- Coaching of parents and caregivers when adjustments are indicated and affirming and praising what they do that engages the child and results in communicative interaction

To minimize costs, groups can be formed for such instruction when appropriate. The Hanen program[15] for parent training is an example of a successful program designed for groups of parents. Other such programs are available for children with special needs and can be obtained through commercial vendors. Most programs of this nature need to be supplemented to address specific needs of a given child and family, but a great deal of well-developed material cast in excellent, well-researched formats is available.

Late Talkers

One of the most rewarding aspects of early communication intervention is seen with children who are late talkers. They are the children who have no other known problems but demonstrate delay in the onset and development of speech. They exhibit, at age 24 months, fewer than 50 words in their expressive vocabularies and have no two-word combinations. They may have had an ear infection once or twice, but they do not have histories of chronic otitis media. Their receptive language appears to be intact.

For such children, a short-term treatment program can be very effective. The program should include child assessment to ensure that the child meets criteria for group IV (risk 0) (see Table 8-2). The program should focus on parent instruction in turn-taking strategies, imitation and expansion of the child's utterances, pretending, and repetition strategies. Striking improvement in late-talking toddlers' communicative abilities usually occurs during or shortly after parent enrollment in such programs.[6] If the children do not have regular opportunities to interact with age peers, participation in a play group, mother's-day-out, or nursery-school program can be indicated. Direct therapy provided by professionals is generally not indicated for these children.

Assistive Technology

For some children, even those who do not have hearing loss, a treatment of choice is early introduction of assistive communication. Early amplification for children who can benefit from it is certainly indicated (see Chapter 10). Toddlers diagnosed with impairments affecting gross motor development and those with oral motor apraxia may be candidates for assistive communication approaches. Depending on the characteristics of the impairments, choices range from introduction of electronic switches for operation of toys (later switch operation can be used with electronic communication devices), the use of simple communication boards constructed to meet the needs of the child at a particular time (e.g., postsurgical hospitalization), early introduction of sign language, pairing adult speech with fingerspelling, or using a total communication approach. This discussion is limited to use of augmentative and alternative communication (AAC) with children whose hearing is intact. See Chapter 10 for information on management of hearing impairments.

Use of AAC may be needed to provide a means of communication for young children whose oral communication skills may be late to develop for physical or psychological reasons, or it may be a long-term process, gradually becoming more sophisticated as the child matures but remains unable to use functional verbal communication. Parents should be informed that research shows that AAC facilitates spoken language rather than impeding it. As Cress[16] comments,

> Children who are having difficulty controlling the muscles involved in the speech/ respiratory process, or who have other neurological or cognitive limitations that affect speech and language, are at risk for developing speech that is intelligible to all listeners. Children's motor systems are still developing in ways that cannot be predicted, and early intervention is too early to give up on further improvement in speech skills. Almost all children who can produce a voice will use sounds in some ways that are interpretable to listeners. When children continue to learn new sounds or new variations on the sounds they are producing, that is a positive sign for their continued vocal development.

Preliminary considerations in choosing AAC methods or devices include the following:

- *Positioning*—Is special positioning necessary to allow range and accuracy of movements required to utilize the method or to operate a chosen device?
- *Signaling method*—Does the child have adequate gross and fine motor development for his or her age? If not, what form of signaling can be used (e.g., eye gaze, switch operation by hand or other body part, vocalization, blowing, sucking). Cress points out that the first "tool" a child learns to control is his own body; operation of other tools requires controlling some type of behavior.
- *Vision*—Does the child have vision impairments? If so, are color, size, sound, or tactile properties of the device critical to its successful use?

Cress states that a nonverbal child should not initially be given a device that is geared to yes-no responses but should be provided AAC that stimulates functional communication from the beginning. Functional communication may be targeted to development of requests for attention or objects, protests, greetings, or commenting (e.g., "want more" or "all done"), all of which typically developing toddlers use.

In addition to the availability of many switch-operated toys and a wide variety of custom switches designed for children with physical limitations, the commercial toy market has a huge array of relatively inexpensive battery-powered "educational toys" designed for very young children. It is helpful for SLPs to be familiar with what is available, because many electronic toys can be adapted quite easily for use as AAC devices.

Children for whom assistive communication therapy is appropriate should experience a high degree of impact when they exert the effort to use the chosen approach. Their partners' responses to their expressions of intent should be prompt and appropriate. Attribution of presumed intent should be offered by the adult when it is apparent that the child is attempting to use the assistive method to communicate. When it is clear that the intent is to express a choice, make a request, offer an observation, convey feelings, affirm or negate, or offer information, it is important that communicative partners verbalize their understanding of the child's intent. This not only recognizes the attempt to convey a particular intent but also allows the child to affirm or deny the partner's interpretation of intent. Typically developing peers enjoy the rewards of affecting events in their lives; that power also enhances the communicative development of atypically developing children.

Use of assistive devices, of course, must be determined in light of the child's apparent cognitive abilities. Development of a sense of cause and effect (e.g., when the water is running, bath time is approaching; when a bottle or feeding equipment appears, a meal is on the way) can indicate a toddler's readiness for introduction to switches that cause toys to do something. Cress cautions, however, that "since even voice output switches can be a means to learn cause-effect, we should tend to limit as far as possible promoting a sense of prerequisites as we consider utilization of assistive devices. To the extent possible, the assistive system should support later verbal communication if it is anticipated that the child will develop it at some point. It should enable the child to communicate with as many individuals as possible. It should be paired with the partner's use of speech so that associations can be established between verbal symbols (e.g., words, phrases) and the symbols used in the assistive method used."

Toddlers, even those who are physically challenged, learn best through play and the interactions of daily living. Thus efforts to support development of communication should be focused on such activities and at a level on which the child is able to function. The reader also may refer to Appendix B, Table B-4, and the suggestions developed by Norris and Hoffman[17] for children functioning below a developmental age of 1 year.

A Word About Toddlers With a History of Brain Injury in Infancy

Children who have a history of brain injury in early infancy appear to need more frequent exposures to language experiences in early childhood to attain normal levels of language ability.[18] Encouraging multiple exposures to such experiences can be viewed as a form of prevention or amelioration of future language problems for which the child is at risk. As time goes on, the need for such added exposure, combined with pressures to master specific material in the classroom under time constraints, can reveal previously unsuspected learning difficulties. Therefore, as these children enter school or center-based programs, continued monitoring is recommended and should be communicated to personnel in those settings.

Approaches When Assistive Technology Is Not Required

For purposes of the following discussion, it is assumed that the child for whom a program is being planned has demonstrated some cognitive ability, has attending behaviors that allow the child to focus on tasks that interest him or her, and has shown some frustration with his or her inability to communicate so that others can understand his or her intent. Such a child may be language delayed or language disordered. Ongoing assessments concurrent with treatment and intervention discriminate between the alternative conclusions as the plan is implemented.

Direct Management

In planning ways to assist a child who has communicative difficulties, the SLP must address the following:

- The child must have experiences to which the symbols of communication can be applied.
- Communicative treatment or intervention should be interwoven with activities of daily living and not be a set of activities set aside for only specific blocks of time.
- Parents and caregivers should be directly involved in ongoing language-stimulation activities with the child.
- The plan of treatment or intervention must include strategies for adult education on how to provide effective interactions that are geared to the child's developmental level.
- Depending on the child's developmental level, language intervention can be directed at some or many of the following items:

Labeling or naming objects, actions, feelings

Attributing meaning to the child's actions

Self-talk to describe one's own actions as they occur

Parallel talk to describe the child's actions as they occur

Providing communicative temptations that increase the probability that the child will attempt to communicate (see Appendix B, Table B-5, for Wetherby's[8] list of communicative temptations).

Making sure the child has a need to talk. Avoid the temptation to supply responses for the child when others ask questions or make comments directed to him or her.

Positioning the child to optimize communicative events. Provide stable seating that minimizes the child's need to focus energies on balance. Place objects within reach if joint attention is desired. Place them just out of reach and stay near the child to optimize the probability of the child's requesting them.

Withholding a desired object until the child attempts to communicate a desire for it. Avoid requiring the child to produce a target word perfectly. Reward attempts to verbalize.

Ensuring the power of communication. Be sure something *happens* when the child communicates; the attempt should have an effect.

Engaging in vocal play. Just producing sounds for the fun of it is interesting to toddlers; varying intonation and stress patterns as the "game" proceeds highlights use of suprasegmental linguistic features. Be sure to imitate the child's vocalizations, taking turns in the vocal play as it progresses. Maintain the child's interest at an appropriate developmental level.

Stimulating approximations of syllabic content. Avoid early attention to articulatory accuracy; focus instead on syllable configurations. This activity also enhances awareness of morphemes that are markers for number, tense, ongoing action, and possession. It also builds awareness of monosyllabic and polysyllabic elements.

Producing meaningful nonspeech sounds such as motor noises, animal noises, and other environmental noises. These are often easier, and sometimes less stressful, vocalizations that are early representations of the objects or actions with which the child is familiar. Such intentional vocalizations also can be modified to include emphasis, to imply a question, or to contrast qualities of loud or soft speech.

Using mutual experiences in play that stimulate communicative interaction, such as splashing at bath time and banging on inverted plastic containers to emulate the bang of a drumbeat or to establish rhythm patterns that can be mirrored in vocalizations or verbalizations. This is sometimes helpful in establishing syllabic configurations.

Simplifying adult language so that its flow is easier for the child to follow (e.g., reduce sentence structure to basic elements, such as "Bobby stand up," "Mary eat cookie," or "Mama go to store").

Accompanying verbalization with gestures or signs. This is helpful even for some children who are not hearing impaired and especially for those who may have oral apraxia, pervasive developmental disorder (PDD), or suspected central auditory processing difficulties.

Pairing speech with music or rhythm by singing, clapping, and speaking to phrase cadence.

Enlisting the assistance of all members of the family to interact with the child using the strategies that have been selected to interweave communicative stimulation throughout the day's activities.

Providing affective vocal models that show the child in play activities how to express frustration and anger, as well as pleasure. A fact that is poorly understood is that children who do not have symbolic means to express their emotions essentially have two choices: withdraw or act out. Acting out often results in the interpretation that the child has a behavior problem rather than a communication problem.

Using or adapting techniques designed for children with hearing impairment when appropriate. Many activities recommended for hearing-impaired children include appropriate techniques for language delayed and impaired children. Multisensory stimulation and use of household objects and activities (e.g., responding to the ring of a phone or doorbell, listening for the whistle of the tea kettle) to focus joint attention are examples.

Following the child's lead and demonstrated interests. By their nature, toddlers are explorers and do not have lengthy attention spans. As their attention is attracted by objects and activities, be responsive to the naturally occurring shifts and move along with them to implement appropriate communicative activities.

Utilizing Adamson and Bakeman's Communication Play Protocol (CPP), research with toddlers who had a variety of severe developmental disabilities yielded significant results.[19–21] The minimally verbal toddlers increased their attempts to communicate verbally and vocally under two play contexts with a familiar adult: the *requesting context* and the *commenting context.* Although the researchers used only 5-minute play intervals for purposes of collecting data, the play activities listed in Table 9-2 could be extended for as long as the child's interest is sustained for purposes of intervention strategies to increase language output.

TABLE 9-2
Communication Play Protocol: Eliciting Communicative Interactions With Toddlers—Requesting and Commenting Scenarios*

Requesting Activities

"Help Me" Play With a Toy Scenario

Suggestions:

1. Although you know what the child wants from among the available toys, wait for a request. You might blow up a balloon and then let the air out when the child is attending to it; wait to see if the child requests a repetition. If a request is not made within several seconds, blow the balloon up again and let the air out of it.

2. Blow a series of bubbles and then put the cap back on the bottle and place it in front of the child on the table. Wait to see if the child initiates a request to repeat the activity.

"I Want" That Toy on the Shelf Scenario

Suggestions:

1. The child notices toys located on a shelf too high to reach. You help get the desired one down but only after you've pretended not to understand what the child wants.

2. Readily agree to help, but give the child the wrong toy. Finally, give the right one to the child after noting the child's response to the "error."

3. If the child doesn't pay much attention to the toys, try to direct attention to them without indicating a specific one. Let the child play with one of the toys for a minute and then "put it away" on the shelf and see if the child requests help in retrieving it—or another toy.

Commenting Activities

Visit to the "Art Gallery" Scenario

Suggestions:

1. Together with the child, enjoy looking at the pictures displayed around the room. Try to attract the child's attention to each of the pictures. After looking at all of them, return to the picture the child seemed to like best and then to the least-liked one. Comment on the pictures and try to engage the child in responding in some way without asking direct questions.

2. One of the pictures has a nonsense label attached to it. Comment that it reminds you that the picture is of a "hodfern" that goes "brockety-brock." Monitor the child's reaction.

What's in "The Container" Scenario

Suggestions:

1. Sitting at a table or on the floor, empty the container one object at a time As each object is removed, share it for a while before getting another out, commenting on its properties (form, function, color, usual place it might be found).

2. Name each object and play with it for a while before taking out another one.

3. Imitate what the child does with the object; try to get the child to imitate what you do with it.

Modified from Adamson LB, Bakeman R: *The communication play protocol for toddlers,* technical report 8, Atlanta, Ga, 1998, Developmental Laboratory, Department of Psychology.

*The purpose of the play is to encourage the child to communicate with facial expressions, sounds, and gestures. A method of documenting communicative means and intent should be selected in advance of conducting the scenarios. It is helpful to use a video camera so that analysis of the child's communicative acts can be conducted after the session. Toys used in the "Help Me" scenario might be bubbles, two balloons, play house or farm, Legos, an insert puzzle, and a bus with people figures. For the "I Want" scenario, use a toy clock, plush toy, favorite toy brought from home. For "The Container," use a closed box or jar filled with five small age-appropriate objects such as a stuffed animal, vehicle, pretend food, utensil. For the "Art Gallery," six framed greeting card sized pictures of individual animals, infants, or vehicles are placed around the room at different heights (one on a table). One "nonsense picture" is placed so that the child is facing the camera when viewing it; it is also labeled with a nonsense word. These suggestions may be modified, but they are a good starting point to elicit communication during the scenarios shown above.

Parents and caregivers can be provided with training to use such scenes in the course of their regular play times with their children to promote communication development. Another means of promoting mutual enjoyment during playtime while enhancing the probability of increased communicative attempts by the child is "floor time."[23] This approach promotes the adult's participation in and copying whatever the child exhibits interest in doing during play. The adult can initially simply mimic what the child is doing, then add a comment or label, and acknowledge and gradually expand on the child's utterances when they appear. Joint attention in manipulating an object, performing an action, or series of actions, humming or making noises, copying facial expressions or gestures, marching or other activities initiated by the child can be a vehicle to support vocalizing and verbalizing. The SLP should provide an explanation that play is a natural and interesting activity through which to promote communicative development so that the parents realize there is a legitimate purpose to their participation and to the configuration of that participation.

Yoder and Warren[24] describe the methods used in Prelinguistic Milieu Teaching (PMT) and Responsive Prelinguistic Milieu Teaching (RPMT). The first method (PMT) relies on a 1:1 adult:child ratio, whereas the RPMT method utilizes an adult and a group of age peer children. Both methods are accomplished in play situations.

Ongoing Assessment as Treatment or Intervention Planning

Ongoing assessment of the child's overall development and communicative skills should guide the SLP and family in selecting appropriate goals for a given time frame. Whether the child's needs dictate use of assistive communication; development of basic concepts; development of oral-motor or other physical competencies necessary to communicative skills; collaboration with other professionals in management of persistent sucking, swallowing, and feeding problems; development of auditory awareness and joint attention; or other targets, the SLP can help parents capitalize on the rich opportunities for stimulation that exist in daily activities.

▼ SUMMARY

Many strategies can be used to assist children in acquiring communication skills, but the SLP who selects wisely from the approaches listed in this chapter can help the family and caregivers get started on a constructive program. The SLP needs to monitor progress, confer frequently with the family, evaluate circumstances as they change, and adjust the prescribed program as needed.

For most children, progress will occur if the following are true:

1. There are a sufficient number of attempts at communication; if there are not, increasing the attempts becomes a goal.
2. The child has a sense of security from knowing his or her attempts will be accepted and responded to by those with whom communication is attempted.
3. Communication is a part of most daily activities and is not an effort restricted to "therapy" or "speech" time.
4. The effort to communicate has results and a perceived effect.

It is impossible to guarantee that children entrusted to the care of an SLP will achieve optimal communicative functions and succeed thereby in being physically, mentally, and emotionally healthy. However, our pledge to these children and their families is to work with them and with our professional colleagues to make possible that which is within our ability to achieve.

▼ **REFERENCES**

1. Brazelton TB: Assessment in early infancy as an intervention. In Gilderman D, et al, editors: *The health care/education relationship,* Chapel Hill, NC, 1981, Technical Assistance and Development System, p 3.
2. Coleman PP, et al: Consultation: applications to early intervention, *Infants Young Child* 4(2):41, 1991.
3. Banigan RL: Memorandum to the author, 1991.
4. Barrera M, Rosebaum P: The transactional model of early home intervention, *Infant Ment Health J* 7:112, 1986.
5. Moxley-Haegert L, Serbin LA: Developmental education for parents of delayed infants: effects on parental motivation and children's development, *Child Dev* 54:1324, 1983.
6. Schober-Peterson D, Cohen M: Facilitating parent-child interactions. Paper presented at the ASHA Conference, Atlanta, Ga, November 1991.
7. Crais E, Roberts J: Decision making in assessment and early intervention, *Lang Speech Hear Serv Sch* 22:25, 1991.
8. Wetherby A: Infants and toddlers with special needs. Syllabus accompanying presentation at the Alton Ochsner Clinic Continuing Medical Education Program, New Orleans, May 1996.
9. Wetherby AM, Prizant BM: *Communication and symbolic behavior scale (CSBS),* Normed edition, Chicago, 1993, Applied Symbolix.
10. American Speech-Language-Hearing Association: Packet of reports on treatment outcomes, Rockville, Md, 1997, American Speech-Language-Hearing Association. (Available from ASHA, 10801 Rockville Pike, Rockville, MD 20852.)
11. Kayser HR: Bilingual language development and language disorders. In Battle DE: *Communication disorders in multicultural populations,* ed 3, Boston, 2002, Butterworth-Heinemann, pp 205–232.
12. Sparks S: Assessment and intervention with at-risk infants and toddlers: guidelines for the speech-language pathologist, *Top Lang Disord* 10:43, 1989.
13. Zeanah CH Jr, Mammen OK, Lieberman AF: Disorders of attachment. In Zeanah CH, Jr, editor: *Handbook of infant mental health,* New York, 1993, Guilford Press, p 332.
14. Letourneau N: Fostering resiliency in infants and young children through parent-infant interaction, *Infant Young Child* 9:36, 1997.
15. Maolson A: *It takes two to talk,* ed 3, Toronto, 1992, Hanen Center Publications.
16. Cress CJ: Speech/phonological intervention for young non-speaking children with limited sound inventories. Seminar presented at the American Speech-Language-Hearing Association conference, New Orleans, Nov 16, 2001.
17. Norris JA, Hoffman PR: Comparison of adult-initiated vs. child-initiated interaction styles with handicapped prelanguage children, *Lang Speech Hear Serv Sch* 21:28, 1990.
18. Keefe KA, Feldman HM, Holland AL: Lexical learning and language abilities in preschoolers with perinatal brain damage, *J Speech Hear Disord* 54:395, 1989.
19. Kubitz KR, et al: Communication play exchanges of toddlers with severe developmental disabilities. Poster session presented at the American Speech-Language-Hearing Association conference, New Orleans, Nov 16, 2001.
20. Adamson LB, Bakeman R: Viewing variations in language development: the communication play protocol, *Augmented and Alternative Communication* (Newsletter for ASHA Division 12) 8:2–4, 1999.
21. Adamson LB, et al: Autism and joint attention: young children's responses to maternal bids, *Applied Dev Psychol* 22:439–453, 2001.

22. Adamson L, Bakeman R: The communication play protocol manual for toddlers: technical report 8, Atlanta, Ga, 1998, Developmental Laboratory, Department of Psychology.
23. Greenspan SI: A developmental approach to problems in relating and communicating in autistic spectrum disorders and related syndromes, *SPOTLIGHT Top Dev Disabilities* 1(4):1–6, 1998.
24. Yoder PJ, Warren SF: Relative treatment effects of two prelinguistic communication interventions on language development in toddlers with developmental delays vary by maternal characteristics, *J Speech Lang Hear Res* 44:224–237, 2001.

CHAPTER 10

HABILITATION AND COMMUNICATION DEVELOPMENT IN HEARING-IMPAIRED INFANTS AND TODDLERS

Thomas G. Rigo

Hearing loss has a multidimensional effect on the communicative and social-emotional development of infants and toddlers. A hearing deficit early in life impairs the normal acquisition of speech and language. The communication problem can, in turn, cause learning and social difficulties, reduce academic performance, and limit vocational opportunities. The successful remediation of these potential deficits requires the collaborative efforts of speech-language pathologists, audiologists, physicians, social workers, psychologists, educators of the deaf, and family members. This chapter discusses the effects of early hearing loss on communication ability and the procedures used to facilitate the development of speech and language. It focuses on those topics that relate directly to the typical functions of the speech-language pathologist (SLP) and audiologist within the interdisciplinary framework.

▼ EFFECT OF HEARING LOSS ON ORAL COMMUNICATION ABILITY

Sensory Perception

Speech sounds are composed of a combination of subphonemic features that give each sound its individual perceptual identity. Hearing loss disrupts the perception of speech by distorting or limiting the auditory reception of these features.

When a hearing loss occurs after language has developed (postlingual onset), a listener often is able to compensate for a loss of sensory input by predicting the likely components of a message. Once an elemental amount of sensory information is received, an understanding of the rules of language and the use of contextual and situational cues allow the listener to make predictions about the likely structure and content of the message. The acoustic pattern need not be processed in detail; its analysis proceeds only so far as is necessary to confirm the accuracy of the anticipated linguistic patterns.

When a hearing deficit occurs before language is acquired (prelingual onset), the loss of sensory information has a more disruptive effect. A young child, unable to predict how a message evolves, must analyze sensory input in more detail to acquire and comprehend oral language. If this input is degraded substantially by hearing loss, the acquisition of language auditorily may not be possible. As such, the handicap associated with a hearing loss depends not only on its severity but also its time of onset.

Auditory Reception

Vowels. Vowels are intense phonemes and account for much of the energy in the long-term spectrum of speech. Their identification requires the reception of the first and second vowel formants (F1 and F2, respectively). F1 frequency location is related inversely to the degree of articulatory constriction. It ranges from 250 Hz for high vowels to 850 Hz for low vowels. F2 frequency location is related to the front-back place of production. It ranges from 850 Hz for back vowels to 2800 Hz for front vowels.[1] As a general rule, the amplitudes of vowel formants decrease as their frequency locations increase.

Hearing loss most often affects the reception of F2. F1 is more likely to remain audible, because it is higher in intensity and lower in frequency. Both formants should remain audible to children with mild-to-moderate hearing impairments. Severe hearing loss above 1000 Hz limits the reception of F2. Because F2 for front vowels is lower in intensity and higher in frequency, they are more vulnerable to distortion than are back vowels. Severe-to-profound hearing loss across all frequencies impairs the reception of both F1 and F2 formants.

Consonants. The perception of consonants requires the reception of acoustic cues associated with voicing, manner of production, and place of production. The primary voicing cue is the presence or absence of fundamental frequency, located in the 100 to 250 Hz frequency range.[1] Secondary features, such as voice onset time and phoneme duration, extend the frequency range of voicing cues to the 2000 Hz region. Fundamental frequency is an intense cue and remains audible to all but severe-to-profound hearing-impaired listeners.

Each class of consonants (i.e., semivowels, nasals, fricatives, stops) contains an acoustic cue associated with its manner of production. Semivowels are distinguished by a formant-like energy pattern in the 300 to 400 Hz frequency region. Nasals are characterized by the presence of a band of harmonic energy located at 200 to 300 Hz (nasal murmur). Both fricatives and stops are composed of wide-band, aperiodic acoustic energy that is predominant at frequencies above 1000 Hz. The difference between these two classes of sounds is related to their temporal characteristics. Fricatives are associated with a continuous, steady-state noise pattern.

Stops are characterized by a transient burst of noise.[2] The acoustic cues for semi-vowels and nasals are intense, harmonic, and low in frequency. They remain audible until hearing loss reaches a severe-to-profound level. In contrast, the acoustic cues for fricatives and stops are less intense and aperiodic. Manner confusions between these classes of sounds are more common and occur with lesser degrees of impairment.

Voicing and manner cues alone do not provide a listener with enough acoustic information to identify individual phonemes. For example, the reception of nasal murmur allows the recognition of a sound as a nasal but does not provide sufficient information to determine which nasal phoneme was spoken. The reception of acoustic cues associated with place of production is necessary to distinguish phonemes that share the same manner of production. These cues generally are located at frequencies above 1000 Hz and are, as a group, the least intense of the subphonemic features of speech.[2] The loss or distortion of place of production information is the most common speech-reception deficit experienced by hearing-impaired listeners. Difficulties occur with any degree of hearing loss and typically result in the perceptual confusion of phonemes within a class of sounds.

The reception of the acoustic cues associated with a phoneme does not ensure its accurate identification. Phoneme recognition also requires a listener to distinguish the small acoustic variations that occur among different speech sounds. Sensorineural hearing loss causes not only a loss of audibility but also a reduction of frequency, intensity, and temporal discrimination ability. For this reason, phonemes that are audible but similar acoustically may not be distinguishable to a hearing-impaired child. Discrimination ability cannot be predicted solely on the basis of threshold information. It can be determined, however, by more structured assessment procedures, such as analysis of acoustic confusions, minimal-pairs testing, and age-appropriate measures of speech discrimination.

Visual Reception

Speechreading (or lipreading) enables a person to obtain linguistic information by watching the articulatory movements of a speaker's lips, tongue, and jaw. It can improve the comprehension of speech by providing sensory cues that are unavailable auditorily because of hearing loss or environmental degradation of the acoustic signal. The amount of linguistic information that can be obtained by speechreading is limited because speech is not transmitted visually as efficiently as it is auditorily. Sensory cues are restricted by (1) the poor visibility of many speech sounds; (2) the occurrence of sounds that look alike (i.e., homophones); (3) the rate of speech; (4) articulatory differences among speakers; (5) the effect of coarticulation on the visibility and stability of articulatory movements; and (6) environmental conditions (e.g., lighting, viewing angle, distance from the speaker).[3] Because sensory input is limited, the visual perception of oral language is highly dependent on the speechreader's language competence and inductive ability; that is, a speechreader must be capable of arriving at perceptual and conceptual closures when a substantial part of the sensory code is either missing or ambiguous.

The primary sensory cue that is available visually is place of production. Place information is retrieved by observing the motor patterns associated with the production of phonemes. These patterns can be organized into contrasting groups called *visemes* and are shown in Table 10-1.[3] The viseme groups are arranged separately for vowels and consonants in their order of visibility. Those marked with

TABLE 10-1
Visible Speechreading Movements Under Ideal Viewing Conditions

Movement Pattern	Associated Phonemes
Vowels and diphthongs	
Lips puckered*	/u, ʊ, o͞u, ɝ/
Lips back*	/i, ɪ, e͞ɪ, ʌ/
Lips rounded*	/ɔ/
Lips relaxed to lips puckered*	/a͞ʊ/
Lips relaxed	/ɛ, æ, ɑ/
Lips rounded to lips back	/ɔ͞ɪ/
Lips relaxed to lips back	/a͞ɪ/
Consonants	
Lip to teeth*	/f, v/
Lips puckered*	/w, hw, r/
Lips together*	/p, b, m/
Tongue between teeth*	/θ, ð/
Lips forward*	/ʃ, ʒ, tʃ, dʒ/
Teeth together	/s, z/
Lips back	/j/
Tongue up or down	/t, d, n, l/
Tongue back	/k, g, ŋ/

*Denotes that the movement pattern is highly visible.

an asterisk are highly visible and can be identified accurately by most speechreaders. The other visemes listed are not as easily perceived and may not be distinguishable under less than ideal viewing conditions.

Individual phonemes, with the possible exception of the /ɔ/ and /j/, cannot be identified solely by their visual motor pattern, because many sounds share the same place of articulation. For example, /p/, /b/, and /m/ cannot be distinguished on the basis of visual information only; additional information about their voicing and manner characteristics is needed to discriminate one from the others.

Auditory-Visual Reception

For many hearing-impaired children, the comprehension of speech is not possible under auditory-only or visual-only conditions. Auditory cues are missing or distorted because of the hearing deficit, and visual cues are incomplete because of the inherent limitations of speechreading. However, when speech is processed under an auditory-visual (bimodal) condition, the nonoverlapping cues provided by each modality can be combined to improve message comprehension.

The degree to which bimodal reception improves the comprehension of speech will depend on the severity of the hearing loss and the benefit of amplification. Children with mild or moderate hearing impairments will benefit significantly when speech is processed bimodally because the primary cue that is lost auditorily, place of production, can be retrieved from the visual channel. This bimodal advantage will not be as great for children with severe to profound hearing losses.

Although the same speech cues are available to them visually, the severity of their hearing impairments will prevent the auditory reception of low-frequency linguistic features that are not readily visible. For these children, speech comprehension will depend more heavily on closure ability and may not be possible if auditory reception is not enhanced substantially by hearing aids, cochlear implants, or other sensory devices.

Nonverbal Reception

Nonverbal cues provide significant information about the semantic and pragmatic aspects of a verbal message, the emotional state and attitude of the speaker, and appropriate response behavior. Nonverbal information is transmitted auditorily via the prosodic aspects of speech. The reception of prosodic features is possible if hearing is adequate at frequencies below 750 Hz.[4] Because the acoustic cues are relatively intense, prosodic information will remain at least partially audible until the degree of low-frequency hearing loss approaches a severe to profound level.

Nonverbal information is transmitted most effectively through the visual channel. Visual nonverbal cues include facial expression, eye behavior, body movement, and posture. It is intuitively attractive to assume that hearing-impaired children compensate for their reduced auditory abilities by developing superior sensitivity to visual nonverbal cues. Studies have shown, however, that the hearing-impaired are less able to decode visual nonverbal information than are normal hearers.[5,6] This deficit has been attributed to differences in the processing strategies of normal-hearing and hearing-impaired listeners. The hearing-impaired must monitor a speaker's lips closely to maximize their linguistic reception and, in doing so, may lose nonverbal information located peripheral to the lip region. Even when registered iconically, attention restrictions may limit the extent to which these peripheral cues can be processed. In contrast, a normal hearer is less dependent on lipreading, leaving the visual modality free to attend to and process nonverbal information in a more comprehensive manner.

Oral-Language Characteristics

Most children with congenital or prelingual hearing loss exhibit delays or deficiencies in the acquisition of oral language. Problems can occur in all areas of language, including morphology, syntax, semantics, and pragmatics.

The oral-language deficits of hearing-impaired children are related primarily to the severity of hearing loss, although skills vary among children with similar audiograms. Other factors of influence include the time of onset of the hearing loss, discrimination skills, the timing and benefit of amplification, and the ability to tolerate and use incomplete sensory data.[7]

The oral language problems of hard-of-hearing children increase with the degree of hearing loss but generally do not approach the deficits that typically occur with profound impairment. Language-acquisition patterns are similar for normal-hearing children and those with mild hearing loss, and for children with moderate hearing loss and severe hearing loss.[8] The oral language difficulties of hard-of-hearing children can, in most cases, be remediated successfully if intervention is provided early and with strong family support. For many deaf children, however, the lack of sufficient sensory input prevents the acquisition of language auditorily.

TABLE 10-2
Common Oral-Language Characteristics of Hearing-Impaired Children

Vocabulary and word-class usage
  Reduced vocabulary
  Restricted knowledge of word classes, including the following:
    Overuse of nouns and verbs
    Omission or restricted use of function words
Semantics
  Restricted use of semantic operations
  Restricted use of abstract language forms
  Difficulty with words with multiple meanings
Syntax
  Omission or restricted use of bound morphemes
  Restricted knowledge of verb forms
  Overuse of subject-verb-object sentence structures
  Reduced sentence length
  Restricted knowledge and use of complex sentence forms
  Reduced syntactic quality (word omissions, inversions, substitutions, and
    additions)
  Agrammatical sentence forms
Pragmatics
  Passive communication style (reduced initiation of verbal interaction)
  Difficulty sustaining and repairing conversations
  Provision of ambiguous or uninformative responses

The oral language deficits of hard-of-hearing children also differ qualitatively from those demonstrated by deaf children. Hard-of-hearing children usually exhibit a language delay rather than a language disorder. That is, they acquire language in a normal developmental sequence but at a slower rate than their normal-hearing peers. They may also demonstrate premature plateaus of development, particularly in the morphosyntactic area. In deaf children, deviant language forms can accompany severe language delay. Their knowledge of words and meanings may be irregular and related more to teaching curricula than to natural language experience. Their productions may be characterized by agrammatical and nonsentence forms, such as omissions of major sentence constituents, absent or incorrect morphological markers, and asequential word orders.[2,9] The common oral language deficits of hearing-impaired children are listed in Table 10-2.

Speech Characteristics

Severe-to-Profound Hearing Loss
The vocalizations of deaf and normal-hearing children cannot be differentiated until the onset of babbling. Profoundly impaired children are not likely to enter the babbling stage. Severely impaired children may demonstrate limited babbling behaviors, but, if so, their vocalizations will differ from those of normal-hearing

children in both quantity and quality. Hearing infants typically exhibit an increase in speech-like sounds and a decrease in nonspeech sounds with age, but both types of vocalizations decline in children with significant hearing losses shortly after babbling begins. Hearing-impaired babies evidence a smaller variety of consonant sounds and produce fewer multisyllabic utterances than hearing babies. They tend to produce a high proportion of vocalizations containing glides and glottal stops.[10,11]

The vocalizations of profoundly and severely impaired children will depend on the quality of their auditory experience. The early preverbal behaviors of the deaf generally consist of auditory and vocal elements, gestural elements, and observation of the speaker. With early and proficient use of hearing aids or cochlear implants, a primarily auditory and vocal style can develop. However, when sensory devices are delayed or provide little benefit, auditory and vocal behaviors decrease and visual and gestural behaviors predominate.[12]

The speech of deaf children is characterized by severe and multiple deficits that involve both segmental and suprasegmental aspects. As a group, their speech intelligibility is poor, although it varies widely among individuals. Most studies have found the intelligibility of deaf speakers to be 20% to 40%.[9] Deviant speech characteristics are due mainly to the loss of auditory feedback but also can be caused by poor respiratory control and excessive laryngeal and articulatory tension. The common characteristics of the speech of the deaf are listed in Table 10-3.

Mild-to-Moderate Hearing Loss

Although any degree of hearing loss can cause errors of speech production, the speech of hard-of-hearing children resembles the productions of normal-hearing children more closely than that of the profoundly or severely impaired. Most hard-of-hearing children produce intelligible speech. Their voice quality, suprasegmental production, and vowel articulation is comparable to normal-hearing children. The majority of speech errors involve the articulation of conso-nants and consonant blends. Sounds of low intensity, high frequency, or short duration are most commonly affected. Errors of substitution and distortion predominate, although other types of errors occur frequently and include omission of final consonants; decreased production of voiced fricatives; and limited use of voiced, back, lingual consonants.[8,9,13]

▼ AURAL HABILITATION

The primary goal of aural habilitation is to maximize the receptive and expressive communication abilities of hearing-impaired children. Remediation activities can include parent counseling and education, the fitting of hearing aids or other sensory devices, sensory training (auditory and visual), the development of language in oral or manual form, and the development of speech.[14]

Meeting Parental Concerns Through Counseling and Education

For parents, the initial diagnosis of their child's hearing loss is a time of shock and confusion. Their emotional reactions during this period may be similar to the

TABLE 10-3
Common Speech Characteristics of Deaf Children

Suprasegmental
  Pitch and intensity characteristics
    Inappropriate vocal pitch (usually higher than normal)
    Pitch breaks
    Phonetically linked pitch breaks (usually on high vowels)
    Monotone voice
    Inappropriate vocal intensity (too loud or too soft)
    Inability to vary vocal intensity across speaking situations
    Faulty stress pattern (may stress all vowel nuclei)
  Temporal characteristics
    Slow speaking rate
    Abnormal pause behavior (both between and within phrase)
    Increased duration of speech sounds and segments
  Voice quality
    Harshness, breathiness, and hypo- or hypernasality may occur alone or in combination
Segmental
  Vowels and diphthongs
    Substitution (most often involving tense/lax or near-neighbor vowels)
    Neutralization
    Reduction of diphthongs; diphthongization of vowels
    Nasalization
  Consonants
    Omissions
      Word position (most often on word-final consonants)
      Place of production (most often on back consonants)
    Manner substitutions
      Nasal/oral
      Voice/voiceless
      Stop for fricative (due to articulatory overconstriction)
    Place substitutions (related to visibility factors)
    Distortions
    Poor coarticulatory skills
    Omission of consonant blends
Other Characteristics
  Poor respiratory control
  Glottalization and intrusive voicing
  Exaggerated lip and jaw movement

stages of grief that follow the death of a loved one: denial, guilt and anger, bargaining, depression, and, ultimately, acceptance. The duration of the grieving process will vary considerably but typically encompasses a period of 6 to 12 months.[15] These reactions are normal and should not be avoided, but they may inhibit or delay the parents' active involvement in remediation activities.

Professionals can minimize potential difficulties by understanding and accepting the nature of grief as a coping behavior, by providing the appropriate emotional and educational support at each stage of the grieving process and by coordinating and monitoring the provision of services during this period. The participation of psychologists or social workers, either directly or indirectly, may be necessary. Parent support groups are especially valuable and may be a clinician's most powerful counseling tool. They allow parents to help one another by sharing concerns and experiences, and provide emotional and informational support on a continuous basis.

A substantial amount of information must be communicated to parents to provide for their needs and those of their hearing-impaired children. Counseling and training sessions will be necessary at each stage of remediation. Information should be provided in a clear, candid manner and with a minimum amount of technical jargon. Demonstration and hands-on practice often will be needed. It should be remembered that parents are attempting to absorb a large quantity of information during a time of emotional stress, frustration, and anxiety. Because of this, it is critical that all educational activities be conducted in a comfortable, empathetic, and tolerant fashion. Parents also should be provided with written materials that review, supplement, and expand upon information that is provided during counseling and training sessions. The topics that should be addressed during parent consultations include the following:

1. The impact of hearing loss on communication, learning, and social-emotional development
2. Accessing emotional and financial support services, child advocacy organizations, and community service agencies
3. Educational, habilitative, and other related services
4. Federal, state, and local regulations regarding service provision to hearing-impaired children
5. Language and communication options and considerations
6. The role of the family in the remediation process
7. The roles and capabilities of the various professionals, organizations, and agencies involved in the remediation process
8. Locating information and support sources: books and written materials, recommended internet sites, resource groups, hearing-impaired organizations
9. Methods for effective parent-child communication
10. Benefits and limitations of hearing aids, cochlear implants, and other sensory devices
11. Hearing aid orientation, use, care, and troubleshooting
12. Parent-child intervention: procedures, techniques, materials, and resources

Hearing Aids

Hearing aid selection and fitting should begin immediately after a child's hearing loss is identified and medical clearance for hearing aid use is obtained. It is an ongoing process that requires close observation of aided behaviors, parental support and involvement, and collaboration among professionals involved in the child's management. Several clinical decisions are made by the dispensing audiologist during the hearing aid selection process, including the type of instrument to be worn, whether binaural or monaural amplification should be used, the ideal electroacoustic characteristics of the device(s), and the way in which hearing aid performance and benefit will be measured. It is probable that fitting adjustments will be necessary, as the child's reaction to and performance with the instruments are monitored during the early period of hearing aid use.

Types of Hearing Aids

Ear-level hearing aids (behind-the-ear [BTE], in-the-ear [ITE], and in-the-canal [ITC]) have replaced the body aid as the instruments of choice for young children. The BTE hearing aid is the most commonly used instrument with the pediatric population. It is preferred over the body aid because it is light-weight, has no external wires, does not amplify clothing noise, and provides auditory reception at the natural head position.[16] Body aids may be necessary, however, for children with poor head control and when the microphone and receiver must be separated to reduce acoustic feedback.

ITE and ITC hearing aids are used less often with young children. Although they can provide adequate power for most degrees of hearing loss, they have limited flexibility and external input capabilities (e.g., direct audio input and telecoil options). Also, the frequent recasing that would be necessary because of the growth of the child's pinna and ear canal is more costly and time-consuming than is the fabrication of new earmolds.[17] Bone conduction hearing aids can be used as a temporary measure for children with congenital anomalies of the pinna or ear canal. They typically are replaced with conventional air conduction instruments after the completion of surgical reconstruction.

Earmolds

Earmolds are designed to deliver amplified signals to the ear canal without substantial acoustic leakage. Significant leakage of sound through or around an earmold will cause acoustic feedback, particularly when ear-level hearing aids are worn. Earmolds are available in a variety of styles that differ in size, weight, and occlusiveness. Body aids and high-gain ear-level aids will require earmolds that fit snugly in the ear canal and fill the concha of the pinna. Smaller, less occlusive earmolds can be worn with mild-gain ear-level instruments. A child's pinna increases in size until about 9 years of age. Because of this, earmolds and the casings of ITE and ITC hearing aids have to be remade every 3 to 6 months for young hearing aid users.

Earmolds are often modified to alter the frequency response of the hearing aid. Common modifications include venting, damping, and horning. Vents can be drilled through the earmold to reduce low-frequency gain. They also increase comfort by allowing aeration of the ear canal. Dampers are filters that can be placed in the earmold tubing to smooth frequency response peaks and reduce the hearing aid's output, primarily in the mid-frequency range. Horning is the progressive increase of the diameter of the sound channel as it passes through the earmold. It has the effect of increasing high-frequency gain.

Earmolds can be made of either hard or soft materials. Soft materials are often used with young children to prevent injury if the child falls or is struck on the ear. Also, a soft earmold provides a tight acoustic seal because body heat causes the material to expand. Semi-hard, nonallergenic earmolds are available for children who have allergic reactions to other types of material.

Binaural vs. Monaural Amplification

Binaural amplification is recommended for children with bilateral hearing loss. This applies to both symmetrical and asymmetrical hearing impairments. The advantages of binaural hearing include (1) improved localization ability and loudness perception; (2) elimination of the head shadow effect; (3) better speech understanding in noisy listening situations; and (4) improved sound quality, spatial balance, and ease of listening.[17,18]

Hearing Aid Orientation

Once amplification has been obtained, it should be introduced in a gradual fashion. Most children accept hearing aids quickly, but some may require a longer period of adjustment. Downs[19] recommended the use of a 6- to 8-week orientation program for young hearing aid users. Others have argued that such schedules draw attention to the hearing aid and lengthen the adjustment process.[20] Rather than adhering to rigid timetables or ignoring them completely, it is best to view orientation recommendations as guidelines that can be shaped to suit a child's particular reaction to hearing aid use.

The factors that should be considered during the adjustment process include (1) the period of time that the hearing aid is worn; (2) the gain-control setting; and (3) the listening situation. Initially, hearing aids should be worn for short periods (e.g., 10 to 20 minutes) several times a day with the gain control at its minimal setting. The time of use should be increased in small steps until the hearing aid can be worn successfully throughout the entire day. The gain control can be increased gradually during the early stages of the adjustment period until its target setting is reached. At first, the hearing aid should be worn in pleasant, reinforcing listening environments that contain minimal levels of ambient noise. Aided listening situations can then be expanded progressively from controlled acoustic environments to those that include a more natural and complex array of auditory stimuli. Parents should be provided with a written orientation plan that includes time guidelines and practical examples of appropriate listening situations.

Use and Care of Hearing Aids

A hearing aid can be an intimidating device, and its use can seem awkward at first. Because of this, a significant amount of training, encouragement, and technical support from the dispensing audiologist and other clinicians is necessary during the early period of intervention to ensure that the hearing aid is being used and maintained properly. Every caregiver in regular contact with a young hearing aid user should be taught the following:

1. The parts of a hearing aid (e.g., microphone, on-off switch, volume control, battery compartment, earmold, and tubing)
2. The correct insertion of the battery; how long it lasts; how to check its voltage; precautions for its safe use
3. The correct insertion of the earmold and how to keep it clean
4. The proper position of the volume control
5. The causes of acoustic feedback and what to do if it occurs
6. What can damage a hearing aid (e.g., impacts, high temperatures, moisture, excessive dirt or dust, hair spray)

The condition and performance of a hearing aid should be monitored on a daily basis. A routine check also should be conducted by clinicians before each therapy session. This is particularly important in light of the consistent (and disappointing) findings of a number of investigations concerning the condition of hearing aids worn by school-age children. These studies, conducted over a 30-year period, found that 27% to 92% of children's hearing aids are malfunctioning at any given time.[21]

Some equipment is needed to carry out a hearing aid check, including a battery tester, a hearing aid stethoscope or listening mold, a brush and wire loop to remove cerumen from the earmold, and a hand syringe to clean the tubing of the earmold. A complete hearing aid check consists of the following:

- A visual inspection of the hearing aid, tubing, and earmold.
  Check hearing aid switches.
  Check tubing for stiffness, holes, or cracks.
  Check earmold for cerumen and moisture.
- A battery check.
  Check battery voltage.
  Check battery contacts for corrosion.
  Check that battery door is closed securely.
- A listening check.
  Check the quality of amplified sound.
  Check for excessive noise, intermittent signals, and acoustic feedback while tapping the casing of the hearing aid and rotating the volume control.
  Check for a smooth increase in gain as the volume control is rotated.

Parents can solve many of the problems that inevitably occur by learning simple troubleshooting techniques. Common problems include the use of batteries that are dead, weak, or inserted improperly in the battery compartment; switches turned to incorrect settings; and earmolds that are too small, inserted incorrectly, or blocked by cerumen or moisture. Most problems can be solved without visits to the dispenser's office by providing parents with troubleshooting charts and procedures.

Alternative Sensory Devices

Cochlear Implants

In most sensorineural hearing losses, it is the hair cells of the inner ear that are nonfunctioning rather than the fibers of the auditory nerve. The benefit provided by hearing aids can be insignificant for many profoundly hearing-impaired patients because of the extent of hair-cell damage. A cochlear implant is designed to bypass the nonfunctioning hair cells by applying electrical stimulation directly to the fibers of the auditory nerve. The system consists of an external microphone, a speech-processing unit, a transmitting wire or coil, and a surgically implanted receiver-stimulator and electrode array.

To be considered for implantation, a child must be profoundly hearing impaired and obtain no significant benefit from hearing aids (i.e., the inability to use aided hearing for speech perception). The child must be at least 12 months of age before implantation, primarily to permit time for diagnosis, evaluation, and determination of hearing aid benefit. Additional nonauditory criteria can include normal intelligence, the absence of additional handicaps that can affect the success of the implant, and evidence of family support.[18] The anatomical factors that influence selection and postsurgical success include the patency of the cochlea and degree of neural survival.[22]

Speech-perception abilities vary greatly among children with cochlear implants and can range from limited sound detection to open-set word recognition. The success of an implant is related most closely to (1) the age at which deafness occurred; (2) the duration of deafness before implantation; (3) the neural survival in the cochlea; (4) the coding strategy used by the speech processor; (5) the child's rehabilitation; and (6) the level of parental and educational support.[22,23] Generally, the largest improvements have been observed in adults and children with postlingual hearing loss. Although most children with congenital or prelingual hearing impairments benefit from cochlear implants, they are slower to acquire auditory skills and can require 1 to 2 years of implant use before demonstrating improvements in speech perception.[24] Performance improvements have been measured for a range of behaviors, including sound detection, pattern recognition, preverbal communication, closed- and open-set speech recognition, speechreading, and speech production.[25-27]

Vibrotactile Sensory Aids

Vibrotactile aids transduce auditory signals into vibratory patterns on the skin. They are a noninvasive alternative for deaf children who derive negligible benefit from conventional amplification. Both single-channel and multichannel devices are in use. Single-channel aids provide primarily suprasegmental information and segmental voicing cues. Multichannel systems (or vocoders) provide these same low-frequency cues and also can transmit high-frequency components of speech, including frication and other manners of production cues.[28,29]

Although vibrotactile devices have been shown to improve the speechreading abilities, early vocal behaviors, phonetic repertoires, and syllabic productions of young deaf children,[30,31] they require teaching and learning strategies that are different from those used with auditory devices such as hearing aids and cochlear implants. Often, children can only receive training and follow-up services in specialized centers that are limited in number and removed from school settings.[28] These difficulties have prevented the extensive use of vibrotactile instruments in the deaf population.

Communication Methodologies

A variety of communication methodologies are being used to facilitate the language development of hearing-impaired children. The major approaches are outlined in Table 10-4. Each method has its proponents and detractors, but no single method has proven to be best for all children. As Davis and Hardick[2] explained, "the major decision for infants is whether or not the child should be exposed to some form of manual communication … in addition to spoken language" (p. 158).

In the 1970s, total communication (TC) replaced oralism as the most common communication methodology used in educational programs for the hearing impaired. Debate continues, however, between oral and TC practitioners about the use of manual communication and its effect on the development of oral language. Oral proponents argue that the simultaneous use of speech and signs inhibits the development of speech perception and production skills. TC proponents maintain that the early establishment of language, regardless of teaching modality, serves to facilitate the development of oral communication. Empirical investigations have

TABLE 10-4
Communication Methodologies for Hearing-Impaired Children

Methodology	Description
Oral English	Reception and expression of language via speech
	Auditory reception can be supplemented by speechreading, other visual cues, or both
Unisensory method (also known as *acoustic, auditory,* or *acoupedic*)	Uses auditory input only for speech perception
	Lipreading is discouraged until the child has shown the ability to use audition effectively
Oral method (also known as *auditory, verbal-oral,* or *oral-aural*)	Uses audition and speechreading for speech perception
Rochester method (also known as *neo-oralism* or *visible speech*)	Uses fingerspelling to supplement audition and speechreading for speech perception
Cued speech	Uses eight hand shapes and four hand positions (32 cues) to supplement audition and lipreading for speech perception
	Cues allow homophonous words to be distinguished and clarified
Manually coded English (also known as *sign systems*)	Reception and expression of language via formal gestures, fingerspelling, signs that represent oral English in manual form, or any combination of these
	Manual symbols are produced in English word order and can be accompanied by common word endings
	Several sign systems have been developed, including Seeing Essential English (SEE$_1$), Signing Exact English (SEE$_2$), and Signed English
American sign language (also known as *ASL* or *AMESLAN*)	The natural language of the deaf community
	ASL differs from English at all structural levels, having its own morphology, syntax, and lexicography
Bilingual-bicultural approach	An educational approach advocated by members of the deaf culture
	Recognizes ASL as the natural language of the deaf, encourages its use, and teaches oral English, manually coded English, or both as a second language
Total communication (also known as *TC*)	A philosophy, rather than a specific methodology
	Uses any and all communication methods that prove successful for a particular child
	In practice, TC programs typically employ the simultaneous use of speech and manually coded English for reception and expression of language
Deaf-blind methods	Uses the tactile reception of speech motor patterns, fingerspelling, or signs
	Speech movements are monitored by placing a hand on the face and neck of the speaker (Tadoma method)
	Fingerspelling and signs are monitored by placing hands on the hands of the sender

failed to clarify these issues. Some studies have measured superior oral language abilities in children from oral programs,[32,33] whereas others have suggested that the use of a simultaneous communication technique is not a detriment to the development of oral-language skills.[34,35]

There is a general consensus that a unisensory or multisensory oral English method is most appropriate for hard-of-hearing children. For deaf children, however, the selection of the ideal educational approach is not as clear cut. The oral language potential of deaf children depends not only on the amount of residual hearing but also on the age of onset, the age of identification and initiation of intervention, and the benefit provided by sensory devices. Other nonauditory factors can be of significant influence, including the child's cognitive ability, the existence of other handicapping conditions, the level of family support, and the types and quality of programs that are available in the child's community.[2]

Quantitative scales are available to assist parents and professionals in the selection process. The Deafness Management Quotient uses a weighted assessment of residual hearing, central intactness, intellectual factors, family constellation, and socioeconomic condition to arrive at recommendations regarding oral versus TC placement.[36] The Spoken Language Predictor Index evaluates hearing capacity, aided performance, language competence, nonverbal intelligence, family support, and speech communication attitude to determine the degree to which speech, signs, or both should be emphasized.[37]

The majority of tests designed to evaluate the language abilities of normal-hearing children can be used with the hearing impaired. There are, however, potential shortcomings to this approach. First, there are a limited number of standardized tests that assess the unique language deficits associated with hearing loss. Second, the effects of auditory confusions, speechreading, and short-term memory for signs on test-taking ability are not fully understood and can confound the validity of particular instruments to varying degrees.[38] For these reasons, a battery of informal and formal measures should be used to evaluate the language abilities of hearing-impaired children. The specific tests and procedures that are used to assess the language skills of infants and toddlers are described in Chapter 8 and in Appendices A and B. A detailed review of language intervention procedures for infants and toddlers is presented in Chapter 9.

Development of Sensory Skills

Auditory Training

Normal-hearing children acquire auditory skills naturally and early in life in response to continuous auditory stimulation. By 6 months of age, hearing babies can attend to speech at conversational levels, localize the source of sounds, recognize differences in vocal tones, and discriminate the various acoustic features of the speech signal. By 1 year of age, they have developed enough auditory and linguistic ability to recognize their names, familiar words, and simple instructions. The normal developmental sequence of auditory skills is shown in Table 10-5.

Hearing loss can prevent or delay the acquisition of auditory skills by depriving a child of auditory stimulation. The effect of hearing impairment on auditory development depends on its severity and time of onset. Children with severe to

TABLE 10-5
Normal Developmental Sequence of Auditory Skills During the First Year of Life

1. *Reflexive:* Child responds reflexively to suprathreshold sounds (e.g., startle, initiation or cessation of activity, stirring or arousal from sleep, eye widening or blink, crying).
2. *Attending and alerting:* Child attends to environmental sounds and voices. Listening attitude, searching behavior, and changes in facial expression may be seen.
3. *Localization:* Sources of sounds can be identified. Child may turn or move toward sounds.
4. *Distance hearing:* Infant localizes and attends to sounds at varying distances.
5. *Gross environmental discrimination, identification, and comprehension:* Child can associate environmental sounds with their sources. May point to, manipulate, or imitate sound sources.
6. *Vocal discrimination, identification, and comprehension:* Child can discriminate and associate gross vocal sounds, words, and phrases with their sources and meanings.
7. *Speech discrimination, identification, and comprehension:* Speech sounds can be distinguished and comprehended. Perceptual skills for vowels precede those for consonants.

profound impairments do not acquire auditory skills without sensory devices and intervention. Hard-of-hearing children can acquire some basic auditory behaviors naturally (e.g., auditory attention, localization), but the development of more sophisticated skills is delayed until amplification is obtained.

The goal of auditory training is to maximize the receptive abilities of hearing-impaired children by developing their listening skills to the fullest extent. Several approaches to auditory training have been developed and include the Carhart method,[39] traditional approaches,[40] the acoupedic method,[41] the cognitive auditory method,[42] and the verbo-tonal method.[43] Each approach is based on the normal developmental sequence of auditory skills, but the approaches differ in their degree of structure, manner of delivery and reinforcement, and use of supplemental sensory devices.

The auditory training of infants and toddlers is most effective when it is conducted during normal daily activities. As a child's skills develop, structured activities can be incorporated into the remediation program to facilitate the growth of advanced auditory functions (e.g., sequential memory, closure, selective attention). Home-based intervention requires the informed participation of family members. They should be familiar with the developmental sequence of auditory behaviors as well as therapeutic techniques and materials. A variety of auditory training programs are available commercially. Many are either written for parents or can be adapted for their use.

Visual Training

Most educational methodologies encourage the use of speechreading to maximize the receptive abilities of hearing-impaired children. Few, however, incorporate structured visual training into the early stages of intervention. As Hipskind[44] explained, "there is a tendency to allow this aspect of rehabilitation to develop naturally in conjunction with the acquisition of auditory, speech, and linguistic skills" (p. 150).

Although visual training is not formalized early in remediation, steps can be taken during this period to maximize the reception of visual linguistic cues. Ophthalmological testing should be conducted as early as possible. Visual acuity must be within normal limits or corrected to normal limits to enable the reception of the subtle articulatory movements of speech. Speechreading ability is also affected by distance and viewing angle. Perceptual skills are optimal when speech is received at a horizontal viewing angle of 0 to 45 degrees and from a distance no greater than 10 feet.[45] Proper room illumination must be maintained, and speakers should avoid positioning themselves where light sources cause their faces to be in shadow.

Structured speechreading exercises can be incorporated into remediation as a child's oral language ability develops. Historically, both analytical and synthetic approaches have been used to teach speechreading. Analytical methods concentrate on the visual identification of the individual components of speech (e.g., phonemes, syllables, words). Synthetic methods focus on the comprehension of the general meaning of a message rather than the identification of each component within the message. Most contemporary methods combine these two approaches in their training procedures. An excellent description of the combined approach to speechreading training is presented by Jeffers and Barley.[3]

Speech Training

Speech assessment of hearing-impaired children should focus on three areas of production: suprasegmental skills, segmental skills, and speech intelligibility. Intelligibility testing may not be appropriate for young children with limited speech skills. As a child's expressive ability increases, however, this measure should be incorporated into the assessment battery.

Children must demonstrate the spontaneous and consistent use of voice for communicative purposes before speech skills can be developed. Although an auditory-verbal communication style evolves naturally in most children with mild-to-moderate hearing loss, a concerted effort by parents and clinicians usually is required to sustain the vocal behaviors of children with severe-to-profound impairments. Early vocalizations can be encouraged by involving children in activities that require the frequent use of voice (e.g., verbal play, singing, game playing, imitation of nonspeech sounds). Voice-activated toys and visual devices also can be used to elicit vocal behavior. Any activity that encourages a child to initiate, imitate, or respond to vocalization should be noted and used as a foundation for further training.

Formal speech-training programs use distinctive feature contrasts,[46] word and syllable productions,[47] a hierarchy of segmental and suprasegmental contrasts,[4] or any combination of these to develop the speech skills of hearing-impaired children. Auditory models should be used whenever a child is able to detect and discriminate the acoustic features of the stimulus. Most children, however, require the combined use of auditory, visual, and tactile sensory modalities to acquire and monitor target productions. A variety of techniques can be used to provide supplemental visual and tactile feedback. Electronic and computer-based instruments (e.g., the IBM Speech Viewer III, spectrographic displays, electropalatography, vibrotactile devices) provide detailed visual and tactile feedback for a variety of suprasegmental and segmental characteristics. Simpler, less costly techniques include speechreading, visual prompts and hand cues, and tactile impressions of the breath stream, laryngeal and nasal vibration, and articulator location.

▼ REFERENCES

1. Peterson GE, Barney HL: Control methods used in a study of the identification of vowels, *J Acoust Soc Am* 24:183, 1954.
2. Davis JM, Hardick EJ: *Rehabilitative audiology for children and adults*, New York, 1986, Macmillan.
3. Jeffers J, Barley M: *Speechreading (lipreading)*, Springfield, Ill, 1971, Thomas, p 3.
4. Ling D: *Speech and the hearing impaired child: theory and practice*, Washington, DC, 1976, The Alexander Graham Bell Association for the Deaf.
5. Schiff W, Thayer T: An eye for an ear? Social perception, nonverbal communication, and deafness, *Rehabil Psychol* 21:50, 1974.
6. Rigo TG, Lieberman DA: Nonverbal sensitivity of normal-hearing and hearing-impaired older adults, *Ear Hear* 10:184, 1989.
7. Norlin PF, Van Tasell DJ: Linguistic skills of hearing impaired children, *Monogr Contemp Audiol* 1:1, 1980.
8. Elfenbein JL, Hardin-Jones MA, Davis JM: Oral communication skills of children who are hard of hearing, *J Speech Hear Res* 37:216, 1994.
9. Seyfried DN, Hutchinson JM, Smith LL: Language and speech of the hearing impaired. In Schow RL, Nerbonne MA, editors: *Introduction to aural rehabilitation*, ed 2, Austin, Tex, 1989, Pro-Ed, p 181.
10. Stark RE: Phonatory development in young normally hearing and hearing-impaired children. In Hochberg I, Levitt H, Osberger MJ, editors: *Speech of the hearing impaired: research, training, and personnel preparation*, Baltimore, 1983, University Park Press, p 251.
11. Stoel-Gammon C, Otomo K: Babbling development of hearing-impaired and normally hearing subjects, *J Speech Hear Disord* 51:33, 1986.
12. Tait M, Lutman ME: Comparison of early communicative behavior in young children with cochlear implants and with hearing aids, *Ear Hear* 15:352, 1994.
13. West J, Weber J: A phonological analysis of the spontaneous language of a four-year-old hard-of-hearing child, *J Speech Hear Disord* 38:25, 1973.
14. American Speech-Language-Hearing Association: Preferred practice patterns for the professions of speech-language pathology and audiology: aural rehabilitation, *ASHA* 35:23, 1993.
15. Tanner DC: Loss and grief: implications for the speech-language pathologist and audiologist, *ASHA* 22:916, 1980.
16. Northern JL, Gabbard SA, Kinder DL: Pediatric considerations in selecting and fitting hearing aids. In Sandlin RE, editor: *Handbook of hearing aid amplification. Vol II: Clinical considerations and fitting practices*, San Diego, 1995, Singular Publishing Group, p 113.
17. Mueller HG, Grimes A: Amplification systems for the hearing impaired. In Alpiner JG, McCarthy PA, editors: *Rehabilitative audiology: children and adults*, Baltimore, 1987, Williams & Wilkins, p 115.
18. Northern JL, Downs MP: *Hearing in children*, ed 4, Baltimore, 1991, Williams & Wilkins.
19. Downs M: *The establishment of hearing aid use: a program for parents*, 1967, MAICO Audiology Library Series, p 4.
20. Ross M: Hearing aid selection for preverbal hearing impaired children. In Pollack M, editor: *Amplification for the hearing impaired*, 1975, New York, 1975, Grune & Stratton, p 207.
21. Elfenbein JL, et al:. Status of school children's hearing aids relative to monitoring practices, *Ear Hear* 9:212, 1988.
22. Fryauf-Bertschy H: Pediatric cochlear implantation: an update, *Am J Audiol* 2:13, 1993.
23. Tyler RS: Cochlear implants and the deaf culture, *Am J Audiol* 2:26, 1993.
24. Fryauf-Bertschy H, et al: Performance over time of congenitally and postlingually deafened children using multichannel cochlear implants, *J Speech Hear Res* 35:913, 1992.

25. Dawson PW, et al: Cochlear implants in children, adolescents, and prelinguistically deafened adults: speech perception, *J Speech Hear Res* 35:401, 1992.
26. Dawson PW, et al: A clinical report on speech production of cochlear implant users, *Ear Hear* 16:551, 1995.
27. O'Donoghue GM, et al: Cochlear implants in young children: the relationship between speech perception and speech intelligibility, *Ear Hear* 20:419, 1990.
28. Eilers RE, et al: A longitudinal evaluation of the speech perception capabilities of children using multichannel tactile vocoders, *J Speech Hear Res* 39:518, 1996.
29. Osberger MJ, Maso M, Sam LK: Speech intelligibility of children with cochlear implants, tactile aids, or hearing aids, *J Speech Hear Res* 36:186, 1993.
30. Steffans ML, et al: Early vocal development in tactually aided children with severe-profound hearing loss, *J Speech Hear Res* 37:700, 1994.
31. Boothroyd A: Special issue: auditory and tactile presentation of voice fundamental frequency as a supplement to speech reading, *Ear Hear* 9:6, 1988.
32. Geers AE, Moog JS: Speech perception and production skills of students with impaired hearing from oral and total communication education settings, *J Speech Hear Res* 35:1384, 1992.
33. Hyde MB, Power DJ: The receptive communication abilities of deaf students under oral, manual, and combined methods, *Am Ann Deaf* 137:389, 1992.
34. Caccamise F, Hatfield N, Brewer L: Manual/simultaneous communication research: results and implications, *Am Ann Deaf* 123:803, 1978.
35. Grove C, Rodda M: Receptive communication skills of hearing-impaired students: a comparison of four methods of communication, *Am Ann Deaf* 129:378, 1984.
36. Downs MP: The deafness management quotient, *Hearing and Speech News* Jan-Feb 1974.
37. Geers AE, Moog JS: Predicting spoken language acquisition of hearing impaired children, *J Speech Hear Disord* 42:84, 1987.
38. Moeller MP, Osberger MJ, Morford JA: Speech-Language assessment and intervention with preschool hearing-impaired children. In Alpiner JG, McCarthy PA, editors: *Rehabilitative audiology: children and adults*, Baltimore, 1987, Williams & Wilkins, p 163.
39. Carhart R: Auditory training. In Davis H, Silverman R, editors: *Hearing and deafness*, ed 2, New York, 1960, Holt, Rinehart & Winston, p 368.
40. Erber NP: *Auditory training*, Washington, DC, 1982, Alexander Graham Bell Association for the Deaf.
41. Pollack D: *Educational audiology for the limited hearing infant*, Springfield, Ill, 1970, Thomas.
42. Grammatico L: The development of listening skills, *Volta Rev* 77:303, 1975.
43. Guberina P: *Studies in the Verbo-Tonal system*, Columbus, Ohio, 1964, The Ohio State University Press.
44. Hipskind NM: Visual stimuli in communication. In Schow RL, Nerbonne MA, editors: *Introduction to aural rehabilitation*, ed 2, Austin, Tex, 1989, Pro-Ed, p 125.
45. Caccamise F, Meath-Lang B, Johnson D: Assessment and use of vision: critical needs of hearing-impaired students, *Am Ann Deaf* 26:361, 1981.
46. Bennett C: Articulation training of profoundly hearing-impaired children: a distinctive feature approach, *J Commun Disord* 11:433, 1978.
47. Abraham S, Werner F: Efficacy of word training vs. syllable training on articulatory generalization by severely hearing-impaired children, *Volta Rev* 87:97, 1985.

CHAPTER 11

MARKETING WHAT WE HAVE TO OFFER: WHY? HOW?

Frances P. Billeaud

M arketing is a constant challenge for communicative-disorders specialists. It is a very important facet of the array of professional responsibilities the speech-language pathologist (SLP) assumes, and one in which few university training programs provide instruction. In this era of managed care with its emphasis on reduction of costs, often accomplished by restricting the use of specialists, marketing what we have to offer to administrative entities, managed care organizations, and consumer groups is a task for which we must develop skills. Koyanagi and Lorber[1] have provided an excellent set of suggestions and guidelines in this regard in their article, "Can managed care meet the mental health needs of very young children?" Their practical suggestions are applicable across other infant-toddler-family service provision areas.

Marketing does not have to be expensive or glitzy. It must serve a clear purpose (e.g., promote a new program, increase use of an existing service, educate peer professionals about issues in communicative development and its relationship to their own specialties, or inform parents that early intervention with infants and toddlers is effective). It must meet the needs of both the marketer and the target audience. It must be delivered in a format that is appealing, direct, informative, and accessible to the target audiences. The first task, then, is to identify the prospective audiences and determine how to reach them most efficiently. The next thing to do is to decide what message(s) to deliver: what the audience needs to know, what degree of detail is necessary, what approach and medium are likely to be most productive and what level of language should be used.

Marketing tools include the SLP's business card; short topic-specific informational sheets, pamphlets, or brochures; cover letters directed to a specific person or group when reports are transmitted; presentations to professional peer groups; displays or programs provided at events such as health fairs; videotapes; personal visits to key personnel (e.g., administrators, prospective or existing referral sources); and short articles submitted to in-house newsletters, community newspapers, or periodical publications of organizations. Marketing tools also include appearances on television or radio programs to provide information about communicative development in children, how to handle particular disorders, and how to access parent resources.

Organized (as opposed to haphazard) marketing takes time but is an essential part of conducting a professional practice. It can yield benefits that range from improved understanding of the services SLPs offer to increased referrals from professional colleagues, and from increased visibility in the community to improved use of services for infants and toddlers at risk for communication disorders.

More specifically, in keeping with the focus of this book, targeted marketing efforts should be directed at expanding the use of services for infants and toddlers with or at risk for communicative disorders and at improving the understanding of the purpose of those services among administrators, peer professionals, and parents. Such efforts can be organized around the services themselves or around the targeted age groups.

▼ MARKETING THE SPEECH-LANGUAGE PATHOLOGIST'S SERVICES FOR NEWBORNS

Rehabilitation units in hospitals usually have SLPs on staff. The same is not true of most neonatal intensive care units (NICUs), although increasing numbers of SLPs are being hired for that environment. An increasing body of literature is available on the advantages of multidisciplinary teams that include the SLP in the NICU. In attempting to establish a presence on such teams, a specialized marketing effort must be implemented with the medical staff and the hospital administration.

Newborns admitted to the NICU are often small, sick, and fragile. Resolution of the health problems is the primary concern of the medical staff. Recognition of that fact assists the SLP who wishes to establish a presence in the NICU and in knowing how to approach the marketing effort. Sparks and colleagues[2] suggested that the SLP have a specific plan in mind when meeting with the medical staff to discuss involvement in the NICU: (1) Establish that the clinician has a role on the health care team; (2) explain biological and caregiving conditions that place communication development at risk and how those conditions interact; (3) explain principles of communicative assessment within the context of the developmental assessment process; (4) explain principles of intervention with this population; and (5) introduce prevention as a role for clinicians in the NICU. Written information should be provided about the benefits of achieving optimal outcomes for patients and reduced costs associated with developmental care.

Nurse-practitioner Lee McKenzie[3] stressed the importance of approaching the busy NICU staff initially as an interested observer who is there to learn the system. She suggested that the "nontraditional" professional who seeks to be a part of the NICU team should ask for information about caregiving provided by a key staff member (she suggested that it be a nurse). It is important to know the jobs of those who work on the NICU and to stay out of the way as they conduct routine procedures. Showing genuine interest, avoiding violation of professional space, learning the routines and the chain of command, and being a "presence" that becomes recognized on the unit, McKenzie suggested, go a long way toward making the staff receptive to listening to what you have to offer.

Sparks and colleagues[2] echoed this advice: "To participate in the NICU, clinicians must establish credibility by studying medical conditions, gain expertise by working with pediatric patients, and be willing to commit time. It is also advantageous to be able to assist with feeding." The latter, of course, also requires specific training.

If it is difficult to schedule conferences with the staff members of newborn care units, videotaped presentations lasting no more than 10 to 20 minutes can be a way to reach key personnel. Banigan[4] (1991) used this technique in working with hospital pediatric staff members for some time. It has also been the author's experience that colleagues in pediatrics, obstetrics, and gynecology departments enjoy having such in-service materials available to them for use in the doctors' lounge during lulls in their schedules or to take home for viewing at a convenient time. Nurses also seem to appreciate the convenience of this approach.

Research should be done by the SLP regarding the hospital's stated position, if any, on what constitutes quality care for all patients. If there is a multihospital corporate structure, do other hospitals in the corporate system use SLPs on their NICU staffs? Would inclusion of the SLP on *this* hospital's NICU team be advantageous to the hospital administration in terms of accrediting criteria, community marketing efforts, or attracting desired medical staff personnel?

Preparing a concise proposal for administrative and medical staff review is required at the appropriate time. Supporting information can be included as attachments or exhibits when the proposal is presented for consideration.

▼ MARKETING SERVICES FOR INFANTS AND TODDLERS IN THE COMMUNITY

Not all babies who are at risk for communicative disorders are graduates of NICUs. Many are discharged from well-baby nurseries or are born at home and are never in a hospital nursery. Maternal- and child-health clinics in the public sector or private pediatric practices may be the SLP's first point of contact with these infants and their parents. The communicative disorders specialist who wishes to work with the infant-toddler-family population should be familiar with the federally funded Early and Periodic Screening, Diagnosis, and Testing [EPSDT] program provided by public Maternal and Child Health Services. The Early and Periodic Screening, Diagnosis, and Testing program is responsible for conducting regular, comprehensive health screenings, including screening for communication problems for children from birth through the school years. Marketing services to the administrators of such programs is advisable. An example of a tool that can be used in such an effort is shown in Table 11-1. Providing multiple copies with a request that they be circulated to the nursing staff is a means of getting information to personnel who work with the population on a daily basis, and the "sampler" could serve as a means of raising the awareness level among nurses about risk identification for communication disorders.

Other important community agencies serving young children include medical clinics, early-intervention programs, private practices, social-service agencies,

TABLE 11-1
A Sampler of Etiologies Associated with Communicative Disorders in Infants and Toddlers

Hearing impairment
  Congenital hearing loss (genetic, syndromes, infections, anomalies)
  Transitory hearing loss (i.e., persistent, chronic episodes of otitis media; viral and bacterial illnesses; noise-induced problems; acute trauma)
  Acquired or adventitious hearing loss
    Iatrogenic (e.g., ototoxic drugs)
    Etiologically traced to illnesses (especially viral infections) or injuries
Delayed or disordered receptive language development
  Mental retardation
  Hearing impairment (see above)
  Other sensory impairments (especially severe vision impairments)
  Metabolic disorders (e.g., phenylketonuria)
  Syndromes not identified with chromosomal anomalies (e.g., fetal alcohol syndrome)
  Psychiatric disorders (e.g., psychopathologies such as autism, pervasive developmental disorder)
  Chromosomal disorders (e.g., fragile X syndrome)
Delayed onset of speech without obvious receptive language impairment
  Structural anomalies (e.g., cleft palate, choanal atresia)
  Neurophysiological and neurobehavioral organization disorders (e.g., cerebral palsy, oral apraxia, sequelae of prenatal cocaine exposure)
  Environmental factors (e.g., abuse or neglect, unusual child-rearing practices that discourage speech or language development, lack of experience or poor speech models)
  Attention deficit disorder with or without hyperactivity
  Idioglossia (associated with multiple births)
Disordered development of speech or language
  All factors listed in sections above
  Neuropathologies (e.g., brain damage, facial or glossal nerve paralysis)
  Psychopathologies (e.g., autism, schizophrenia, pervasive developmental disorder not otherwise specified, childhood disintegrative disorder)
  Regression or interrupted development (e.g., trauma, degenerative or progressive disease processes)
  Laryngeal pathologies (e.g., vocal cord stridor, laryngeal web, papillomatosis, damage residual to prolonged or repeated intubation, prolonged tracheostomy with resulting paresis of the vocal cords)
  Velopharyngeal incompetence or insufficiency and other structural anomalies of the oral and laryngeal mechanism
  Language-learning disability (novel within the index family)

preschools and child care centers, and public-health programs. This diversity obviously indicates that marketing efforts must be targeted to the specific entity, its consumer group(s), or both. Knowing the structure of the agency, the composition of its staff, programmatic goals, mission statements, and administrative philosophy is important to devising a successful marketing effort.

Many SLPs in private practice provide complimentary consultative services to their colleagues in private pediatric, otorhinolaryngology, plastic surgery, neurology, and family practices. It is highly unlikely that those medical practitioners will, on their own, seek information about the roles of SLPs with infants and their families. An excellent list of suggestions for interacting with pediatricians is provided by Richardson,[5] who is a pediatrician and former president of the American Speech-Language-Hearing Association (ASHA).

The role of the SLP or audiologist seems to assume more visibility after the expected age of speech onset is reached (i.e., 12 to 14 months), possibly because parents voice their own heightened concerns at or around that time. Unfortunately, there are some health care professionals who persist in advising families to wait until the child has reached the age of 3 years before taking steps to determine why speech has not emerged, especially if the child does not exhibit signs of cognitive deficits or physical anomalies.[5-7] It is obvious that we cannot relax our efforts to keep the professional community and parents advised of the importance of communication competence to the child's cognitive, emotional, social, and educational development.

Having on hand copies of recommended practices or position statements from professional organizations of professional colleagues in related disciplines is recommended. Excerpts from those documents authored by their professional peers relating to communication assessment and referral can be provided to practitioners. Your familiarity with their literature is also likely to establish confidence in your professionalism and strengthen bonds among members of the team. In addition to ASHA, key organizations that have published position papers and practice guidelines include:

- American Academy of Pediatrics[8-14]
- The Interdisciplinary Council on Developmental and Learning Disorders[15]
- American Academy of Neurology[16]
- Child Neurology Society[16]

▼ ONGOING MARKETING STRATEGIES

Marketing is a continuous process in which the SLP remains involved over the course of association with an agency or practice. Different goals and objectives are promoted at different times using different marketing tools. Some of the means by which the SLP can communicate effectively with professional colleagues and parent groups about the importance of early attention to communicative development include the following:

- Presentation at team or staff meetings or meetings of parent groups (seek invitations to targeted groups.)
- Circulation to colleagues or posting at the workplace of a "fact of the week" (or "day" or "month") regarding some aspect of child development, costs associated with care, assessment tips, new referral resources in the community
- Notices of useful Internet sites related to the interests of colleagues
- Short videotaped presentations prepared for viewing by team members at their convenience
- Distribution of reprints or copies of pertinent articles from professional journals to key associates with an informal note indicating that you think the colleague may be interested in the topic (depending on circumstances, highlighting passages may be appropriate.)
- Short articles prepared for in-house newsletters or other publications

- Participation in seminars, workshops, and staff development activities (be visible to colleagues at professional gatherings of this nature.)
- Following up on your referrals to other specialists by note, letter, phone, or personal visit
- Requesting permission to attend in-service programs put on for colleagues in related fields and then being there (a shared knowledge base is important.)
- Asking for input from colleagues about standards of care or management of a particular condition or problem; valuing their experience and expertise and letting them know that you do
- Acknowledging your awareness of the contributions of practitioners in other disciplines (e.g., Brazelton, Greenspan, Capute and Accardo, and Shonkoff and colleagues in medicine; outstanding contributors in psychology and other fields)
- Being visible to professional colleagues and community groups; introducing yourself by your professional title; providing your business card to people at appropriate times
- Sending short thank-you notes for professional courtesies; letting your colleagues know you notice and appreciate their assistance, encouragement, and interest
- Participating in events sponsored by agencies and organizations that support child development.

ASHA has developed specific materials to assist practitioners in devising marketing plans and identifying appropriate marketing tools.[17–20] See Appendix C, Table C-3, for information on obtaining these publications from ASHA.

▼ CONCLUSION

The first 36 months of life are the child's most critical developmental period. The rapid and interrelated changes that occur across physical, cognitive, social, and behavioral parameters are integral to development of the communication system. The communication system, in turn, facilitates other areas of maturation and growth and is the foundation on which school success relies. Early identification of children with atypical development is essential if the most effective management is to be a possibility.

Clinical experience and research efforts of professionals who represent many disciplines provide a developing body of information that assists in providing appropriate services to affected children and their families. Selected materials from that body of information are provided in the glossary and appendices that follow this chapter, which are designed to serve as a practical clinical reference. They are also meant to be a resource for practitioners, a stimulus for further exploration of the emerging literature of the field. They also may supply information for marketing efforts described in this chapter. The materials included address the following areas:

- Terminology used in serving pediatric populations (Glossary)
- Selected developmental norms and expectations; assessment materials (Appendix A)

- Infant feeding and oral motor information; intervention materials (Appendix B)
- Lead agencies in 50 states; addresses of selected national organizations (Appendix C)
- A guide to useful Internet sites (Appendix D)

▼ REFERENCES

1. Koyanagi C, Lorber M: Can managed care meet the mental health needs of very young children? *Infant Young Child* 10:38, 1997.
2. Sparks SN, et al: Infants at risk for communication disorders: the professionals' role with the newborn. Short course presented at American Speech-Language-Hearing Association Convention, Boston, November 1988.
3. McKenzie L: How to start a grassroots multidisciplinary neonatal intervention team. Presentation at Region IV Interagency Coordinating Council's Multidisciplinary Conference on Handicapped Infants and Toddlers, Lafayette, La, October 1990.
4. Banigan R: Letter to author, Nov 29, 1991.
5. Richardson SO: Pediatrics. In Haller RM, Sheldon N, editors: *Speech pathology and audiology in medical settings*, New York, 1976, Stratton Intercontinental Medical Books, p 37.
6. Alt E: Speech delay predictive of later problems [letter to the editor], *Exceptional Parent* 20:8, 1990.
7. Moon E: Speech delay predictive of later problems [letter to the editor], *Exceptional Parent* 20:7, 1990.
8. American Academy of Pediatrics. Policy statement: Advanced practice in neonatal nursing (RE9257), *AAP News* 9(7):17, 1992.
9. American Academy of Pediatrics: Policy statement: role of the primary care physician in the management of high-risk newborn infants, *Pediatrics* 98(4):786–788, 1996.
10. American Academy of Pediatrics: Policy statement: shaken baby syndrome: rotational cranial injuries—clinical report, *Pediatrics* 108(1):206–210, 2001.
11. American Academy of Pediatrics: Policy statement: role of the pediatrician in family-centered early intervention services, *Pediatrics* 107(5):1155–1157, 2001.
12. American Academy of Pediatrics: Policy statement: assessment of maltreatment of children with disabilities, *Pediatrics* 108(2):508–512, 2001.
13. American Academy of Pediatrics: Policy statement: noise: a hazard for the fetus and newborn, *Pediatrics* 100(4):724–727, 1997.
14. American Academy of Pediatrics: Policy statement: the physician's role in the diagnosis and management of autistic spectrum disorder in children, *Pediatrics* 107(5): 1221–1226, 2001.
15. Interdisciplinary Council on Developmental and Learning Disorders: ICDL clinical practice guidelines: redefining the standards of care for infants, children, and families with special needs, Bethesda, Md, 2000, ICDL Press. Also available for free download-ing at http://www.icdl.com.
16. Quality Standards Subcommittee of the American Academy of Neurology and the American Academy of Neurology: Practice parameter: screening and diagnosis of autism, *Neurology* 55:468–479, 2000.
17. American Speech-Language Hearing Association: *Marketing manual: a resource guide*, Rockville, Md, 1996, ASHA.
18. American Speech-Language Hearing Association: *Physician education program kit*, Rockville, Md, 1991, ASHA.
19. American Speech-Language Hearing Association: *Speech-language pathology marketing kit, person to person: making a difference*, Rockville, Md, 1991, ASHA.
20. American Speech-Language Hearing Association: *Marketing to multicultural audiences kit (speech-language pathology)*, Rockville, Md, 1992, ASHA.

NORMAL DEVELOPMENT AND INFANT ASSESSMENT TOOLS

▼ CONTENTS

Table A-1: Weight Conversion From Pounds and Ounces to Grams

Table A-2: The Cranial Nerves

Table A-3: Language and Brain Growth from Birth to 2 Years

Table A-4: Six Major Events in Central Nervous System Maturation, Neural Abnormalities, and Neuropsychological Consequences That Can Occur During Central Nervous System Maturation

Table A-5: Primitive and Postural Infantile Reflexes of the First Year

Table A-6: Infantile Oral Reflexes

Table A-7: Diagnostic Guide: Implications for Normal and Deviant Patterns of Language Development

Table A-8: Pragmatic Development in Infants and Toddlers

Table A-9: High-Risk Criteria for Referral, Assessment, and Management in Infant Feeding, Sucking, and Swallowing Disorders

Table A-10: Neonatal Assessment for Feeding and State Organization

Table A-11: Oral-Motor and Swallow Assessment and Intervention for Infants with Craniofacial Anomalies

Figure A-1: Risk History for Infants and Toddlers (Billeaud)

Figure A-2: Sample Form for Hospital-Based Multidisciplinary Evaluation (Louisiana Region II ICC Multidisciplinary Evaluation Project)

TABLE A-1
Weight Conversion From Pounds and Ounces to Grams

OUNCES

	0	1	2	3	4	5	6	7	8	9	10	11	12	13	14	15
0	0	28	57	85	113	142	170	198	227	255	283	312	340	369	397	425
1	454	482	510	539	567	595	624	652	680	709	737	765	794	822	850	879
2	907	936	964	992	1021	1049	1077	1106	1134	1162	1191	1219	1247	1276	1304	1332
3	1361	1389	1417	1446	1474	1503	1531	1559	1588	1616	1644	1673	1701	1729	1758	1786
4	1814	1843	1871	1899	1928	1956	1984	2013	2041	2070	2098	2126	2155	2183	2211	2240
5	2268	2296	2325	2353	2381	2410	2438	2466	2495	2523	2551	2580	2608	2637	2665	2693
6	2722	2750	2778	2807	2835	2863	2892	2920	2948	2977	3005	3033	3062	3090	3118	3147
7	3175	3203	3232	3260	3289	3317	3345	3374	3402	3430	3459	3487	3515	3544	3572	3600
8	3629	3657	3685	3714	3742	3770	3799	3827	3856	3884	3912	3941	3969	3997	4026	4054
9	4082	4111	4139	4167	4196	4224	4252	4281	4309	4337	4366	4394	4423	4451	4479	4508
10	4536	4564	4593	4621	4649	4678	4706	4734	4763	4791	4819	4848	4876	4904	4933	4961
11	4990	5018	5046	5075	5103	5131	5160	5188	5216	5245	5273	5301	5330	5358	5386	5415
12	5443	5471	5500	5528	5557	5585	5613	5642	5670	5698	5727	5755	5783	5812	5840	5868

TABLE A-2
The Cranial Nerves

Number	Name	Summary of Function
I	Olfactory	Smell
II	Optic	Vision
III	Oculomotor	Innervation of muscles to move eyeball, pupil, and upper lid
IV	Trochlear	Innervation of superior oblique muscle of eye
V	Trigeminal	Chewing and sensation to face
VI	Abducens	Abduction of eye
VII	Facial	Movement of facial muscles, taste, salivary glands
VIII	(Vestibular) acoustic	Equilibrium and hearing
IX	Glossopharyngeal	Taste, swallowing, elevation of pharynx and larynx, parotid salivary gland, sensation to upper pharynx
X	Vagus	Taste, swallowing, elevation of palate, phonation, parasympathetic outflow to visceral organs
XI	Accessory	Turning of head and shrugging of shoulders
XII	Hypoglossal	Movement of tongue

From Love R, Webb W: *Neurology for the speech-language pathologist,* ed 3, Boston, 1996, Butterworth-Heinemann, p 140.

TABLE A-3
Language and Brain Growth From Birth to 2 Years

Age	Language Milestones	Brain Weight in Grams
Birth	Crying	335
3 months	Cooing and crying	516
6 months	Babbling	660
9 months	Voicing intonated jargon	750
12 months	Approximating first word	9225
18 months	Early naming	1024
24 months	Making two-word combinations	1064

From Love R, Webb W: *Neurology for the speech-language pathologist,* ed 3, Boston, 1996, Butterworth-Heinemann, p 257.

TABLE A-4

Six Major Events in Central Nervous System Maturation, Neural Abnormalities, and Neuropsychological Consequences That Can Occur During Central Nervous System Maturation

Major Events and Time Period (Listed in Sequential Order)	Etiology of Neural Abnormalities	Neuropsychological Consequences*
1. Dorsal induction (18–26 gestation days)	Disorders of neural tube closure	Meningomyelocele and anencephaly, profoundly impaired
2. Ventral induction (4–10 gestation wk)	a. Brain fails to make normal cleavage	Holoprosencephaly, seizures, profoundly impaired
	b. Cyst separates cerebellar hemispheres	Mental retardation, other brain anomalies
3. Proliferation of neurons (2–4 gestation mo)	a. Head size 2–3 SD below mean, arrested cell division, chromosome abnormality	Microcephaly syndromes, mild to moderate mental retardation, possible cleft lip and cleft palate
	b. Early cessation of cell division	Microcephaly, fetal alcohol syndrome, cognitive impairments
4a. Migration of neurons (8 gestation wk)	Bilateral cleft of cerebral hemispheres, all six cortical layers not formed	Schizencephaly, multiple congenital abnormalities, seizures, sensorimotor deficits
4b. Migration of neurons (11–13 gestation wk)	Smooth brain, few gyri, all six cortical layers not formed, neurons in abnormal locations	Lissencephaly, profoundly impaired, seizures, microcephalic, most die in infancy
4c. Migration of neurons (2–5 gestation mo)	Failure to develop fibers crossing between cerebral hemispheres	Agenesis of corpus callosum, developmentally delayed, seizures
4d. Migration of neurons (4–5 gestation mo)	Multiple small shallow convolutions on brain surface, neurons in abnormal location	Polymicrogyria, possible mental retardation and seizure disorder

From Hallett T, Proctor A: Maturation of the central nervous system as related to communication and cognitive development, *Infants Young Child* 8:3, 1996. Copyright © 1996 by Aspen Publishers.

*Communication, speech, and/or language disorders and cognitive deficits are associated with the neuropsychological consequences(s).

SD, Standard deviation.

TABLE A-5
Primitive and Postural Infantile Reflexes of the First Year

Reflex	Response
Asymmetric tonic neck reflex	Infant extends limbs on chin side and flexes on occiput side when turning head
Symmetric tonic neck reflex	Infant extends arms and flexes legs with head extension
Positive support reflex	Infant bears weight when balls of feet are stimulated
Tonic labyrinthine reflex	Infant may retract shoulder and extend neck and trunk with neck flexion; tongue thrust reflex may occur
Segmental rolling reflex	Infant may roll trunk and pelvis segmentally with rotation of head or legs
Galant reflex	Infant arches body when skin of back is stimulated near vertebral column.
Moro's reflex	Infant may adduce arm and move it upward, followed by arm flexion and leg extension

From Love R, Webb W: *Neurology for the speech-language pathologist*, ed 3, Boston, 1996, Butterworth-Heinemann, p 278.

TABLE A-6
Infantile Oral Reflexes

Reflex	Stimulus	Age of Appearance	Age of Disappearance
Rooting	Oral area being touched	Birth	3–6 mo
Suckling	Nipple in mouth	Birth	6–12 mo
Swallowing	Bolus of food in pharynx	Birth	Persists
Tongue	Tongue or lips being touched	Birth	12–18 mo
Bite	Pressure on gums	Birth	9–12 mo
Gag	Tongue or pharynx being touched	Birth	Persists

From Love R, Webb W: *Neurology for the speech-language pathologist*, ed 3, Boston, 1996, Butterworth-Heinemann, p 288.

TABLE A-7
Diagnostic Guide: Implications for Normal and Deviant Patterns of Language Development*

	Normal Pattern of Language Development	Deviant Pattern of Language Development in the Clinical Population
Rate	Rapid, samples changing every 3 wk	Slow, consecutive samples similar
Jargon	Intermittent, ceases by 27 mo	Predominant feature continuing beyond 30 mo
Echoing	Intermittent, ceases by 29 mo	Predominant feature continuing beyond 36 mo
Single words	Varies by 12–18 mo	Only nouns beyond 24 mo
Nonverbal cues	Primarily on words or word phrases	Consistent for negative or questions beyond 30 mo
Verbal play	Ceases by 29 mo	Continuing beyond 36 mo
Verbal experimentation	Primarily for phrases and constructions	None or limited
Concepts		
Social terms	By 24 mo	None by 30 mo
Body parts	By 22 mo	None by 24 mo
Numbers	By 20 mo	None by 24 mo
Colors	By 35 mo	None by 42 mo
Announcing action	By 25 mo	None by 30 mo
Self-correcting errors	By 36 mo	None by 48 mo
Commands 100 utterances	By 23 mo	Not by 24 mo
Single words decrease as sentences increase	From 18–23 mo	No decrease of single words by 24 mo
Developmental Sentence Scoring (DSS) becomes valid	By 28 mo	Not valid by 30 mo
DSS and mean sentence length (MSL)	Not growing together, illness affecting only MSL	Growing together, illness affecting DSS
Growth of complexity exceeds growth in length	By 36 mo	Not by 42 mo
Half of sentences correct	By 36 mo	Not by 42 mo
Sentence types	Using declaratives, imperatives, interrogatives by 36 mo	Using only declaratives beyond 36 mo
Simple, compound, complex sentences	By 36 mo	Only simple sentences beyond 36 mo
Past tense		
Irregular	By 29 mo	None by 30 mo
Regular	By 34 mo	None by 36 mo
Overgeneralization	By 36 mo	None by 40 mo
Future tense	By 30 mo	None by 30 mo
Indefinite pronouns		
It, this, that	By 18 mo	None by 24 mo
One, some, other	By 24 mo	None by 24 mo
Somebody, something	By 36 mo	None by 36 mo

TABLE A-7
Diagnostic Guide: Implications for Normal and Deviant Patterns of Language Development*—Cont'd

	Normal Pattern of Language Development	Deviant Pattern of Language Development in the Clinical Population
Personal pronouns		
You	By 27 mo	None by 30 mo
They	By 34 mo	None by 42 mo
He, those	By 36 mo	None by 36 mo
We	By 36 mo	None by 42 mo
Verbs		
Can + verb	By 31 mo	None by 36 mo
Are, will, do + verb	By 36 mo	None by 48 mo
Am + verb + -ing	By 36 mo	None by 48 mo
Negatives		
Can't, don't used in sentences	By 36 mo	None by 36 mo
Conjunction and connecting objects and sentences	By 36 mo	None by 36 mo
Questions		
Who? what? where?	By 27 mo	None by 30 mo
Where + subject + -ing	By 36 mo	None by 36 mo
What + subject + -ing	By 36 mo	None by 42 mo

From Trantham CR, Pederson JK: *Normal language development: the key to diagnosis and therapy for language-disordered children,* Baltimore, Md, 1976, Williams & Wilkins, p 33.
*The normal pattern column gives the upper age limit of the normal range; the deviant pattern column indicates strikingly different patterns characteristic of language-impaired children.

TABLE A-8
Pragmatic Development in Infants and Toddlers

0–12 Months	1–2 Years	2–3 Years
1. Attempts to imitate the gestures and vocalizations of adults	1. Uses nonverbal communication to signify intent:	1. Ideational options—learning to express own experience of the phenomena of the external world and the internal world of own consciousness
2. Uses vocalizations in play for self-amusement	To request (reaching toward the object)	Learns to be an observer. Begins to use language as a way of talking about the real world
3. Uses telegraphic devices (rising intonation, vocalization with specifications of desires, negating, imperatives, interrogatives) accompanied by gestures and intonation markers	To draw attention to object (pointing, showing)	2. Interpersonal communication. Begins to participate in conversational situations. Learns to adopt a role to express opinions and personality. Dialogue begins
4. Uses onomatopoetic speech (words that sound like the object to mean the object)	To draw attention to self (vocalizing)	3. Can make what he or she says operational in the communicative context
5. Uses perlocutionary behaviors—signals issued by one person that have an effect on the listener that is not necessarily intended (e.g., crying, laughing)	To request transfer (reaching toward another person)	4. Begins to use definite versus indefinite articles (i.e., *the* versus *a* or *an*). Often uses *the* incorrectly. Assumes the listener knows what he or she is talking about
6. Crying takes on different meanings; is directive for parent and later for child (angry, hungry, cranky). Used to communicate events and needs of infant	To show dislike (falling tone [intonational pattern])	5. Can judge quality of language 50% of the time (e.g., polite versus impolite). Does not use consistently
7. Uses illocutionary behavior—signals to carry out some socially organized action (i.e., intentional communication)	To show disappearance (slapping or waving)	6. Uses more action identity tags (e.g., "bow wow," "meow," "choo-choo")
8. Picks up an object and shows it	To show rejection (negative head shake)	7. Some role playing is possible. Takes caregiver's place (e.g., if the mother says, "I can't," the child says, "yes, you can")
9. Uses pointing to pick things out and to obtain someone's attention	To indicate pleasure (surprise, recognition, smile)	
	2. Performatives emerge—child uses language with communicative intent; the child may know what is wanted, but the meaning is not necessarily clear to the listener	
	3. Presuppositions also emerge—common shared information regardless of phonetic information; child uses expressions that have shared meaning to both speaker and listener	
	4. Begins talking about the inanimate world	

10. Uses gestures communicatively and starts to perceive reactions (making sure listener is attentive before continuing)
11. Responds to pointing as a communicative gesture (looks in direction adult is pointing instead of focusing on that individual's face or hand)
12. Uses pointing to learn new vocabulary—people in the environment label things for the child
13. Realizes vocalizations of intonation and articulation have meaning for adults, so borrows some of their sounds ("mama," "dada") and also makes up own meanings for vocalizations. They have content and expression
14. Nonverbal vocalizations have functions:
    (1) Instrumental "I want" (satisfies personal needs)
    (2) Regulatory "Do it" (seeks to control behaviors of others)—interactional, personal, heuristic, imaginative

5. Uses of early words to signify communicative intent:
   Requesting ("milk")
   Possession ("mine")
   Imperatives ("up")
   Problems ("hurt")
   Statements ("shoe")
   Give objects ("gimme")
   Locations ("there")
   Desires ("I want")
6. At one-word stage—expresses only what's new to child. At two-word stage—expresses new information and given information (uses vocal stress to tell which is which)
7. Vocabulary—transition from own language to adult language; learns that certain sounds have certain meanings
8. Dialogue—acquires a grammatical structure; can be both speaker and listener; learns some rules of discourse ("when someone talks, you should listen")
9. Uses increasing tone in inflectional pattern
10. Literally interprets the things heard; can't play with words
11. Verbal turn-taking
12. Functions; mathetic; pragmatic; informative

8. Repetition used for:
   Answering questions (e.g., Do you want milk? "Milk.")
   Commenting (e.g., We're having hot dogs. "Hot dogs.")
   Affirming (e.g., We're building a fire. "Oh, go build fire.")
   Self-informing (e.g., We're cooking sausages.")
   Querying (e.g., Put that on top. "On top?")
   Imitating (e.g., Hi. "Hi." I'm a good cook. Yes, the greatest. "The greatest.")
   Reverse directions of an order (e.g., You do it. "No, you do it.")
   Reverse directions of an information question (e.g., Where's the spoon? "Mommy, where's the spoon?")
   Clarification of an utterance (e.g., Fab. "Fab, what you mean?")
9. Acquires morphemes—Uses concepts of past and present inconsistently
10. At two-word stage: Word combinations are used to express these functions:
    Identification (e.g., "See doggie.")
    Location (e.g., "Book there.")
    Repetition (see above)
    Nonexistence (e.g., "All gone thing.")
    Negation (e.g., "Not wolf.")
    Possession (e.g., "My candy.")
    Attribution (e.g., "Big car.")
    Question (e.g., "Where ball?")
11. Functions: ideation, interpersonal, textual

From Shulman BB: *Pragmatic development chart*, Mobile, Ala, 1991.

TABLE A-9
High-Risk Criteria for Referral, Assessment, and Management in Infant Feeding, Sucking, and Swallowing Disorders*

High-Risk Criteria

Prematurity (26 wk or less)
Small for gestational age
Apgar of less than 7 at 5 min
Seizures
Sepsis or meningitis
Phototherapy or transfusion
Ventilator therapy
Prolonged hypotonia or hypertonia beyond 24 hr
Recurrent apnea
Congenital anomalies
Congenital or perinatal infections
Poor endurance for feeding
Abnormal or poor suck
Fussy, overstimulated, or disorganized baby
Drug or alcohol abuse (maternal)
Post extracorporeal mechanical oxygenation
5%–7% loss of birth weight

Sequence for Assessment

Gather birth history
Handle infant to assess tone
Elicit oral reflexes
Assess non-nutritive suck
Apply intervention techniques to establish the best possible performance in all areas
Gather information from parents:
  Is this a typical feeding?
  What is the child's feeding usually like?
  Is the child gaining weight appropriately?
  How long does a feeding usually take?
  How much does the child usually eat at one feeding?
  How does the child deal with solid foods?
  What is the child's sleep and awake pattern like?

*Candidates for feeding assessment are infants who meet identified high-risk criteria. The criteria listed here are those used at the Mapleton Center in Boulder, Colo. They were developed by Beth Landry Murphy as part of the Neonatal Assessment of Feeding and State Organization.

TABLE A-10
Neonatal Assessment for Feeding and State Organization

Name: _____   Parent or guardian: _____
DOB: _____   Date of initial assessment: _____
Chronological age: _____
Corrected age: _____
Apgar: 1 _____   2 _____
O_2: _____
Weight: _____
Significant medical history

Course of Feeding

IV: _____
Gavage: _____   How often? _____
Breast: _____
Bottle: _____   Nipple used: _____
Receiving therapeutic treatment? _____

Oral Reflexes

Reflex	Method to Elicit	Pass	Fail
Root open	Stroke front of lips	Mouth opens or suck begins	No opening or suck is seen
Root open and turn (integrated at 3 mo)	Stroke side of cheek	Head turns to side stroked, and mouth opens with or without suck	No head turning and no open or suck is seen
Suck initiation	Place finger in mouth	Suck begins strong and immediate	No suck is initiated, or suck is weak
Swallow	Give small amount of milk or observe during feeding	Swallow is immediate after three or four sucks	Swallow is not seen after seven or more sucks
Hand to mouth	Observe child	Hand to mouth is seen purposively without assistance or wrapping	Hand to mouth is not seen
Bite	Place finger in mouth	No bite is felt	Bite is felt
Gag	Observe during above procedures and during feed	Gag is not observed, or a weak gag may be seen	Gag is observed

Techniques to Improve Oral Motor Function

Techniques to facilitate oral reflexes
To reduce bite:
   Rub gums in four quadrants; wait for swallow
To reduce gag:
   Use firm pressure when touching
   Massage cheeks in small circles
   Use finger and place some milk in buccal pocket then massage cheek
   Rub gums with milk on finger or nipple
   Gradually and firmly stroke the tongue from back to front at midline
   "Walk" back on tongue

Continued

TABLE A-10
Neonatal Assessment for Feeding and State Organization—Cont'd

Techniques to Improve Oral Motor Function—Cont'd

To improve root and open:
   Touch lip with bottle, nipple, or finger and give a long pause to allow mouth to open
   Place small amount of fluid on lip and wait for open and possibly suck
   Press firmly in the palm of the baby's hand (palmomental reflex)
To increase hand to mouth:
   Swaddle infant
   Keep infant's shoulders and arms rolled forward
   Assist hand to mouth to console baby

Techniques to improve jaw control and movement
Stroke massage forward from back of jaw to front
Apply quick, firm taps under chin
Flexed body position
Give jaw stabilization when feeding by placing finger under jaw

Techniques to improve normal tongue position and movement
Stroke tongue from back to front at midline and sides
"Walk" back on tongue
Let baby suck on your finger when non-nutritive sucking; if tongue is humped, apply firm
   pressure to midtongue blade
To continue tongue movement, apply firm strokes under chin and move finger back to front

Techniques to improve lip movement
Massage cheeks and lips
Snap lips
Lip flicks
Hold cheeks and pull forward with nippling
Give jaw support
Keep the infant's head flexed forward and chin tucked

Techniques to Improve Coordination

Use tongue, jaw, and lip techniques
Reduce all external stimulation
If the child is 3–4 mo or older, provide a distraction, especially if initiation is difficult
   (e.g., television, music, toy)
Provide rhythm with movement
Determine the baby's rhythm and try to impose a rhythm depending on skill level
Pump the bottle then pause, remove the bottle or tip it back until the baby swallows
Allow pauses when the infant is panting, disorganized, or fatigued
Impose pauses in the feed as above
Try a Haberman feeder if swallow is good but suck is poor due to initiation, suction, or
   expression difficulties
Experiment with a variety of nipples. Give a preemie nipple if weak suck and fatigue are
   factors
A cardiac baby may nipple better when positioned in more extension
Hold baby at an incline of less than 45 degrees

From Landry MB: *Neonatal assessment of feeding and state organization,* Boulder, Colo, 1990, NAFSO.

TABLE A-11
Oral-Motor and Swallow Assessment and Intervention for Infants With Craniofacial Anomalies

All neonates have two basic needs to sustain life: respiration and nutrition. An interdisciplinary team is needed to deal with the complex issues presented by infants with craniofacial anomalies. The speech-language pathologist (SLP) has a major role on the team as decisions are made regarding management of oral-motor function, which underlies later speech development. The SLP's role also includes contributing information and guidance regarding early communicative development, much of which occurs during the infant's feedings. The outline below highlights issues that must be addressed in providing appropriate care to infants who have craniofacial anomalies.

I. Interdisciplinary team for feeding
   A. Neonatologist: overall status
   B. Otolaryngologist: airway
   C. Nutritionist: dietary issues
   D. SLP: oral-motor function and communication
   E. Occupational therapist: positioning and tone
   F. Nursing: primary feeding
   G. Maxillofacial: consideration of prosthesis
   H. Social worker: family issues

II. Assessment
   A. Tone (overall and oral-motor)
   B. Cleft
   C. Neurologic status (e.g., alertness, evidence of sequelae of syndromes, structural anomalies)
   D. Communication and bonding
   E. Structure (e.g., tracheoesophageal fistula, syndromic/structural anomalies)

III. Oral-motor assessment
   A. Lips, mandible, tongue, and palate for symmetry, strength, and coordination
   B. Cleft factors: width, length, location, surrounding structures, and tissues
   C. Oral-motor function correlated with anatomy
      1. Generation of negative intraoral pressure
      2. Movement against nipple
      3. Deficits matched to feeding devices

IV. Oral feeding guidelines (stable airway and neurologically normal)
   A. Upright position
   B. Haberman feeder (Medela, Inc., P.O. Box 386, Crystal Lake, IL 60014; phone: [800] 435-8316), which allows infant or feeder to control flow of milk with a specially designed valving system.
   C. Large X-cut nipple with careful placement
   D. Frequent burping
   E. Small frequent feedings (i.e., 30 min maximum)
   F. Applying external pressure to cheeks and mandible
   G. Rule of thumb for quantity at 1–2 wk of age: 30 cc (3 oz)/1b/day

V. Breast feeding with cleft
   A. Isolated cleft lip: some success
   B. Isolated cleft palate: usually difficult
   C. Complete cleft lip and palate: very difficult

VI. Palatal feeding prostheses
   A. Indications
      1. Large bilateral cleft lip and palate
      2. Insufficient seal with nipple
      3. Feeding problems for longer than 2–3 weeks

Continued

Table A-11
Oral-Motor and Swallow Assessment and Intervention for Infants With Craniofacial Anomalies—Cont'd

VI. Palatal feeding prostheses—Cont'd
  B. Purposes
    1. Aid in deglutition
    2. Aid in correct tongue position
    3. Enhance sucking pattern
    4. Prevent collapse of arches
    5. Ease burden on nursing staff
  C. Precautions
    1. Irritation of mucous membrane
    2. Edema of mucous membrane
    3. Not an aid in preventing otitis media
    4. Replacement needed with growth
    5. Oral hygiene

VII. Nonoral feeders
  A. Airway compromise (Robin malformation sequence)
    1. *U*-shaped palatal cleft
    2. Micrognathia
    3. Glossoptosis
    4. Upper-airway obstruction
  B. Prematurity (low birth weight with neurologic impairment)
    1. Depressed sucking reflex
    2. Weak suck (trisomy 21 syndrome, Mobius' sequence, Arnold-Chiari malformation, clefting)
    3. Uncoordinated suck (central nervous system asphyxia, Arnold-Chiari malformation)

VIII. Types of nonoral feeding
  A. Orogastric feeding
  B. Nasogastric feeding
  C. Gastrostomy

IX. Treatment for nonoral feeders
  A. Oral-motor stimulation
    1. Stroking rhythmically
    2. Nonnutritive sucking
  B. Goals with tube feeders
    1. Improved postural control
    2. Improved pharyngeal airway control
    3. Touch and movement used communicatively
    4. Response to normalization
    5. Rhythmic suck, swallow, and respiratory pattern
    6. Reduction of gastroesophageal reflux
    7. Improved tone and movement in face
    8. Use of lips and tongue to explore environment
    9. Sound-play facilitation
    10. Total communication approach in learning environment

X. Feeding in the postoperative period
  A. Lip surgery
    1. Cup into side of mouth away from cleft
    2. Syringe with soft tubing
    3. Breast feeding

TABLE A-11
Oral-Motor and Swallow Assessment and Intervention for Infants With Craniofacial Anomalies—Cont'd

X. Feeding in the postoperative period—Cont'd
   B. Palate surgery
      1. Cup feeding (duration variable per surgeon)
      2. No chewable food
      3. No pacifiers, straws, spoons, forks, or "tippy" cups
   C. Sequence for texture changes
      1. First 4–6 mo: formula
      2. Between 4 and 6 mo: strained baby food
      3. 10–11 mo: lumpy foods (these are more difficult to introduce if delayed to 14–16 mo)

From Arvedson JC: Presentation given at the 1990 ASHA Convention, Seattle, November 1990.
Sources:
A. Finger IM, Guerra LR. Provisional restoration in maxillofacial prosthetics, *Dental Clinics of North America* 1989;3:435, 1989.
B. Morris S, Klein MD: *Prefeeding skills*, Austin, Tex, 1987, Pro-Ed.
C. Weatherly-White RCA: Surgical timing and postoperative feeding in the cleft-lip child. In Kernahan DA, Rosenstein SW, editors: *Cleft lip and palate: a system of management*, Baltimore, 1990, Williams & Wilkins.
NOTE: See also Rothschile MA, editor: *Otologic Clin North Am Syndromic Congenital Anomalies Head Neck* 33(6), 2000 and Wolf LS, Glass RP: *Feeding and swallowing disorders in infancy: assessment and management*, Tucson, Ariz, 1992, Communication Skill Builders.

Name of child: _____ DOB: _____
Gestational age at birth: _____ Birth weight: ____g *or* ____lbs ____oz
Where delivered? _____ Apgar at 1 min: _____ 5 min _____
By whom delivered? _____ Birth order in family: _____
Type delivery: Vgn _____ C-sec _____ Brch _____Ftlng _____ Stargaze _____
        Multiple _____ (# of sibs _____) Other_____
List known complications: _____
Parent(s) name(s): _____
        _____ Natural   _____ Adoptive   _____ Foster
Mailing address: _____
Home address: _____
Phone: _____(H) _____ (Mo.B) _____ (Fr.B)
Child's present physician(s): _____ Address: _____
Name and position of person completing this form: _____
Who referred child/family here? _____
Services being requested:_____

Did mother receive regular prenatal care? _____Y   _____N

Potential Risk Factor Checklist

Verify presence or absence of every item. Enter annotations for any "yes" item; provide specifics from interview, medical records, or both; attach information to this form as necessary.

Maternal Factors	*Yes*	*No*	*Annotations*
Previous preterm births	_____	_____	_____
Repeated miscarriages	_____	_____	_____
Miscarriage adjacent to this Pregnancy	_____	_____	_____
Stillbirth(s)	_____	_____	_____

▼ **Figure A-1**   Risk History: Long Form

Maternal Factors	Yes	No	Annotations
Unexplained fetal or neonatal deaths (e.g., sudden infant death syndrome)	_____	_____	_____
Cervical incompetence	_____	_____	_____
Placental abnormalities	_____	_____	_____
Genetic disease or chromosomal disorders	_____	_____	_____
Infections in first trimester	_____	_____	_____
Blood group problems (i.e., Rh incompatibility)	_____	_____	_____
Toxemia of pregnancy	_____	_____	_____
Unexplained bleeding	_____	_____	_____
Significantly high or low blood pressure	_____	_____	_____
Maternal diabetes	_____	_____	_____
Maternal seizures	_____	_____	_____
Medications, drugs, or alcohol	_____	_____	Please specify: _____
Other conditions	_____	_____	What and When: _____

Labor, Delivery, and Perinatal Factors	Yes	No	Annotations
Abnormal length of pregnancy	_____	_____	Term: _____
Long or short labor	_____	_____	Length: _____
Instruments used at delivery	_____	_____	
Low birth weight (LBW) or very low birth weight (VLBW)	_____	_____	<2500 g _____ <1500 g _____ <1000 g _____
Intrauterine growth retardation	_____	_____	_____
Hyperbilirubinemia (jaundice)	_____	_____	_____
Meconium staining or aspiration	_____	_____	_____
Central nervous system disorders	_____	_____	_____
Abnormal muscle tone	_____	_____	Hypotonicity _____ Hypertonicity _____ Asymmetry _____
Breathing problems	_____	_____	Hypoxia _____ Anoxia _____ Cyanosis _____
Oxygen supplement	_____	_____	For how long? _____
Abnormal head size	_____	_____	Macrocephaly _____ Microcephaly _____ Asymmetry _____
Convulsions	_____	_____	When? _____ Type: _____
Apnea	_____	_____	_____
Excessive irritability	_____	_____	_____
Abnormal reflex patterns	_____	_____	
Respiratory distress	_____	_____	BPD _____ Other: _____
Gastrointestinal problems	_____	_____	_____
Poor sucking and swallowing	_____	_____	_____
Orogastric or nasogastric feeding	_____	_____	_____
Poor weight gain (e.g., failure to thrive)	_____	_____	_____
Neonatal infections (e.g., human immunodeficiency virus, cytomegalovirus, sepsis, TORCH)	_____	_____	What? _____
Generalized edema	_____	_____	_____
Intracranial hemorrhage	_____	_____	Grade III _____ Grade IV _____
Congenital anomalies	_____	_____	List: _____
NICU admission?	_____	_____	Length of stay: _____
Postnatal drug exposure	_____	_____	To what? _____
Medications administered	_____	_____	Specify: _____
Surgeries performed	_____	_____	Specify: _____
Other conditions and observations worthy of note	_____	_____	Specify: _____

▼ **Figure A-1** *Cont'd*

Developmental Factors	Yes	No	Annotations
Serious illnesses	_____	_____	What: _____ When:_____
Serious trauma or injury	_____	_____	What: _____ when: _____
Inattention to sounds	_____	_____	At what age? _____
Known ear infections	_____	_____	When? _____ Treament:_____
Inattention to visual stimuli	_____	_____	At what age? _____
Known visual impairment	_____	_____	Age DX'd: _____Type: _____

Delayed Pattern of Development Relating to Specific Factors	Yes	No	Annotations
Motor skills	_____	_____	_____
Social skills	_____	_____	_____
Speech and language skills	_____	_____	_____
Adaptive behavior	_____	_____	_____
Failure to thrive	_____	_____	_____
Clinical manifestation of undiagnosed anomaly?	_____	_____	_____
Sleep disturbances	_____	_____	_____
Eating, chewing, or swallowing disorders	_____	_____	_____

Other Factors	Yes	No	Annotations
Family HX for genetic or educational problems (e.g., learning disability, reading problems, mental retardation)	_____	_____	Specify: _____
Exposure to environmental hazards (e.g., metals, toxic fumes)	_____	_____	_____
Handicapped sibling	_____	_____	_____
Other handicapped relatives	_____	_____	_____
Known allergies	_____	_____	_____
Physical abuse or neglect	_____	_____	_____

Psychosocial Factors	Yes	No	Annotations
Low family income	_____	_____	_____
Educational level of mother	_____	_____	Last grade completed: _____
Emotional abuse or neglect	_____	_____	_____
Little or no opportunity for stimulation	_____	_____	_____
Low intelligence	_____	_____	_____
Speech or language impairment	_____	_____	_____
Vision impairment	_____	_____	_____
Other (list):	_____	_____	_____

Other comments and observations to be considered:

_____
_____
_____
_____
_____

List other pertinent reports received:

_____
_____
_____
_____
_____

List other pertinent reports to be obtained and from whom:

_____
_____
_____
_____
_____

▼ **Figure A-1** *Cont'd*

Child's name: _____ DOB: _____ Date of evaluation: _____
Parent(s) name(s): _____ Birth weight: _____g Gestational age: _____
Address: _____ Phone: _____
Hospital family service coordinator: _____
School system contact: _____
Primary medical provider (after hospital discharge): _____
_____ meets criteria for services under Part H of the Infant and Toddler
      (child's name)   Act due to the following:

Criteria A

Established medical condition
    _____ Genetic disorder
              Specify: _____
    _____ Congenital or neonatal
              infections or infections
              with a high probability of
              resulting developmental
              delay
              Specify: _____
    _____ Sensory impairment
              Specify: _____

Developmental

Screening done in neonatal intensive care unit

Screening	Date	Results
PKU	_____	_____
T_4/TSH	_____	_____
(thyroid		
profile)		
Hbg. Elect	_____	_____
Vision	_____	_____
Cranial	_____	_____
Ultrasound	_____	_____

Criteria B

Biologically at risk
    _____ Birth weight less than 1000 g
    _____ Birth weight less than 1250 g
              with complicating factors
              requiring level III neonatal
              intensive care unit care
    _____ Hypoxic ischemic
              encephalopathy
    _____ Intraventricular hemorrhage
              grade III or IV or
              periventricular leukomalacia
    _____ Technology dependence that
              is likely to result in later
              developmental delay
    _____ Exposure to known
              teratogens or drugs and
              findings on effects
    _____ Chronic or degenerative
              orthopedic conditions,
              neurological conditions, or
              both that have a high
              probability of developmental
              delays
              Specify: _____

Status of child's developmental functioning in the following areas: physical status (i.e., motor, vision, hearing), cognitive, language and speech, self-help:
_____
_____
_____
_____

Identification of Family's and Child's Strengths and Needs

Family's strengths as related to enhancing their child's development:
_____
_____
_____
_____

Family's needs as related to enhancing their child's development:
_____
_____
_____
_____

Child's needs:
_____
_____
_____
_____

▼ **Figure A-2** Sample form for Hospital-Based Multidisciplinary Evaluation. From the Louisiana Region II Interagency Coordinating Council Multidisciplinary Evaluation Project, Baton Rouge, La, 1992.

Individualized Family Service Plan Considerations

———— Family service coordinator
———— Early interventionist
———— Counseling
———— Nutritionist
———— Diagnostic and programmatic assessment
———— Referral to: ————————————————
———— Other: ——————————————————
————————————————————————
————————————————————————

Additional Comments

————————————————————————————————
————————————————————————————————
————————————————————————————————
————————————————————————————————
————————————————————————————————

Evaluation Participants

—————————————————   —————————————————
Parent(s)   Physician

—————————————————   —————————————————
Social worker   Nurse

—————————————————   —————————————————
Other   Other

Hospital-to-Home Discharge Planning: Individual Family Service Plan

Child Medical Needs

Pediatrician: ————————————   Ophthalmologist: ————————————
Cardiologist: ————————————   Neurologist: ———————————————
Audiologist: —————————————   Orthopedist: ——————————————
Pediatric surgeon: ————————   Geneticist: ————————————————
Home health: ———————————   Lab follow-up: ———————————————
Home monitoring: —————————   Respiratory support: ————————————

Child Educational Needs

Nutritional consultation: —————————   Occupational therapy: ————————————
Physical therapy: ——————————   Speech therapy: ———————————————
Developmental assessment: ————————   Educational programming: ———————————

Discharge Planning Participants
The following participated in this individualized family service plan:
Signature   *Title*   *Agency*   *Date*

————————————————————————————————
————————————————————————————————
————————————————————————————————
————————————————————————————————

Hospital-to-Home Discharge Planning: Individualized Family Service Plan

Child's name: ——————————————————————————————
Family: ———————————————————————————————————

Family needs   **Date**   **Person responsible**
————— Family service coordinator
————— Community service information
————— Parent training
————— Transportation
————— Financial
————— Other needs

Special instructions:

▼ **Figure A-2** *Cont'd*

APPENDIX B

ASSESSMENT AND INTERVENTION TOOLS AND PROCEDURES

▼ CONTENTS

Table B-1: Expanded List of Tools for Assessment of Early Communication Skills

Figure B-1: Infant-Toddler Checklist for Communication and Language Development

Figure B-2: Cue Questions in Assessment of Communicative Means and Functions

Table B-2: Assessment Framework for Parents and Professionals: Identifying Areas of Child Competency and Difficulty

Table B-3: Assisting Parents to Identify and Describe Their Child's Areas of Competency and Difficulties

Table B-4: A Method for Describing Interaction Styles of Handicapped Prelanguage Children

Table B-5: Communicative Temptations

Table B-6: Strategies for Communication Enhancement from the CSBS Model

TABLE B-1
Expanded List of Tools for Assessment of Early Communication Skills

(See Chapter 7 for list of assessment tools for children suspected of having autism spectrum disorders and Chapter 8 for a basic list of assessment tools.)

Instrument	Reference	Features	Recommended Age Group
Assessment of Preterm Infant Behavior (APIB)	Als et al, 1982[1]	APIB was initially designed to be the downward extension of the Neonatal Behavioral Assessment Scale and requires training to administer appropriately.	APIB is used to assess behaviors of premature infants in the hospital setting.
Battelle Developmental Inventory (BDI)	Newborg et al, 1984[12]	BDI uses observation, structured interaction, and caregiver interviews to determine the child's developmental levels across many developmental domains, including communications.	Birth–8 yr
Bayley Scales of Infant Development	Bayley, 1993[2]	This assessment tool compares behaviors of newborns with norms derived from scores of normally developing age peers. It is recommended for infants without known anomalies.	2–30 mo
Clinical Linguistic and Auditory Milestones Scale (CLAMS)	Capute and Accardo, 1978[6]	The format is similar to a physician's standard growth chart. CLAMS is designed for use by physicians during child's office visits with parent acting as informant. CLAMS follows trajectories of communication skill development. The profile indicates whether the child is meeting expected milestones or is lagging behind and in need of referral for assessment.	Birth–24 mo
Denver Developmental Screening Test-II	Frankenberg and Dodds, 1990[8]	This assessment tool requires administration by a certified examiner or supervision by a certified examiner. Criterion-referenced items assess development across modalities, including communication.	2 wk–6 yr

Early Language Milestones	Coplan, 1984[7]	This assessment tool uses parent report, observation, and elicitation of behaviors to assess level of communicative development (receptive and expressive).	Birth through 3 yr
Hawaii Early Learning Profile	Furono et al, 1987[9]	This assessment tool compares infant development skills with those expected of age peers. It covers a range of developmental areas, including communication.	Birth through 3 yr
Neonatal Behavior Assessment Scale (2nd edition) (NBAS)	Brazelton, 1984[3]	A trained examiner is required to administer this infant behavior assessment tool. NBAS uses case history and elicited responses to physical and sensory stimuli, along with evaluation of infant state and neurological status, to determine the child's status.	Appropriate only for newborn, full-term infants.
Receptive Emergent Expressive Language-2 (REEL-2)	Bzoch and League, 1991[4]	This screening tool uses parent report to gauge the child's expressive language skills. It follows the format of the Vineland Social Maturity Scale.	1 mo–3 yr
Reynell Developmental Language Scales	Reynell and Gruber, 1969[13]	This assessment tool uses observation, picture and object identification, and object manipulation to assess language abilities.	1–6 yr
Sequenced Inventory of Communicative Development	Hedrick et al, 1984[10]	This assessment tool uses parent report, picture and object identification, and object manipulation to evaluate the child's communicative skills.	4 mo–4 yr
The Southern California Ordinal Scales of Development	California State Department of Education, 1984[5]	Separate scales assess various aspects of child development. The Developmental Scale of Communication comprises one unit.	Recommended ages are not specified.
Test of Early Language Development-2 (TELD-2)	Hresko et al, 1991[11]	TELD-2 evaluates receptive and expressive language abilities, including content of language and word forms. It employs a one-to-one situation that presumes child's ability to engage in joint attention and ability to follow simple directions.	2 yr–7 yr, 11 mo

▼ REFERENCES

1. Als H et al: Assessment of preterm infant behavior (APIB). In Fitzgerald HE, Lester BM, Yogman MW, editors: *Theory and research in behavioral pediatrics,* Vol 1, New York, 1982, Plenum, p 233.
2. Bayley N: *Bayley scales of infant development,* San Antonio, Tex, 1993, The Psychological Corporation.
3. Brazelton TB: *Neonatal behavioral assessment scale (NBAS),* White Plains, NY, 1984, March of Dimes Materials and Supplies Division.
4. Bzoch KR, League R: *Receptive expressive emergent language test (REEL),* ed 2, Austin, Tex, 1991, Pro-Ed.
5. Diagnostic School for Neurologically Handicapped Children and California State Department of Education: *Southern California ordinal scales of infant development,* Sacramento, Calif, 1984, Foreworks.
6. Capute A, Accardo PJ: Clinical linguistic and auditory milestone scale (CLAMS), *Clin Pediatr* 17:847, 1978.
7. Coplan J: *Early language milestone scale (ELM),* Tulsa, Okla, 1984, Modern Education Corporation.
8. Frankenberg WK, Dodds JB: Denver developmental screening II (Denver II), Denver, 1990, Ladaca Project and Publishing Foundation.
9. Furono S, O'Rilley K, Inatsuka T: *Hawaii early learning profile (HELP),* Palo Alto, Calif, 1987, Vort Corporation.
10. Hedrick DL, Prather EM, Tobin AR: *Sequenced inventory of communicative development (SICD),* Los Angeles, 1984, Western Psychological Corporation.
11. Hresko WP, Reid DK, Hammill DD: *Test of early-language development (TELD-2),* ed 2, Austin, Tex, 1991, Pro-Ed.
12. Newborg J, Stock J, Wnek L: *Battelle developmental inventory,* Allen, Tex, 1984, DLM/Teaching Resources.
13. Reynell JK, Gruber CP: *Reynell developmental language scales,* Los Angeles, 1969, Western Psychological Services.

Child's Name: _____ Date of Birth: _____

Filled out by: _____ Date filled out: _____

Instructions for Caregivers: This checklist is designed to identify different aspects of development in infants and toddlers. Many behaviors that develop before children talk may indicate whether or not a child will have difficulty learning to talk. This checklist should be completed by a caregiver when the child is between **6 and 24 months of age** to determine whether a referral for an evaluation is needed. The caregiver may be either a parent or other person who nurtures the child daily. Please check all the choices that best describe your child's behavior. If you are not sure, please choose the closest response based on your experience. **Children at your child's age are not necessarily expected to be able to do all the behaviors listed.**

Emotion and Use of Eye Gaze

1. Do you know when your child is happy and when your child is upset? ❏ Not Yet ❏ Sometimes ❏ Often
2. When your child plays with toys, does he/she look at you to see if you are watching? ❏ Not Yet ❏ Sometimes ❏ Often
3. Does your child smile or laugh while looking at you? ❏ Not Yet ❏ Sometimes ❏ Often
4. When you look at and point to a toy across the room, does your child look at it? ❏ Not Yet ❏ Sometimes ❏ Often

▼ **Figure B-1**   Infant/Toddler Checklist for Communication and Language Development.

Use of Communication

5. Does your child let you know that he/she needs help or wants an object out of reach? ❐ Not Yet ❐ Sometimes ❐ Often
6. When you are not paying attention to your child, does he/she try to get your attention? ❐ Not Yet ❐ Sometimes ❐ Often
7. Does your child do things just to get you to laugh? ❐ Not Yet ❐ Sometimes ❐ Often
8. Does your child try to get you to notice interesting objects—just to get you to look at the objects, not to get you do anything with them? ❐ Not Yet ❐ Sometimes ❐ Often

Use of Gestures

9. Does your child pick up objects and give them to you? ❐ Not Yet ❐ Sometimes ❐ Often
10. Does your child show objects to you without giving you the object? ❐ Not Yet ❐ Sometimes ❐ Often
11. Does your child wave to greet people? ❐ Not Yet ❐ Sometimes ❐ Often
12. Does your child point to objects? ❐ Not Yet ❐ Sometimes ❐ Often
13. Does your child nod his/her head to indicate yes? ❐ Not Yet ❐ Sometimes ❐ Often

Use of Sounds

14. Does your child use sounds or words to get attention or help? ❐ Not Yet ❐ Sometimes ❐ Often
15. Does your child string sounds together, such as uh oh, mama, gaga, bye bye, bada? ❐ Not Yet ❐ Sometimes ❐ Often
16. About how many of the following consonant sounds does your child use: ma, na, ba, da, ga, wa, la, ya, sa, sha? ❐ None ❐ 1–2 ❐ 3–4 ❐ 5–8 ❐ over 8

Understanding of Words

17. When you call your child's name, does he/she respond by looking or turning toward you? ❐ Not Yet ❐ Sometimes ❐ Often
18. About how many different words or phrases does your child understand without gestures? For example, if you say "where's your tummy", "where's daddy", "give me ball", or "come here", without showing or pointing, your child will respond appropriately. ❐ None ❐ 1–3 ❐ 4–10 ❐ 11–30 ❐ over 30

Use of Words

19. About how many different words does your childuse meaningfully that you recognize (such asbaba for bottle; gaggie for doggie)? ❐ None ❐ 1–3 ❐ 4–10 ❐ 11–30 ❐ over 30
20. Does your child put two words together (such as more cookie; bye-bye daddy)? ❐ Not Yet ❐ Sometimes ❐ Often

Use of Objects

21. Does your child show interest in playing with a variety of objects? ❐ Not Yet ❐ Sometimes ❐ Often
22. About how many of the following objects does your child use appropriately: cup, bottle, bowl, spoon, comb or brush, toothbrush, washcloth, ball, toy vehicle, toy telephone? ❐ None ❐ 1–2 ❐ 3–4 ❐ 3–4 ❐ over 8
23. About how many blocks (or rings) does your child stack? **Stacks:** ❐ None ❐ 2 blocks ❐ 3–4 blocks ❐ 5 or more blocks
24. Does your child pretend to play with toys (such as feed a stuffed animal, put a doll to sleep, put an animal figure in a vehicle). ❐ Not Yet ❐ Sometimes ❐ Often

▼ **Figure B-1** *Cont'd*

	Crying	Aggression	Tantrums/Self-Injury	Passive Gaze	Proximity	Pulling Other's Hands	Touching/Moving Other's	Face	Grabs/Reaches	Enactment	Removes Self/Walks Away	Focalization/Noise	Active Gaze	Gives Object	Gestures/Pointing	Facial Expression	Shakes "No"/Nods "Yes"	Intonation	Inappropriate Echolalia	Appropriate Echolalia	One-Word Speech	One-Word Signs	Complex Speech
Requests for affection and interaction. What if child wants:																							
Adult to sit near?																							
Peer to sit near?																							
Adult to look at him or her?																							
Adult to tickle him or her?																							
To be cuddled or embraced?																							
To sit on adult's lap?																							
Other bids for interaction?																							
Requests for adult action. What if child wants:																							
Help with dressing?																							
To be read a book?																							
To play ball or a game?																							
To go outside?																							
To go to a specific place?																							
Other?																							
Requests for object, food, or things. What if child wants:																							
An out-of-reach object?																							
A door or container opened?																							
A favorite food?																							
To turn on music, radio, or TV?																							
To have keys, toys, or a book?																							
Other?																							
Protest. What if:																							
A common routine is dropped?																							
A favorite food or toy is taken away?																							
The child is taken for a ride without having a desire to do so?																							
Adult terminates interaction?																							
Child is required to do something he or she does not want to do?																							
Declaration or comment. What if child wants:																							
To show you something?																							
To tell you about something?																							
Other																							

▼ **Figure B-2** Cue Questions in Assessment of Communicative Means and Functions. (Reprinted with permission from Schuler S et al: Assessment of Communicative means and functions through interview: assessing the communicative abilities of individuals with limited language, *Semin Speech Lang* 10:51, 1989.)

TABLE B-2
Assessment Framework for Parents and Professionals: Identifying Areas of Child Competency and Difficulty*

Infant Abilities	Parent Abilities	Components of the Interaction
Responsiveness	Parent's awareness of	Predominant affect
Signaling	the child's development	Affectional change
Communication	Parent's ability to function	Initiation of interaction
Cognitive	in the larger environment	Continuation of interaction
Motor	Level of parenting skills	Pace
Emotional	Meaning of the disabling	Turn-taking
Social	condition to the parents and	Use of communicative
Temperament	parent's ability to understand	modalities
Appearance	the condition	

From Hanson MJ, Krentz MS: *Supporting parent-child interactions: a guide for early intervention program personnel*, San Francisco, 1986, University of San Francisco, Department of Special Education.

TABLE B-3
Assisting Parents to Identify and Describe Their Child's Areas of Competency and Difficulties

NOTE: Together, parents and professionals review videotaped interactions of the parent and child during teaching, feeding, and play situations. Answers to the following questions are explored with the parent after the tape has been reviewed:

1. What are the specific areas of competence and the areas that create difficulties?
2. What is the impact of this difficulty on the other partner?
3. Are there specific dynamics of the interaction that need to be addressed, such as turn taking, synchrony, or timing?

After the questions have been answered, interventions can be designed with a specific focus as follows:

1. Targeting the specific behavior of one or the other partner (parent or infant) and trying to change it
2. Targeting the partner's response to the behavior and trying to change it
3. Targeting specific aspects of the interaction for change

▼ STRATEGIES FOR ADAPTATIONS IN THE RELATIONSHIP

Stage I: Regulation of Biological Patterns

Major emphasis: Determine whether the child is over- or undersensitive to the environment and help parent to facilitate child's optimum state.

Continued

TABLE B-3
Assisting Parents to Identify and Describe Their Child's Areas of Competency and Difficulties—Cont'd

Alerting

Commenting and sharing observations: The parent and professional together note whether the infant is passive with low arousal, has a tendency not to make demands of the environment, and/or has muted distress and hunger cues. Conversely, they note if the infant is overly sensitive to outside stimuli with a preponderance of crying behavior, easily shifting states, gaze aversion, and/or an inability to be consoled. Is the parent confused about the infant's signals? Do the partners have very different paces?

Serving as baby's interpreter: Carefully observe the infant's cues and help parents understand the meaning of these cues. Watch for baby's cues that mean "I've had enough" or "I want more."

Guiding

Informing: Discuss how premature birth or disabling conditions can affect state control. Help parents to distinguish different states. Help parents identify engagement cues (cues that begin or maintain an interaction; e.g., looking, smiling, or touching) and disengagement cues (cues that indicate that the baby wants to stop the interaction; e.g., gaze aversion, arching, turning, or crawling away). Help the parent communicate with a "neurologically sensitive" child by using fewer modalities (e.g., using only voice rather than voice, vision, and kinesthetic means). Help parents with a passive child exaggerate their affectual expressions so that the child becomes more interested and alert.

Reframing: Help parents who experience the gaze aversion of their child understand that this is not rejection but an attempt to control an overload of environmental stimuli. Help parents understand that their efforts to feed the child at a fast pace may be motivated by the positive desire to make sure the child has adequate caloric intake and help to decrease the parent's anxiety about this.

Commenting on unique qualities: Help the parents see the child apart from the handicap by mentioning special characteristics or competencies. Help parents to realize the child's uniqueness, such as being sensitive to change in the environment, so that the parents may make additional observations of their own. Comment on the child's qualities to balance the parents' perceptions of the child.

Modeling: Model decreasing stimuli to the "neurologically sensitive" child. Model exaggerated play with the more passive child. Model vocalizing to the child during feedings and play. Model communicating with the child through different modalities.

Experimenting: Try approaching a neurologically sensitive child in a variety of ways.

Highlighting: Comment on the child's positive reactions to the parent. Comment on the parents' sensitivity to the child's cues.

Stage II: The Development of Preferential Attachment Behavior and a Focused Relationship

Major emphasis: Seeing whether both partners are developing an attachment and recognizing ways in which they are forming their relationship.

Alerting

Commenting and sharing observations: Note whether the infant is competent enough to signal attachment and how she or he does it. Observe whether parents respond contingently to the infant.

Serving as baby's interpreter: Comment on the baby's need for specific attachments.

TABLE B-3
Assisting Parents to Identify and Describe Their Child's Areas of Competency and Difficulties—Cont'd

Guiding

Informing: Help the parents know the typical attachment behaviors. Help the parents to know how their child may demonstrate different attachments because of the impairment. Alert parents to baby's withdrawal cues.

Reframing: Interpret baby's protests upon separation as the child's growing attachment to the parent. Interpret separation protest as the indication of a special relationship with the parent.

Commenting on unique qualities: Help the parents to see and accept the divergence between their child's preferential attachment behaviors and what might be more typical. Help the parents understand how they may find it disappointing or difficult if a child cannot show varied or intensive attachment behaviors, such as following or vocalizing, because of the disabling condition. Comment on the more subtle ways the child shows attachment behaviors.

Modeling: Model alternative ways of communicating with the infant, such as through touch or kinesthetically. Model social play with the baby.

Experimenting: See if various physical factors, such as different positioning, visual range, lighting, and so on, can be changed so that they help the baby to be more responsive.

Stage III: Consolidating Positive Interactions and Developing a Communicative Context

Major emphasis: Seeing whether child and parent develop as partners and communicate reciprocally.

Alerting

Commenting and sharing observations: Note whether the infant engages in reciprocal behavior. Observe whether the infant responds to gestures and vocalizations and whether the infant initiates these behaviors and then expects a response.

Serving as baby's interpreter: Comment on the baby's attempts to respond reciprocally. Comment on the baby's need for response to their initiations to feel competent.

Guiding

Informing: Provide information to the parents about the need for predictability and repetition for a communicative context to be established. Help the parents to see how the child's motor, speech, or cognitive impairments can make it difficult for the child to develop a communicative context. Help the parents find the areas of reciprocal behavior in which the child has the most ease and competence.

Reframing: Help the parents to see the child's initiating behavior and the growing intentionality as indication of a growing sense of self.

Commenting on unique qualities: Note the unique qualities a child brings to the task of communicating or comment on the specific ways a child attempts to respond to the parent. Note the parents' adaptability in communicating with their child.

Modeling: Model extended social play for the parent. Model ways of responding to the baby's initiations. Model turn-taking and extending the communication sequence.

Experimenting: Try a range of affective expressions and note the child's responses. Try different paces of interaction with the child to see if the child responds more if more time is given.

Highlighting: Note the development of the relationship and more specifically the growing communication abilities between the partners. Note the most effective ways the baby communicates (vision, vocalizations, or gestures).

Continued

TABLE B-3
Assisting Parents to Identify and Describe Their Child's Areas of Competency and Difficulties—Cont'd

Stage IV: Growing Differentiation of the Partners in the Relationship

Major emphasis: Looking for the child's growing sense of self and the parents' encouragement of this.

Alerting

Commenting and sharing observations: Note the ways in which the child shows his or her growing independence. Is it across all areas of development (emotionally, cognitively, motorically)? Can the parents facilitate the child's autonomy? How do the parents feel about the child's growing independence?

Serving as baby's interpreter: Comment on the child's autonomy. Interpret the child's attempts to resist the parents as an indicator of the child's growing sense of self. Note the child's need for limits to internalize self-regulatory behavior and to be able to be an effective independent agent.

Guiding

Informing: Help the parents identify typical toddler behaviors that indicate the child's growing sense of self. Help parents distinguish the child's emotions as different from their own. Help the parents distinguish appropriate limits for the child. Guide the parents in labeling the child's emotions. Encourage the parents to offer the child appropriate outlets for the child's feelings. Help the parents use verbal means to control their child's behavior.

Reframing: Help parents to see resistant behavior as a sign of the child's autonomy.

Commenting on unique qualities: Help the parents to understand how they feel about the child's independence. Do parents expect too much or too little from the child? Do parents worry about the child's autonomy because of the disabling condition? Comment on child's competence to facilitate the parents' trust in the child.

Modeling: Model appropriate limit setting. Model labeling the child's emotions.

Highlighting: Comment in a positive way on the child's initiative and independent behaviors. Comment on the parents' appreciation of child's growth.

Stage V: Negotiating Separations

Major emphasis: Facilitating and attending to the child's growing ability to function apart from the parents.

Alerting

Commenting and sharing observations: Note the times and conditions when the parent and child are separate. Observe the quality of the separation and also the quality of the reunion. Observe the ability of parent and child to communicate from a small distance (e.g., across the room) and observe the modalities (e.g., visually, auditorily) in which they do it.

Guiding

Informing: Help the parents use distal communication with a child, such as voice, gesture, and gaze, when across the room to assure the child of their presence. Help the parents to understand the child's "back-and-forth" refueling behavior (e.g., child walks or looks back and forth to the parent). Help the parents to be able to reassure the child from a distance and not just from close proximity. Acknowledge and discuss the parents' fears about areas in which the child does not function well independently.

TABLE B-3
Assisting Parents to Identify and Describe Their Child's Areas of Competency and Difficulties—Cont'd

Reframing: Help the parents to understand any rejection of closeness by the child as the child's attempt to develop mastery and control.
Commenting on unique qualities: Help the parents to understand any areas in which their child may have difficulty with separation. For instance, if the child cannot use a visual modality to check back in on the parent or cannot practice coming and going due to motor limitations.
Modeling: Model distal communicative behaviors for the parents. Model leave taking, while preparing the child for this verbally. Model tolerating the child's frustration.
Experimenting: If separation is difficult, help the parents experiment with leaving the child with a familiar adult for brief periods of time.
Highlighting: Note the importance of the child's separateness. Note the importance of the parents having time for themselves.

From Hanson MJ, Krentz MS: *Supporting parent-child interactions: a guide for early intervention program personnel*, San Francisco, 1986, University of San Francisco, Department of Special Education.

TABLE B-4
A Method for Describing Interaction Styles of Handicapped Prelanguage Children

The method developed by Norris and Hoffman (1990) to study adult and infant interaction has clinical application for describing aspects of communicative interaction in young handicapped children who do not yet use oral language. The suggested levels and categories of interaction are useful guides in identifying infant behaviors that have communicative function. They can assist in designing effective intervention strategies based on existing abilities spontaneously demonstrated by the child. The six developmental age levels correspond to the substages of sensorimotor development identified by Piaget.

▼ INFANT SCALE OF NONVERBAL INTERACTION

Levels of Interactive Behavior

- *Level I (1- to 3-month rating):* These behaviors occur in response to general stimulation and are usually in *reaction* to the adult's actions or the general environment.
- *Level II (4- to 6-month rating):* These behaviors occur in response to play between people, generally reflecting turn taking but not specific control over others.
- *Level III (7- to 9-month rating):* These behaviors occur when the infant initiates control in the interaction by imitating actions and reacting as participants share interaction with objects.
- *Level IV (10- to 12-month rating):* These behaviors include imitations of actual *functional* actions and conventional gestures or vocalizations; their meaning is usually clear in context.

Continued

TABLE B-4
A Method for Describing Interaction Styles of Handicapped Prelanguage Children—Cont'd

- *Level V (13- to 18-month rating):* These behaviors are directed at getting the adult to share objects or controlling the game so the adult keeps playing.
- *Level VI (19- to 24-month rating):* These behaviors reflect the child's attempts to describe experiences using a combination of short phrases, single words, and jargon; the child often initiates interactions by handing objects to the communication partner.

Categories of Behavior

- Vocalizations, including nonspeech sounds, speech sounds, and words
- Limb actions, including movements and gestures of the hands, arms, legs and feet
- Facial and body postures, including movements of the eyes and mouth and body positioning that are social

Recording Observed Behaviors

The specific type of behavior is recorded according to the following types, listed by developmental level and category.

Level I: 1- to 3-Month Rating
Vocalizations
Undifferentiated vocalizations done in response to general environment rather than a specific stimulus
Generalized squeals or chuckles of pleasure or frustration
Cooing and other vowel vocalizations produced to general stimuli
Responding to others' vocalization with a vocalization in play, not play with objects

Limb actions
Random body movements showing excitement
Startle response
Attracting attention with body movements
Anticipatory activity (excitement when object seen)

Facial and body postures
Maintaining eye contact when interacted with
Smiling or widening eyes when talked to
Looking at people, not in response to play with objects
Visually following people and objects

Level II: 4- to 6-Month Rating
Vocalizations
Social vocalization, including vocalizing when action done to infant, squealing when talked to, crying if disrupted, and laughing to interaction
Vocalizations characterized by intonation changes in cooing; bilabial consonants /p/, /b/, and /m/ produced; repetition of consonant-vowel syllable; and consonants /m/, /b/, /n/, /d/, /g/, /l/, /w/, /h/, /p/, and /t/
Imitating pitch and loudness changes
Vocalizing directly to another person
Vocalizing while playing with toy
Turn taking in vocalizations

TABLE B-4
A Method for Describing Interaction Styles of Handicapped Prelanguage Children—Cont'd

Limb actions
Social refusals, including pulling away and shaking head
Reacting to social negatives with cries and frowns
Wiggling limbs when adult initiates a familiar gesture
Reaching toward another person or close object

Facial and body postures
Showing anticipation, including raising arms to be picked up, moving close to another, and clinging when held
Smiling or frowning at other people, but not because of play with objects
Moving to see what is being shown or looked at
Joint focus to something presented by adult

Level III: 7- to 9-Month Rating
Vocalizations
Attempting to imitate speech sounds (may not be same sounds) and consonant-vowel sequences
Vocalizations show changes in pitch, quality, intensity, rate, and duration
Vocalizing to have toy reactivated or adult do action
Vocalizing at object, then looking to adult and indicating the need for help by a pull, grab, and so on
Imitating nonspeech sounds (e.g., cough, smacking, animals, vehicles)
Imitating words without attaching meaning
Babbling phrases with four or more different syllables, including sounds such as /t/, /d/, /n/, /w/, /f/, /v/, and /l/

Limb actions
Imitating movements like waving arm and patting hand on tray
Pushing away unwanted food, object, or person
Moving limbs to indicate reactivation or recurrence
Grabbing adult's fingers, pulling hand, and so on to indicate recurrence
Performing action for familiar game like pat-a-cake

Facial and body postures
Smiling and laughing when teased or entertained
Pulling back or moving to reject something
Using eye contact to indicate recurrence or help
Moving by leaning over, moving forward, and so on to follow the actions of adults or objects

Level IV: 10- to 12-Month Rating
Vocalizations
Repeating vocalization if it is responded to
Fussing, crying, and having tantrums when desired object is removed
Expressing negative reaction through vocalization
Using single word to label
Imitating a series of sounds said by an adult
Using jargon to toys and people as if talking

Continued

TABLE B-4
A Method for Describing Interaction Styles of Handicapped Prelanguage Children—Cont'd

Limb actions
Pointing to noticed objects
Pointing to parts of objects upon imitation
Imitating actions that are functional (e.g., eating, washing) or repeating modeled action to make event recur
Imitating novel gesture
Extending toy to give without releasing
Gesturing to represent an action (e.g., wiggling hand to get something to move)
Using social gestures like waving bye-bye or shaking head no

Facial and body postures
Wiggling body to continue a movement such as bouncing
Moving body to represent an action (e.g., rocking to represent a rocking toy)

Level V: 13- to 18-Month Rating
Vocalizations
Using five words
Using one word for many meanings
Imitating variety of words
Using jargon mixed with real words

Limb actions
Giving object to adult to get toy to (re)activate
Pointing, reaching, or grabbing objects or toys to indicate wanting them
Repeating actions that produce laughter or attention
Using gestures in combination to indicate wants

Facial and body postures
Imitating facial movement or expression
Leading adult by hand to desired object

Level VI: 19- to 24-Month Rating
Vocalizations
Vocabulary of 10 to 50 words
Imitating two- and three-word combinations
Attempting to describe experiences using jargon mixed with real words
Using a variety of word classes (e.g., actions, agents, attributes)

Limb actions
Handing book or object to be read or shared
Doing a series of related actions
Facial and body postures
Doing own action if other person does not respond

From Norris JA, Hoffman PR: Comparison of adult-initiated vs. child-initiated interaction styles with handicapped prelanguage children, *Lang Speech Hear Sch* 1:28, 34–36, 1990.

TABLE B-5
Communicative Temptations

This activity list is designed to optimize the probability of communicative acts on the part of a child, avoiding the common practice of asking the child to name different objects. Depending on the circumstances, the child's caregiver may be instructed to carry out the activities, or the clinician may do so. The clinician observes the child's communicative means and functions as the activities are in progress. A third person can be used to record responses or to videotape the process for later analysis, freeing the clinician to engage in the activity at hand.

1. Display attractive snack food in a clear plastic sandwich bag. Open bag and begin eating without offering the child any. You may offer some to the mother or accompanying adult. Record child's reaction.
2. Inflate a balloon as child watches. Release it suddenly, allowing it to dart about the room erratically. Retrieve it, and hold it in child's view and wait for response.
3. Inflate a balloon, slowly release the air as child watches, holding it within child's view. Observe and record child's response.
4. Activate a wind-up toy and allow it to run down. Wait for child's response without comment or present the toy to the child and indicate that it is his or her turn to play with it.
5. Hand the child four similar or identical objects (e.g., blocks, plastic figures) to drop into a bucket or box. Provide a different item (e.g., small car or cup) to the child on the fifth occasion. Record reaction.
6. Present a toy or edible the child is known to dislike, offering it assertively. Observe response.
7. Demonstrate how a "clicker" toy (e.g., frog or insect replica with a metal lever on the underside) is operated and allow the child to operate it. Replace the toy with an identical one whose clicker is inoperable and encourage the child to make it work. Observe child's response.
8. Place an attractive toy or preferred food item in a clear plastic jar with a tight-fitting lid. Put the jar in front of the child. Observe response.
9. Place a noise-making object in a brown paper bag and put the bag in front of the child. Observe response.
10. Provide the child with materials to engage in an interesting task (e.g., paper and crayon); "sabotage" the activity by "accidentally" tearing the paper or breaking off the point of the crayon. Observe response.
11. Hold (or have a third person hold) two hand puppets under the table surface. Knock on the table and call the puppets, bringing them out on three consecutive occasions as a pair. On the fourth round, have only one appear. Observe response.
12. Look through age-appropriate books with the child, pointing to pictured objects and looking at the child expectantly.
13. Provide child with a woman's purse or zippered bag containing a set of keys, a mirror, a pencil and pad, or other interesting objects the mother may typically carry. Allow the child to play with the purse, assisting in opening it, if necessary. Observe reaction.
14. Using a piece of waxed paper or a tray as a surface, place the child's hands in a sticky, cold, or wet substance, such as whipped cream, gelatin dessert, Play-Doh flour and water paste, or white glue. Observe response. NOTE: Have a wet washcloth and dry towel to clean child's hands when finished.
15. Engage the child in an activity that requires use of specific materials (e.g., paper, crayon, scissors, cotton balls, glue); have a third person remove an essential item, taking a seat across the room with the object in plain view of the child. Observe reaction.

Continued

TABLE B-5
Communicative Temptations—Cont'd

16. Provide child with paper and a stapler that is loaded with only a few staples. Show child how to use the device without expending the supply of staples. Allow the child to operate the stapler, observing reaction when staple supply is exhausted.
17. Have two identical colored felt-tip markers on hand, one that is operable and the other dry. Allow the child to mark on paper with the one that works, replacing it with the one that does not. Hold the operable one in the child's view or use it to show the child that you have one that makes marks. Observe child's response.
18. Show the child two toy cars or trucks, one of which has a missing wheel. Allow child to play with the intact toy as you operate the one that is broken. Exchange toys with the child as the "game" progresses. Observe reaction.
19. Provide two balls, one with deflated air, first rolling the intact ball back and forth and then exchanging the deflated one for the original. Observe child's response.
20. Engage the child in assembling a puzzle. After the third piece has been placed, present the child with a piece that does not go with that puzzle. Observe response.

Modified from Wetherby A, Prizant BM: The expression of communicative intent: assessment guidelines, *Semin Lang* 10:77–91, 1989; Wetherby A, Prutting C: Profiles of communicative and cognitive social abilities in autistic children, *J Speech Hear Res* 27:364–377, 1984; with supplemental items from Billeaud 1998.)

TABLE B-6
Strategies for Communication Enhancement from the *CSBS* Model

- Adult should follow child's lead by imitating child's behavior and attuning to child's display of affect.
- Use proximity in positioning and presentation of materials to enhance social referencing.
- For low-rate communicators, design environment to provide many communicative opportunities to increase child's rate of communicating; make sure that others wait and look expectantly at child.
- For children with adequate rates of communication, provide natural opportunities for repairs by holding out for a repetition or modification of communicative signal.
- Design environment to provide opportunities for child to communicate for a range of functions:
  1) Behavior regulation
     - During mealtime or snack time, provide opportunities for child to request desired food, to request help opening a container, and/or to protest undesired food
     - During playtime, provide opportunities for child to request desired toy, request help activating toy, and/or protest undesired toy
     - During dressing or bathing, provide opportunities for child to make choices

  2) Social interaction
     - During social games, provide opportunities for child to request beginning or continuation of game
     - When child is distressed or in need of attention, provide opportunities for child to request comfort and call
     - Practice greeting routines when leaving or arriving
     - During turn-taking games, encourage child to show off

TABLE B-6
Strategies for Communication Enhancement From the *CSBS* Model—Cont'd

3) Joint attention
   - Encourage child to give or transfer objects of interest to reference joint attention
   - During activities with a joint focus of attention, plan for observation of novelty and change to provide opportunities for child to comment and request needed information by waiting and looking expectantly
- Use a facilitative interaction style to acknowledge child's communicative intention and expand on his or her communicative behavior or model a more sophisticated communicative means.
- Provide natural opportunities to "up-the-ante" by holding out for more sophisticated means to express communicative functions that are solidly established in child's repertoire.
- Provide opportunities to engage child in appropriate use of objects and to model play at appropriate level for child during a variety of symbolic and constructive play experiences.
- Provide developmentally appropriate activities and use areas of relative strength to enhance areas of weakness (e.g., types of play, communicative functions); when play demands are more difficult for child, minimize communicative demands, but model and prompt developmentally appropriate behaviors.

From Wetherby A: Strategies for Communication Enhancement from the CSBS Model. Presented November 6, 2000 at the Louisiana Speech-Language-Hearing Association 2000 Convention, Baton Rouge, La (p. 15 of handout).

APPENDIX C

ADMINISTRATIVE
REFERENCES

P lease refer to Appendix D for detailed information on other Internet sites of importance to professionals and families.)

▼ CONTENTS

Table C-1: List of Part C Agencies for States and Jurisdictions of the United States

Table C-2: List of Names and Addresses for Pertinent National Organizations

Table C-3: Reference List for Position and Policy Statements and Practice Guidelines of Various Professional Organizations

TABLE C-1
Part C Agencies for States and Jurisdictions of the United States*†

State/Jurisdiction	Lead Agency
Alabama	Rehabilitation Services
Alaska	Health and Social Services
American Samoa	Health
Arizona	Economic Security
Arkansas	Human Services/Developmental Disabilities
California	Developmental Services
Colorado	Education
Commonwealth of Northern Mariana Islands	Education
Connecticut	Mental Retardation
Delaware	Health and Social Services
District of Columbia	Human Services
Florida	Health (Children's Medical Services)
Georgia	Human Resources/Division of Health
Guam	Education
Hawaii	Education
Idaho	Health and Welfare/Developmental Disabilities
Illinois	Human Services
Indiana	Family and Social Services
Iowa	Education
Kansas	Health and Environment
Kentucky	Human Resources/Mental Health–Mental Retardation
Louisiana	Health and Hospitals
Maine	Education
Maryland	Education
Massachusetts	Public Health
Michigan	Education
Minnesota	Education
Mississippi	Health
Missouri	Education
Montana	Public Health and Human Services
Nebraska	Co-lead: Education Health and Services
Nevada	Human Resources
New Hampshire	Health and Human Services
New Jersey	Health and Senior Services
New Mexico	Health/Developmental Disabilities
New York	Health
North Carolina	Health and Human Services/Division of Public Health, Women's and Children's Health Section
North Dakota	Human Services
Ohio	Health
Oklahoma	Education
Oregon	Education
Palau	Education
Pennsylvania	Public Welfare
Puerto Rico	Health

TABLE C-1
Part C Agencies for States and Jurisdictions of the United States*†—Cont'd

State/Jurisdiction	Lead Agency
Rhode Island	Health
South Carolina	Health and Environmental Control
South Dakota	Education
Tennessee	Education
Texas	Interagency Council on Early Childhood Intervention
Utah	Health
Vermont	Co-lead: Education Human Services
Virgin Islands	Health
Virginia	Mental Health/Mental Retardation/SAS
Washington	Social and Health Services
West Virginia	Health and Human Services
Wisconsin	Health and Social Services
Wyoming	Health

*Federated States of Micronesia and the Republic of Marshall Islands are not currently eligible for this federal program. List current as of 2001; updates, if any, available from the NECTAS web site (http://www.nectas.nc.edu/partc/ptclead.asp).
†Addresses and phone numbers for agencies often change unexpectedly; consult directories of state agencies at their Internet web sites or through telephone directory assistance services.

TABLE C-2
National Organizations

The following organizations are resources for answers to specific questions; guidance in obtaining services; and assistance in locating credentialed professionals, information, and printed materials relating to specific conditions.

Alexander Graham Bell Association for the Deaf
3417 Volta Pl. NW
Washington, DC 20007
(202) 337-5520

Alliance of Genetic Support Groups
38th and R Streets NW
Washington, DC 20057
(202) 625-7853

American Academy for Cerebral Palsy and Developmental Medicine
2405 Westwood Ave., Suite 205
P.O. Box 11083
Richmond, VA 23230
(804) 355-0147

Continued

TABLE C-2
National Organizations—Cont'd

American Academy of Pediatrics
141 Point Blvd. NW
P.O. Box 927
Elk Grove Village, IL 60009
(312) 288-5005

American Brittle Bone Association
1256 Merrill Dr.
Marshalton
West Chester, PA 19380
(215) 692-6248

American Cleft Palate Educational Foundation
331 Salk Hall
University of Pittsburgh
Pittsburgh, PA 15261
(412) 681-9620

American Council for the Blind
1010 Vermont Ave. NW, Suite 1000
Washington, DC 20005
(202) 393-3666
(800) 424-8666

American Foundation for Maternal and Child Health
439 E 51st St.
New York, NY 10022
(212) 759-5510

American Occupational Therapy Association
P.O. Box 1726
Rockville, MD 20850-4375
(301) 948-9626

American Physical Therapy Association
1111 North Fairfax St.
Alexandria, VA 22314
(703) 684-2782

American Society for Deaf Children
814 Thayer Ave.
Silver Spring, MD 20910
(301) 585-5400

American Speech-Language-Hearing Association
10801 Rockville Pike
Rockville, MD 20852-3279
(800) 638-8255

American Association for the Care of Children's Health
3615 Wisconsin Ave. NW
Washington, DC 20016
(202) 244-1801

TABLE C-2
National Organizations—Cont'd

Association for Persons with Severe Handicaps
7010 Roosevelt Way NW
Seattle, WA 98115
(206) 523-8446

Association of Birth Defect Children
3526 Emerywood Ln.
Orlando, FL 32806
(305) 859-2821

Center for Birth Defects Information Services
Dover Medical Building
P.O. Box 1776
Dover, MA 02030
(508) 785-2525

Cornelia de Lange Syndrome Foundation
60 Dyer Ave.
Collingsville, CT 06022
(203) 693-0159

Epilepsy Foundation of America
4351 Garden City Dr., #406
Landover, MD 20785

International Association for Infant Mental Health
Psychology Research Building
Michigan State University
East Lansing, MI 48824-1117

March of Dimes Birth Defects Foundation
1275 Mamoroneck Ave.
White Plains, NY 10603
(914) 428-7100

National Association for Retarded Citizens
2501 Ave. J
Arlington, TX 76006
(817) 640-0204

National Association for Sickle Cell Disease, Inc.
4221 Wilshire Blvd., Suite 360
Los Angeles, CA 90010
(213) 936-7205
(800) 421-8453

National Association for the Visually Handicapped
22 West 21st St., 6th Floor
New York, NY 10010
(212) 889-3141

Continued

TABLE C-2
National Organizations—Cont'd

National Down Syndrome Society
141 Fifth Ave.
New York, NY 10010
(212) 460-9330
(800) 221-4602

National Easter Seal Society
2023 West Ogden Ave.
Chicago, IL 06612
(312) 243-8400

National Information Center for Handicapped Children and Youth
P.O. Box 1492
Washington, DC 20013
(703) 522-0870

National Institute of Child Health and Human Development
9000 Rockville Pike
Bldg. 31, Room 2A32
Bethesda, MD 20205
(301) 496-4143

National Neurofibromatosis Foundation
70 W 40th St., 4th Floor
New York, NY 10018
(212) 460-8980

National Organization for Rare Diseases
P.O. Box 8923
New Fairfield, CT 06812
(203) 746-6518

National Retinitis Pigmentosa Foundation
1401 Mount Royal Ave.
Fourth Floor
Baltimore, MD 21217
(800) 638-2300

The Autism Society of America
7910 Woodmont Avenue, Suite 300
Bethesda, MD 20814-3067
(301) 657-0881

National Tay-Sachs and Allied Diseases Association
92 Washington Ave.
Cedarhurst, NY 11516
(516) 569-4300

Osteogenesis Imperfecta Foundation, Inc.
P.O. Box 838
Manchester, NH 03105
(516) 325-8992

TABLE C-2
National Organizations—Cont'd

Parents of Premature and High Risk Infants International, Inc.
33 West 42nd St.
New York, NY 10036
(606) 277-0008

Prader-Willi Syndrome Association
5515 Malibu Dr.
Edina, MN 55436
(612) 933-0113

Sensory Aids Foundation
399 Sherman Ave., Suite 12
Palo Alto, CA 94306
(415) 329-0430

Spina Bifida Association of America
1700 Rockville Pike, Suite 540
Rockville, MD 20852

United Cerebral Palsy Associations
66 E 34th St.
New York, NY 10016
(212) 481-6300

Zero to Three: National Center for Infants, Toddlers and Families
2000 M Street, NW, Suite 200
Washington, DC 20036
(202) 638-1144

TABLE C-3
Reference List for Position and Policy Statements and Practice Guidelines of Various Professional Organizations

The following documents should be in the library of professionals who serve infants and toddlers with special needs and their families. Many, if not all, of the documents are available on-line from the indicated sources and also may be obtained directly from the sponsoring organizations. The documents provide practitioners with information about responsibilities, ethical guidelines, and best practices to be expected among team members who work with the target population and who represent a range of disciplines.

1. The Interdisciplinary Council on Developmental and Learning Disorders: *Clinical Practice Guidelines: Redefining the Standards of Care for Infants, Children, and Families with Special Needs.* This document is endorsed by organizations of speech-language pathologists, developmental pediatrics, neurology, occupational therapy,

Continued

TABLE C-3
Reference List for Position and Policy Statements and Practice Guidelines of Various Professional Organizations—Cont'd

physical therapy, psychology, social work, special education, and child psychiatry. Available on-line for viewing and downloading at www.icdl.com. Also available from The Interdisciplinary Council on Developmental and Learning Disorders, 4938 Hampden Lane, Suite 800, Bethesda, MD 20814 (Ph: 301-656-2667).

2. American Speech-Language-Hearing Association, National Joint Committee on Learning Disabilities: *Communication Based Services for Infants, Toddlers, and Their Families,* May 1989. Available from ASHA, 10801 Rockville Pike, Rockville, MD 20852-3279. Also available on-line at www.asha.org.

3. American Speech-Language-Hearing Association: The roles of speech-language pathologists in service delivery to infants, toddlers, and their families. *ASHA* 32 (suppl 2):4, 1990. Also available from www.asha.org.

4. American Academy of Pediatrics. Policy statement: The role of the primary care pediatrician in the management of high-risk newborn infants, *Pediatrics* 98(4):786–788, 1996. Also available from www.aap.org/policy/pe000786.html.

5. American Academy of Pediatrics: Role of the pediatrician in family-centered early intervention services, *Pediatrics* 107(5):1155–1157, 2001.

6. American Academy of Neurology: Practice parameter: screening and diagnosis of autism. Report of the quality standards subcommittee of the American Academy of Neurology and the Child Neurology Society, *Neurology* 55:468–479, 2000. Also available from QSS, American Academy of Neurology, 1080 Montreal Ave., St. Paul, MN 55116 (Ph: 1-800-879-1960). NOTE: This statement has been endorsed by the American Academy of Audiology, the American Occupational Therapy Association, the American Speech-Language-Hearing Association, the Autism National Committee, Cure Autism Now, the National Alliance for Autism Research, and the Society for Developmental Pediatrics.

7. American Academy of Pediatrics, Committee on Children with Disabilities: Technical report: The pediatrician's role in the diagnosis and management of autistic spectrum disorder in children, *Pediatrics* 107(5):1221–1226, 2001. Also available at www.pediatrics.org/policy/re060018.html.

8. American Academy of Pediatrics: Policy statement—Noise: a hazard for the fetus and newborn, *Pediatrics* 100(4):724–727, 1997. Also available at www.aap.org/policy/re9728.html.

INTERNET RESOURCES FOR PROFESSIONALS AND FAMILIES

This table is provided as a timesaving device for locating information often sought by practitioners and families. The author's annotations may assist in selecting sites that are of particular interest for specific needs. The arrangement of the sources given in the table is as follows:

- Search engines and metasites for conducting far-flung research on a topic
- Organizations and libraries that provide both general and specific information
- Governmental sites that pertain to federal laws and other legal information
- Sites listed alphabetically by syndrome, condition, or diagnosis
- Sites listing pertinent medical codes for diagnosed conditions (for billing purposes and for sharing information with insurance entities, medical records, and colleagues)

Readers should be aware that web addresses change from time to time. Host sites may or may not provide the new URL (address) when such is the case. The prefix "http://" may be needed to access certain sites if the computer being used is not programmed to automatically add the prefix before "www." when required. The reader should double-check URL extensions (e.g., ".com, .edu, .org, .net, .med"); new extensions have been approved for use in 2002 and subsequent years.

Resources	URL
Search Engines and Metasites	
Google—Speedy; searches many databases; highly recommended as a starting place	**http://www.google.com**
Metacrawler—Searches several databases	**http://www.metacrawler.com**
NCBI—Features 200+ pages of related links listed under search term "disability"; provides access to over 11 million Medline citations; full text articles	**http://www.ncbi.nlm.nih.gov/PubMed/**

Continued

275

Resources	URL
Search Engines and Metasites—Cont'd	
Mamma—General website with an excellent search capability similar to google but faster to access	http://www.mamma
Medscape— Features links to many medical sites	http://www.medscape.com
Alta Vista	http://www.altavista.com
Yahoo	http://www.yahoo.com
Look Smart	http://www.looksmart.com
Lycos	http://www.lycos.com
Hot Bot	http://www.hotbot.com
Galaxy	http://www.galaxy.com
Achoo Health Explorer	http://www.achoo.com
Health A to Z	http://www.healthatoz.com
Search COM Health and Medicine— Site features include updates of new metasearch domain names	http://www.search.com
Education Resource Information Center (ERIC)—This Council for Exceptional Children (CEC) site also has links to the National Parent Information Network and other useful sites	http://www.cec.sped.org
Medpulse	http://www.medpulse.com
Libraries and General Information Resources	
Medical information online	http://www.medicalonline.com
Division of Early Childhood of the CEC	http://www.dec-sped.org
National Education Resource Information Center (ERIC)—Search page for information on clinical, diagnosis, developmental disabilities, early identification, prenatal care, symptoms of individual disorders, and educational diagnosis	http://ericae.net/scripts/ewiz/amain4.asp
Disability Links—Rich resource for links to information for families and professionals	http://wa.gov/dshs/iteip/ links.html#Disability
National Center on Children and Youth with Disabilities (NICCHY)—Provides information about how to obtain therapy services by state	http://www.nicchy.org
National Library of Medicine (NLM)	http://www.nlm.nih.gov
NLM list of serials indexed for online web users	http://www.nlm.nih.gov/tsd/ serials/lsiou.html
NLM list of serials recently included, changed names or discontinued from listing	http://www.nlm.nih.gov/tsd/
Neonatology—Excellent resource with links to related sites	http://www.neonatology.org
Vanderbilt Interactive Pediatric Digital Library	http://www.mc.vanderbilt.edu/peds/pidl
Web Net Lit—Journal collection similar to Medline	http://www.webmedlit.com

Resources	URL
Libraries and General Information Resources—Cont'd	
World Health Organization—Provides much information re: international classification of diseases and disabilities as well as links to related sites	http://www.who.int/icidh
Pediatric Database (PEDBASE)—Describes over 550 childhood conditions and diseases; excellent resource for such information	http://www.icondata.com/health/pedbase/pedlynx.htm
Federal Laws and Legal Information	
Individuals with Disabilities Education Act (IDEA)	http://www.ed.gov/offices/ (NOTE: use search option "IDEA" and select from options)
Americans with Disabilities Act (ADA)	http://adainfo.org
Federal Resource Center	http://www.dscc.org/frc/idea_law.htm
Special Education Laws—Excellent resource for text of laws and links to federal agencies; message boards; bookstore; current news; site is updated frequently	http://www.specialedlaw.net/index.mv
Google—Use Google search site and enter search terms such as "disability law" or "I.D.E.A." or "special education law" and select from among site options provided	http://www.google.com
Apraxia/ Dyspraxia/ Developmental Apraxia of Speech (DAS)	
DAS article for parents	www.apraxia-kids.org/slps/marquardt.html
Attention Deficit-Hyperactivity Disorder	
Children and Adults With Attention-Deficit/Hyperactivity Disorder (CHADD)—Association founded by concerned parents; provides extensive information re: diagnosis and treatment of attention deficit/hyperactivity disorder, sometimes identified in the toddler years	http://www.chadd.org
Autistic Spectrum Disorder (PDD, Asperger Syndrome, PDD-NOS)	
First Signs—Dedicated to informing physicians and parents about early warning signs of autism and other developmental disorders. The goal is the earliest possible identification and intervention for children at risk; good information on children ages newborn to 3 yr with disabilities	www.firstsigns.org
Families for Early Autism Treatment—Support and advocacy for families with autistic children; offers free daily online newspaper that focuses on autism and has an active list serve	www.feat.org
Autism Society of America	http://www.autism-society.org

Continued

Resources	URL
Autistic Spectrum Disorder (PDD, Asperger Syndrome, PDD-NOS)—Cont'd	
National Alliance for Autism Research (NAAR)—Dedicated to finding the causes, prevention, treatment and cure of autistic spectrum disorders; unites families and researchers to fund and accelerate autism research	www.naar.org
Autism Research Institute—Bernard Rimland's site	http://www.autism.org/
Autism Resources—John Wobus' site for parents; products and publications; links to 50 key sites	http://www.autismresources.com
Bio-Medical—Information network—Links to biomedical articles and data	http://www.autism-biomed.org
Autism/PDD Resources Network—Excellent site with links to hundreds of others; good for families and professionals	http://www.autism-pdd.net
National Institute of Neurological Diseases and Stroke	www.ninds.nih.gov/health_and_medical/ disorders/autismshortdoc.htm#toc
Psychcrawler—Sponsored by the American Psychological Association; enter "autism in search area for array of information	http://www.psychcrawler.com
Autism/Asperger Syndrome—Support for families; links to multiple sites; information	http://www.thelaughtongroup.com/ pddsupport/index.html
The National Institute of Mental Health—Resource for a variety of publications about autism	http://www.nimh.nih.gov/publicat/autism. menu
Web of Care—Features articles for home caregivers; animated caregiving skills	www.webofcare.com/autism/html
Autism Network for Dietary Intervention	http//:www.autismNDI.com
The Feingold Dietary Program	http//:www.feingold.org
Gluten-Free Diet Information	http//:www.gfcfdiet.com
Cure Autism Now—Provides links to other autism interest groups and information on research and grants	http://www.cureautismnow.org
Patient Centers—Links to information for families of persons with PDD	http//:www.patientcenters.com
National Center on Birth Defects and Developmental Disabilities	http://www.cdc.gov/ncbddd/default.htm
Birth Defects	
International Clearinghouse for Birth Defects Monitoring Systems (ICBD)—Multiple links re: information on birth defects; good site for both parents and professionals	http://www.icbd.org/link.htm
National Center on Birth Defects and Developmental Disabilities	http://www.cdc.gov/ncbddd/default.htm
Pediatrician's role with ASD—American Academy of Pediatrics site (policy statement)	http://www.aap.org/policy/re060018.html

Resources	URL
Cerebral Palsy	
Cerebral Palsy Information Center—Information ranging from legal to resources	http://www.CerebralPalsyInfoCenter.com
National Institutes of Health—Information page and links to other sites	http://www.ninds.nih.gov/health_and_medical/disorders/cerebral_palsy.htm
United Cerebral Palsy (UCP)	http://www.ucp.org#
Web of Care—For families of children with cerebral palsy	www.webofcare.com/cerebralpalsy.html
National Information Center for Children and Youth with Disabilities—Lists resources (government, education, and organizations) by state with mailing addresses and phone numbers	www.nichcy.org/
National Organization for Rare Diseases—Numerous links and printable fact sheets	http://www.rarediseases.org/cgi-bin/hord
A.I. Dupont Institute—Excellent review of condition and answers to frequently asked questions	http://gait.aidi.udel.edu/res695/homepage/pd_ortho/clinics/c_palsy/cpweb.htm
Cleft Palate and Craniofacial Disorders	
Greg and Catherine's Cleft Palate Information Page—Useful links for parents	http://www.acay.com.au/~gsm/clefts.htm
Smiles—Support group for families of children with cleft palate	http://www.cleft.org
Cleft Palate Foundation—Extensive list of links to pertinent organizations	http://www.cleftline.org
Cochlear Implants	
Cochlear Implants Tutorial from the National Institutes of Health	www.nidcd.gov/health_pubshb/coch.htm
Where Do We Go from Hear? Extensive list of links to information on cochlear implants and other information re: hearing impairment; user-friendly site	http://www.gohear.org/link/link.html
Cochlear Implant Association, Inc.—Links to many pertinent sites re: resources, contacts, organizations, manufacturers	http://www.cici.org
Effects of Cochlear Implants Early in Life	http://www.aamc.org/newsroom/bulletin/umich/010102.htm
Communication Disorders	
Communication Disorders and Sciences Home Page—Judith Kuster's home page for audiologists and SLPs; site has numerous links for communication disorders (CODI) professionals and parents; is updated frequently	http://www.mankato.msus.edu/dept/comdis/kuster2/welcome.html
American Speech-Language-Hearing Association—Information for consumers and professionals	http://www.asha.org

Continued

Resources	URL
Drugs and Pharmacology (NOTE: Also search Google.com by condition/disease name for commonly prescribed drugs)	
MedScape Drug Database	http://www.medscape.com/druginfo
RX LIST—Extensive information on prescription drugs; search by condition or by prescription drug name	http://www.rxlist.com
Family and Parent Resources (Resources re: specific disabilities listed below under name of disability)	
National Parent Network on Children with Disabilities—Provides numerous links	http://www.npnd.org/links_resources.htm
Parents Helping Parents—Provides access to information about specific conditions, programs, organizations, and ways to communicate with other families whose children have the same condition; articles of interest change frequently	http://www.php.com
The Unicorn Children's Foundation—Provides information about specific conditions involving communication disorders and links to other sites; also a quick screening tool for concerned parents of children 1–3 years of age	http://www.eunicorn.com/index
Special Needs—An excellent source of books about children with special needs	http://www.spcialneeds.com
Association of Birth Defect Children—Fact sheets; parent matching; links and more	http://www.birthdefects.org/
Federation for Children with Special Needs—Massachusetts organization; updates on disability issues and links	http://www.fcsn.org/
Med Help International—Patient medical information center	http://www.medhelp.org/
Zero to Three—Excellent resource for information on cognitive, physical, and social development of infants and toddlers	http://www.zerotothree.org/parent.html
Special Education Laws—Excellent resource for test of laws and links to federal agencies; message boards; bookstore; current news; site is updated frequently	http://www.specialedlaw.net/index.mv
Genetics (See also syndromes and disorders listed by name)	
Mendelian Inheritance in Man—Classic site	http://www.ncbi.nlm.nih.gov/omim/
Genetic Alliance—International coalition of 300+ consumer and health professional organizations; links to information and support groups	http://www.geneticalliance.org
Genetic diseases links	http://www.geneletter.org
Association of Birth Defect Children—Features a parent matching service; extensive links	http://www.birthdefects.org/
Health and Disabilities (See also syndromes and diseases listed by name)	
National Center for Birth Defects and Developmental Disabilities	http://www.cdc.gov/ncbddd/dh

Resources	URL
Health and Disabilities (See also syndromes and diseases listed by name)—Cont'd	
Interdisciplinary Council on Developmental and Learning Disorders—Links and annotated information on developmental disorders (DDs)	http://www.icdl.com
Waisman Center—Provides extensive list of links to sites relating to various cognitive and developmental disabilities	http://www.waisman.wisc.edu/ mrsites.html
Kids Health—Physician-approved health and development information	http://www.kidshealth.org
National Health Information Center— English and Spanish texts available	http://www.healthfinder.gov/
Bright Futures—English and Spanish texts; links	http://www.brightfutures.org
Toll-Free Health Hotline Numbers from National Library of Medicine	http://sis.nlm.nih.gov/hotlines
National Library of Medicine— Public Medicine	http://www.ncbi.nlm.nih.gov/PubMed/
Ped Base—Links to information on disorders by name; extensive database on conditions (arranged alphabetically)	http://www.icondata.com/health/ pedbase/pedlynx.htm
List of Disability Organizations and Agencies—Links to government agencies; text of laws and more	http://www.taalliance.org
Disability-specific Websites—Indices and links (arranged alphabetically)	http://www.disserv.stu.umn.edu/disability/
PedINFO—Searches; online journal links	http://www.pedinfo.org
MedScape—Current medical information and search tools for specific conditions	http://www.medscape.com
Pediatrics On Line—Links to many pediatric sites through Medical College of Georgia site	http://www.mcg.edu/PedsOnL/ PedsOnL.Menu.html
Hearing Loss (See also "Cochlear Implants")	
Sites for parents re: hearing loss— Excellent links to many other organizations, resources, and information on communication development and assistive devices	http://www.gohear.org
Free electronic newsletter from Pfizer Pharmaceuticals	http://www.Kidsears.com/
Marion Downs National Center for Infant Hearing—Excellent resource; numerous links	http://www.Colorado.edu/slhs/mdnc/
Medical Conditions and Information (See also "Health and Disabilities"; and "Libraries and General Information Resources")	
Medicine Net—Dictionary of diseases and conditions; database re: treatments, procedures, tests; search "Pediatrics" or "kids health" for detailed information	http://www.medicinenet.com

Continued

Resources	URL
Medical Conditions and Information (See also "Health and Disabilities"; and "Libraries and General Information Resources")—Cont'd	
MT Desk—Medical transcriptionists site; terminology for health professionals	http://www.mtdesk.com
American Academy of Pediatrics Journal—*Pediatrics*	http://www.pediatrics.org/all.shtml
American Medical Association—Sign on to establish a free account, which allows access to the following: search tools, a table of contents and abstracts from the Journal of the Association and other medical journals	http://www.ama-assn.org/
The Merck Manual of Medical Information: Home Edition—Good source of basic information for families on many conditions	http://www.merck.com/pubs/ manual_home/contents/htm
National Institutes of Health—Home page of the NIH provides access to research on specific conditions; use the keyword "childhood" in a general search at this web site	http://www.nih.gov
Galaxy—Links to many sites organized by category; also advanced search option	http://galaxy.einet.net/galaxy/ Medicine.html
Mental Health	
Academy of Child and Adolescent Psychiatry	http://www.aacap.org
Developmental Psychology Links	http://www.socialpsychology.org/
Interscience—Resource for journal articles in infant mental health	http://www3.interscience.wiley.com
Neonatology	
Neonatology on the Web—Links to related sites; excellent resource for parents and professionals	http://www.neonatology.org
American Academy of Pediatrics Reviews of Internet Resources by AAP Fellows	http://www.aap.og/bpi
Cochrane Neonatal Collaborative Review Group—Technical information on many procedures/issues in neonatology and medical management	http://www.nichd.nih.gov/Cochrane.htm
Prematurity	http://www.neonatology.org http://pages.cthome.net/cbristol/ preemies.html
Neurology (See also links through "Libraries and General Information Resources" and Birth Defects listed above)	
NeurologyLinx.com—Extensive information links	http://www.neurologylinx.com/
Pediatric Neurology Links—Excellent site; extensive links list	http://www.waisman.wisc.edu/child-neuro/pediatric-neurology.html

Resources	URL
Nursing	
BrownSON'S Nursing Notes—Outstanding site with many links to useful pediatric information	http://members.tripod.com/~DianneBrownson
Resources for Nurses and Families	http://pegasus.cc.ucf.edu/~wink/home.html#resources
Retardation (See also links shown under "Libraries and General Information Resources" and other organizations listed above)	
The Association for Retarded Citizens in the U.S.	http://www.aamr.org/
Council for Exceptional Children (CEC)—Links to many sites, including the ERIC clearinghouse	http://www.cec.sped.org
Speech and Language Development (see also Communication Disorders)	
American Speech-Language-Hearing Association	http://www.asha.org
Child Development Institute—Select option "disorders"	http://www.childdevelopmentinfo.com/
Syndromes and Congenital Conditions (Author suggests doing a Google search by name for specific syndromes and conditions not listed below)	
Congenital Conditions	http://www.pedinfo.org
The National Fragile X Foundation—Home page provides information and links about fragile x for parents and educators	http://www.fragilex.org/
National Institute on Child Health and Development—Information/facts about fragile x	www.nichd.nin/gov/publications/pubs/fragilextoc.htm
Apert Syndrome—Teeter's Page; information provided in many languages	http://www.apert.org
Fetal Alcohol Syndrome Resources and Materials Guide	http://theArc.org/misc/faslist.html
Prader-Willi Syndrome Association—Home page provides information and numerous links re: PWS	http://www.pwsausa.org
Rett Syndrome—International Rett Syndrome Association	http://www.rettsyndrome.org
National Institutes for Neurological Diseases and Strokes (NINDS) Information Page—Includes fact sheet and links to organizations and web sites	www.ninds.nih.gov/health_and_medical/disorders/rett_.doc.htm
Shprintzen Syndrome (Velocardialfacial Syndrome)—Fact sheet for professionals; information re: support groups; e-mail link to Dr. Robert Shprintzen	http:www.vcfsef.org
Turner Syndrome—Lists clinical and genetic features; links	http://turners.nichd.nih.gov/
Usher Syndrome Links—Information sheets; links to useful resources, organizations	http://www.nidcd.nih.gov/textonly/health/pubs_hb/usher.htm
Williams Syndrome—Information and extensive list of links to other sites and organizations	http://www.williams-syndrome.org

Continued

Resources	URL
Coding Information on Diagnoses and Conditions for Billing and Data Sharing Purposes	
World Health Organization's 2001 International Classification of Functioning, Disability, and Health (ICF)—Classification system adopted by ASHA as the framework for assessment and intervention	http://www.who.int/whosis/icd10/index.html
World Health Organization's International Classification of Disease (ICD)—System to be used in conjunction with the ICF (see previous entry) in coding individual diagnoses	http://www.who/

Abortion Termination of a pregnancy by natural or other means. A *spontaneous abortion* is a miscarriage. An infant born to a mother who has experienced many previous miscarriages, especially if proximal to birth of the index infant, can be at risk for developmental delays.

Acute Having a sudden or unexpected onset, as opposed to being an ongoing or chronic condition.

Additive risk factors Those conditions that, when superimposed on another recognized risk factor, increase the probability that a given individual will experience significant developmental problems; the cumulative effect is likely to be greater than the sum of the potential problems associated with individual risk factors involved.

Adjusted chronological age (ACA) Age a preterm infant would be if he or she had been born at term. The ACA is used in assessing developmental appropriateness of specific skills and milestones at a given point in time. Adjusting chronological age is agreed to be appropriate to 12 months corrected age. Many argue, however, that age adjustments for preterm babies should extend over 24 months to assess the child's development fairly. To compute the ACA, subtract the number of preterm weeks from the actual birth date; the product is the ACA.

Alternative communication Any method of communication designed to take the place of speech (e.g., signing, Rebus symbols, fingerspelling, electronic devices).

Americans with Disabilities Act of 1990 A far-reaching statute that covers individuals with specific disabilities; it provides a wide range of services and protections under federal law.

Amniocentesis A prenatal diagnostic technique in which amnionic fluid is withdrawn from the capsule surrounding the fetus and tested to determine the presence of genetic materials that may result in aberrations. The procedure is generally done at 15 to 20 weeks' gestation.

Anencephaly Literally "without brain," but more accurately referring to a child with a severely malformed, poorly developed brain; associated with profound retardation.

Anomaly Any abnormality of a physical structure; usually used to imply a bad or unfavorable abnormality.

Anoxia Literally "without oxygen"; the term is often used incorrectly to describe the condition of reduced oxygen supply to the brain (i.e., hypoxia). Prolonged reduction in oxygen supply or literal deprivation of oxygen to the brain can cause brain damage or death.

Apnea A cessation of breathing for more than 15 seconds. The condition is common among premature infants and can lead to hypoxia, anoxia, or death. Some premature infants are issued apnea monitors on discharge from the hospital to reduce the chances of infant mortality.

Applied behavioral analysis (ABA) A highly structured language and behavioral therapy intervention approach based on Skinnerian theory and using extended treatment sessions (up to several hours a day) in which classic stimulus-response-reinforcement procedures are rigidly applied. Some use the term *ABA* when referring to an intervention approach devised by Ivar Lovaas.

Aspiration Introduction of solids or liquids into the respiratory system from the oral or nasal cavities; the condition can lead to infection, hypoxia, anoxia, or death. Meconium aspiration is of concern in newborns. Aspiration of any kind reported in a case history signals the need for follow-up information about the incident.

Assessment A term used in different ways in both professional discussions and legal statutes. In the Individuals with Disabilities Education Act, assessment means the process by which it is determined that a complete evaluation of presenting problems is warranted. Under Part C, assessment is used to indicate a multidisciplinary process by which the strengths and needs of an eligible child and the family of the eligible child are determined for the purpose of developing an individual family service plan (IFSP); in this case, the diagnosis may actually follow the assessment. Eligibility for services is determined through the evaluation process as defined under Part C.

Assistive device Any object designed to help an individual compensate for a deficit or disorder; in communicative disorders, the term usually applies to assistive listening devices that help the hearing-impaired cope with the loss of hearing acuity.

Asymmetrical tonic neck reflex (ATN) A normal, primitive reflex pattern in newborns that, if not resolved through maturation, is cause for concern and can indicate significant problems in motor development.

At risk A term indicating that a young child has a greater-than-average chance of having a developmental delay or disorder. The risk can arise from a diagnosed handicapping condition or medical, biological, or environmental factors. Federal legislation (C of PL 205-17) allows states to define and include or exclude certain risk groups as being eligible for services under provisions of the law; hence, eligibility varies from state to state for members of specific risk groups.

Atresia An anatomical anomaly characterized by the absence of a biological opening (e.g., atresia of the external auditory meatus or choanal atresia, both of which are related to disorders of communicative development).

Auditory brainstem evoked response (ABER) testing A form of auditory evoked potential response testing in which the neurophysical behavior of the auditory mechanism is measured.

Auditory evoked potential response (AER) The neurophysiological behavior of the auditory system, which is measured by highly skilled professionals using electrophysiological devices.

Augmentative communication Any method of communicating that involves use of elements other than speech to facilitate intelligibility of the message, including the use of signs, fingerspelling, communication boards, and electronic augmentative devices.

Autism One of several childhood disorders falling under the broader category of pervasive developmental disorder; a serious, probably lifelong, developmental disorder having its origin before age 3 years and characterized by specific behaviors that meet criteria defined in the current revised edition of the *Diagnostic and Statistical Manual* published by the American Psychiatric Association. The condition affects more boys than girls and affects 1 in 500 children in the United States. Communicative impairment is a hallmark feature of the disorder, as are certain social and behavioral problems. It is often accompanied by stereotypical behaviors and tenuous eye contact, which may be the first indications of the need for assessment. Autism is genetic in some cases; the cause is unknown in others.

Autistic spectrum disorder A term used to infer varying ranges of behavioral effects or characteristics found among children diagnosed with any of the pervasive developmental disorders. Children with fewer effects, especially those with more advanced communication skills and social interactions, are likely to have a better prognosis than children who have little or no speech and whose social interactions are profoundly impaired.

Bradycardia Slow heart rate.

Branchial arch disorder Any one of several serious birth defects arising from a disturbance in embryonic development involving the branchial arch structures; such disorders often result in communicative disorders and are identified as specific syndromes (e.g., Turner syndrome) associated with the particular branchial arch affected.

Bronchopulmonary dysplasia (BPD) Damage to lung tissue that is often associated with prematurity because of the preterm infant's underdeveloped respiratory structures and use of the respirator. When tears or holes appear in the lung tissue, the infant is said to have "blown" a lung. In prematurity, BPD is often associated with intraventricular hemorrhage (IVH); the IVH-BPD combination places an infant at very high risk for communicative disorders during the developmental period.

Care plan Any one of several plans designed to provide optimal assistance to a given child or family; examples include the nursing care plan, individualized health care plan, individual family service plan, and individual education plan.

Case management Under Part H of PL 99-457, the process of coordinating all services needed to execute the individual family service plan. The term was replaced with *family service coordination* under PL 102–119 of the Individuals with Disabilities Education Act. *Case management* is also a term used by many professionals to refer to direct therapy activities. The manner in which the term is used is important, and the operational definition at any given time should be clearly understood by those who are working with the child and family because legal ramifications can be involved. Medicaid uses the term *case management* to refer to a specific set of procedures for which providers can charge a fee for services.

Case manager Under Part H of PL 99-457, the designated individual selected from the profession most closely related to the child's disability or handicap who performs the functions of service coordinator; PL 102–119 uses the term *family service coordinator* (FSC) in place of *case manager*. Parents cannot serve as their own service coordinator, but they can serve as another family's FSC. Under other standards, the meaning of case manager is considerably different, usually being restricted to discipline-specific services. Because of the legal implications, it is imperative that practitioners understand how the term is being used and what is being assumed when one agrees to take on the role of "case manager" as defined under any legal statute or implementation guideline.

Cerebral palsy A term used to describe a number of permanent neuromotor impairments acquired before the age of 3 years; subcategories of cerebral palsy that describe the type of neuromotor involvement resulting from specific areas of the brain are spasticity, ataxia, athetosis, rigidity, and mixed. Prematurity and birth trauma are commonly cited etiological factors. Because normal patterns of neuromotor maturation occur over time, it can take up to 2 years to confirm a diagnosis of cerebral palsy. Children with cerebral palsy are at high risk for hearing problems and oral communication difficulties, and many benefit from assistive communication devices.

CHARGE association A collection of physical anomalies that can occur in various combinations and to varying degrees, including coloboma, heart defects, choanal atresia, retarded growth and development, genital hypoplasia, and ear anomalies. Children diagnosed with CHARGE association are at high risk for hearing loss.

Charge nurse The nurse in charge of nursing care in a hospital or health-care unit for a given work shift.

Chorionic villus sampling A prenatal diagnostic technique in which a small sample of placental tissue is removed and used to perform chromosomal analysis. The testing can be done at an earlier gestational point (10 to 11 weeks) than can amniocentesis but is thought to be somewhat riskier to the fetus than the latter procedure.

Chromosomal anomaly or disorder Any one of many physical problems arising from too many, too few, misplaced, broken, or malformed chromosomes. Many syndromes are traced to chromosomal anomalies; many involve communicative disorders (*see* Chapter 3).

Chronic Ongoing or lasting; often used to describe a medical condition associated with communicative impairment (e.g., chronic otitis media).

Complex A collection of features or symptoms that suggest the possibility of a syndrome but lack the complete array of characteristics that would justify diagnosing that syndrome.

Condition A given characteristic or set of characteristics that differentiates a problem from a disease process (e.g., cerebral palsy versus progressive encephalopathy).

Congenital Present at birth.

Consanguineous Related by blood through common ancestors.

Consultation An indirect problem-solving process in which practitioners confer with one or more professional peers, parents, or both for the purpose of bringing their collective expertise to bear on a specific issue or problem.

Continuous positive airway pressure (CPAP) Method of delivering oxygen via nasal cannula, a procedure commonly used for brief periods of time for infants who require supplementary oxygen; extended use can result in physical damage to the respiratory system if pressure is too high.

Cyanosis Blue or dusky appearance of the skin caused by lack of oxygen.

Cytomegalovirus (CMV) A common virus that is detrimental and sometimes lethal to the developing fetus; it can cause birth defects and mental retardation.

Delay Postponement or extended time needed to accomplish a designated activity or skill.

Developmental delay Defined in two ways: (1) a significant lag in attaining developmental milestones or skills attributable to known or unknown factors; (2) lifelong deficits or anomalies that require ongoing provision of training to achieve adaptive behaviors and can require ongoing use of equipment or supportive assistance in personal care. It is essential that the professional understand the manner in which the term *developmental delay* is being used. Infant-toddler legislation (Part C of PL 205-17) allows states to define the term as they wish, and the definition varies significantly from state to state. Families and some professionals use the term to include a functional delay in acquisition of developmental milestones, whereas others use it to define lifelong disabilities.

Developmental disabilities Conditions that are permanent, have a neurodevelopmental basis, and have an effect on functional abilities in the areas of major life activity including but not limited to receptive and expressive language and mobility; the definition also includes, but is not limited to, cerebral palsy, mental retardation, multiple congenital anomalies, autism, and pervasive developmental disorder of childhood, as well as epilepsy, sensory impairments (deafness and blindness), serious learning disabilities, and hyperactivity with attention deficit disorder. Children who meet the legal definition of *developmentally disabled* are entitled to a number of social, medical, and educational services through publicly funded programs. *See* definitions included in the Americans with Disabilities Act of 1990. (Title 42, Chapter 126, USC, Section 12102); it can be accessed at http://www4.law.cornell.edu/uscode/42/ch126.html

Diagnosis In medicine, the act or process of identifying or determining the nature of a disease through examination; also the opinion derived from such examination. In general usage, an analysis of the nature of something or the conclusion reached through such analysis; also, a precise and detailed description of the characteristics for taxonomic classification. The term is often used by medical and allied health practitioners with the modifiers *descriptive*, *differential*, *definitive*, and *presumptive*. The meaning(s) of the term *diagnosis* should be clearly understood and agreed on by members of multidisciplinary teams who, as a result of their various disciplinary orientations, may use the term differently.

Diagnostic and Statistical Manual (DSM) A standard reference work published by the American Psychiatric Association containing descriptions of and criteria for labeling specific psychological and psychiatric disorders. The *DSM* is revised on a regular basis; practitioners should use the most current revision.

Dilantin A drug commonly prescribed for seizure control; if used in pregnancy, the substance can have deleterious effects on the developing fetus.

Disorder A problem or difficulty that persists over time. A disorder can be responsive to appropriate therapeutic management either through resolution of the problem or through compensatory adjustment.

Dysfunction Inefficient operation of an expected function. A dysfunction usually is responsive to appropriate intervention and need not be a permanent condition.

Dysmorphic Abnormal appearance of physical structure(s).

Dysplasia Abnormal growth of a physical structure of the body.

Early and Periodic Screening, Diagnosis, and Treatment (EPSDT) A federally funded program that provides free child-health services to eligible children from birth through 21 years of age.

Early interventionist A person who works with infants and young children who have developmental delays or disabilities or who are at risk for developmental problems and their families. In some states, an early interventionist is more specifically a person with a specific credential who serves as an infant-toddler and family educator. It is important to know the manner in which the term is used in any given state.

Education for the Handicapped Act (EHA) A federal entitlement program (PL 94-142), which established the right to a free, appropriate education in the least-restrictive environment for handicapped students from birth to 21 years of age. It was amended in 1986 to require states to provide educational services to preschool children from 3 to 5 years

of age under Part B (previously a state option) and to encourage provision of comprehensive services to handicapped and at-risk infants and toddlers under Part H (which
remained a state option under IDEA, the 1991 special education entitlement act).

Efficacy Documentation or proof that a particular treatment is more beneficial than it is
harmful.

Efficiency Documentation that a particular treatment is effective in terms of expenditure
of time, personnel, and money (not to be confused with efficacy [*see* Efficacy]).

Eligibility Meeting specified qualification(s) to receive services under state and federal
statutes, rules, and regulations; payment for providing such services hinges on determination of eligibility.

Encephalitis A viral infection that invades the brain tissue; a serious condition that can
result in death or permanent disability.

Encephalocele Opening in the skull through which encased brain matter protrudes.

Encephalopathy A disorder or disease of the brain.

Endotracheal tube (ET) A thin tube inserted through the mouth or nose and into the
trachea to deliver oxygen to the lungs.

Environmental risk The presence of family, community, or social conditions that are
predictive of negative developmental outcomes for infants and young children.

Epilepsy Any one of a range of seizure activities related to electrophysiological functions
of the brain; *see* Seizure.

Etiology The cause or source of a disease or disorder.

Evaluation *See* Assessment.

Exon A portion of DNA that codes for the mature messenger RNA.

Extra-corporeal mechanical oxygenation (ECMO) Delivery of oxygen via a heart-lung
machine to some infants admitted to the neonatal intensive care unit.

Failure to thrive (FTT) A condition diagnosed in the first 2 years of life when a child's weight
drops below the third percentile of growth with no known organic etiology.

Fat pads Extra tissue present in the cheeks of infants born at term and absent in preterm
babies, which assists the infant during sucking and feeding; also called *sucking pads.*

Fetal alcohol effects (FAE) Physical features, behaviors, or both that are associated with
maternal use of alcohol during pregnancy; this term is used when fetal alcohol syndrome
is not fully in evidence.

Fetal alcohol syndrome (FAS) A set of physical traits and behaviors common to children
with a history of prenatal exposure to alcohol. Such children often have limited cognitive
abilities, specific communicative and learning disabilities, and characteristic behaviors, as
well as physical traits that are indicative of the condition. Velopharyngeal inadequacy,
submucous cleft palate, or both are sometimes found in this population.

Focal lesions Pathogenic changes in tissues in a localized area. The term is often used in
reporting results of electroencephalograms (EEGs).

Fontanel Any one of several soft spots on the baby's head between the bony plates of the
skull. Premature fusion of the bones causes limitation of space for the brain to grow and
can result in mental retardation; timing of surgical treatment is crucial to prevention of
mental retardation associated with premature closure.

Full-term The description of the level of maturation of an infant born between
37 and 41 weeks' gestation.

Functional skills Abilities needed to perform activities of daily living.

Gavage feeding Tube feeding using a nasogastric tube leading from the nose or mouth to
the esophagus.

Genetic disorder Any of several disorders arising from autosomal dominant, autosomal
recessive, or X-linked inheritance patterns; *see also* Chromosomal anomaly or disorder.

Gestational age Age of an infant at delivery as calculated from the day of conception to the
date of delivery.

Glabella A smooth prominence on the frontal bone above the root of the nose; the forward
projecting point of the forehead in the midline at the level of the supraorbital ridges.

Glossoptosis Downward displacement of the tongue.

Gravida A term used to specify pregnancy; usually modified by a number
or description (e.g., *primigravida* for first pregnancy and *gravida 4* for fourth pregnancy).

G-tube A feeding tube (surgically attached through the abdominal wall to the stomach) that permits the child to receive nourishment when there are problems with swallowing or with certain anatomical structures of the digestive system; also called a *peg; see also* Nasogastric tube.

Haberman feeder A specially designed infant feeder for use with babies who have cleft palate; it also can be appropriate for other infants with feeding and swallowing problems.

Handicap A condition, often permanent, that interferes with one's ability to perform everyday activities in the customary way; handicaps can be physical, mental, or both.

Human immunodeficiency virus (HIV) The cause of acquired immunodeficiency syndrome, a disease known to affect the nervous system. Congenital HIV places the infant at risk for many problems, including communicative disorders.

Hydrocephalus An accumulation of cerebrospinal fluid in the head; if not relieved, the increased pressure on the brain can cause permanent damage resulting in mental retardation. Treatment is often provided in the form of a surgical shunt to divert the excess fluid to the abdominal cavity where it can be eliminated naturally.

Hyperbilirubinemia Excessive supply of the chemical bilirubin, which if left untreated can cause liver damage and, in extreme cases, brain damage or death; commonly referred to as *jaundice* because of the observable yellow skin or eye tint resulting from the condition.

Hyperextension Overextension of motor movements; when persistent or aberrant, can indicate a physical condition that interferes with typical development of motor functions.

Hypertelorism A condition in which there is an abnormally wide distance between the eyes; can reflect a family trait but is often associated with other anomalies, suggesting a syndrome.

Hypertonia Overly tense body tone; can be a diagnostic sign of motor development problems.

Hypotonia Floppiness of body tone; can be a diagnostic sign of motor or other developmental problems.

Hypoxia Significant reduction of oxygen to the brain; prolonged oxygen deprivation can cause brain damage; *not* synonymous with "anoxia."

Iatrogenic Caused by or from a treatment process (usually an undesirable effect residual to use of a life-saving drug).

Idiopathic toe walking An observable behavior of children without obvious neurological deficits who persistently walk on their toes over a *prolonged* period during the preschool years; may be an early sign of autistic spectrum disorders.

Incidence The rate of *new occurrences* of a condition in a population within a specified period of time; the term is *not* synonymous with "prevalence."

Individual education plan (IEP) The plan required for every school-age child served under federal special education legislation.

Individual family service plan (IFSP) The document that outlines services an eligible infant or toddler and family are to receive under provisions of Part C of PL 105-17. Requirements of the IFSP include a statement of the child's current health status, current levels of functioning in five developmental areas, and strengths and needs; a statement of the family's strengths (resources) and needs (priorities) and the services required to assist the family in enhancing the child's development; expected outcomes; the name of the designated family service coordinator; timelines for provision of services; sources of payment for designated services; and a transition plan.

Individuals with Disabilities Education Act (IDEA) of 1991 The act and its subsequent revisions mandate a free, appropriate education for persons with a wide range of disabilities from birth through 21 years of age.

***International Classification of Diseases* (ICD)** A standard medical reference published by the American Medical Association and used in health care settings. *ICD* codes often appear on billing slips and are used by insurers in connection with reimbursement schedules. (*See also* CPT.)

Intervention A term used to describe the various services that are provided to enhance the development of a child with developmental delays or disabilities or one at risk for disabilities or delays because of specific criteria. The term is used differently by members of different professional disciplines (especially by counselors and psychologists who also may work in substance-abuse programs). Practitioners should ensure that they understand the manner in which the term is used by colleagues. *Early intervention (or developmental intervention)* is the preferred term used in working with infants and toddlers; however, *early intervention* also is used by practitioners to identify interventions offered on recognition of a problem, which can connote a different timeframe than is used by infant-toddler specialists.

Intrauterine growth retardation (IUGR) Failure of the fetus to develop appropriate body size, weight, or both during gestation; a condition often associated with developmental delays and disorders.

Intraventricular hemorrhage (IVH) A condition common to premature infants involving bleeding within the ventricles of the brain. The extent of the bleeding is designated by assignment of a grade: grade I is least extensive, and grade IV is most extensive. Informally referred to as a *bleed*, the condition may resolve itself with no discernible aftereffects. A child with a grade III or grade IV IVH is considered to be at risk for communication problems (and other developmental problems) that can emerge at a later date. IVH is detected by head ultrasound testing.

Intubation Insertion of a tube into the body; endotracheal intubation is the process used to administer certain anesthesias. Repeated or careless intubation can result in damage to the surrounding structures, especially the vocal cords, causing difficulty with phonation.

Jaundice A common condition exhibited by newborns; treated by bilirubin reduction lamps (bililights); *see* Hyperbilirubinemia.

Kernicterus Damage to the nervous system caused by excessive bilirubin in the blood.

Lanugo A covering of fine, downy hair on the fetus; its presence in the newborn is a characteristic of preterm delivery.

Laryngeal hypoplasia Underdevelopment of laryngeal structures; it can have implications for both respiratory function and phonation.

Lead agency The designated state agency responsible for implementation of infant-toddler legislation and coordination of efforts among other state and community agencies and provider groups.

Leukomalacia A serious condition characterized by softening of the white matter of the brain caused by loss of viability and function of the tissue.

Lovaas therapy An intensive and specific program of behavioral therapy requiring 40 hours of intervention per week and used with children who are diagnosed with pervasive developmental disorder or autism; *see* Applied behavioral analysis.

Low birth weight (LBW) Variously defined as birth weight of less than 2500 g, but usually understood to refer to birth weights of less than 1250 g.

Macrocephaly Head circumference larger than normal for age and body size; it can be a family trait or be indicative of hydrocephalus or other significant medical conditions.

Management A course of intervention or treatment provided to prevent or reduce the effects of a condition; often used interchangeably with *treatment* or *intervention*. Members of multidisciplinary teams should discuss and agree on the use of the terms for purposes of their work with infants, toddlers, and families.

Meconium The waste product material excreted by the fetus; aspiration of meconium is a potentially serious perinatal complication affecting the infant's respiratory system. Infections resulting from meconium aspiration can be lethal. Infants with this condition may be at risk for future communication disorders and other developmental disorders.

Medicaid A state-operated, federally funded health program available to infants and toddlers whose parents qualify for eligibility by way of income level or special circumstance, such as admission of the newborn to a neonatal intensive care unit or extremely low birth weight of the infant.

Meningitis Inflammation of the meninges (tissue encasement of the brain and spinal column) caused by viral or bacterial infection; it can result in brain damage, blindness, cerebral palsy, seizures, hearing loss, or mental retardation.

Meningocele Hernial protrusion of the meninges (the three layers of tissue that envelop the brain and spinal cord: dura matter, pia matter, and arachnoid) through a defect in the skull or vertebral column.

Microcephaly Literally "small head"; can be associated with premature fusion of the bones of the skull, which, if left untreated, can restrict brain growth and result in mental retardation.

Microtia A craniofacial anomaly in which the structure of the ear(s) is small; often but not always associated with hearing loss.

Monitors Any of several devices used to measure some aspect of the infant's physiological status (e.g., oxygen intake, apnea, temperature, respiration, heart rate, intake of liquids, composition of blood gases).

Morbidity Illness or disease; rate of occurrence of disease in the population.

Moro reflex A normal primitive reflex. Failure of resolution through maturation of the central nervous system can have diagnostic implications for motor problems.

Myelination Formation of an outer sheath as nerve fibers mature. Failure of myelination is associated with developmental delays and disorders.

Myelomeningocele Hernial protrusion of the cord and its meninges through a defect in the vertebral canal.

Nasogastric (NG) tube A flexible tube inserted through the nose or mouth and esophagus and used to deliver breast milk or formula to infants who have difficulty swallowing.

Necrosis Dying off of tissue cells.

Neonatal intensive care unit (NICU) A specialized hospital nursery facility designed for infants with critical care needs; there are four levels, representing increasing capabilities to handle complex medical care of newborns. Sophistication of equipment and staff increases as the levels increase. Level I must provide adequate staff to resuscitate infants born in the delivery room, stabilize sick infants before transfer to Level II, III, or IV units, continue care for healthy infants until discharge, and continue special care for sick infants transferred from Level II, III, or IV NICUs. Level II must have personnel to provide all services listed for Level I units plus intermediate care for infants born in the hospital's high-risk delivery facilities. Level III must provide personnel to serve normal and high-risk infants, including resuscitation, stabilization, and continuing care for sick infants transferred from Level I and Level II facilities. Level IV units must have facilities and trained staff to perform the most advanced medical and surgical procedures (e.g., organ transplants).

Neonate Newborn infant through age 28 days.

Neural tube defect A general term inclusive of myelomeningocele, meningocele, spina bifida, and anencephaly.

Neurodevelopmental treatment (NDT) *See* Sensory integration therapy.

Nonverbal communication Any form of communication that does not use spoken words.

Norm-referenced scales assessment Measures that compare a child's performance to that of typical age peers.

Occiput The back of the head.

Osteogenesis imperfecta A syndrome in which bones are susceptible to fracture; deafness can be a coexisting condition.

Ototoxin Any chemical or substance that damages the auditory nerve and consequently has the potential to impair hearing.

Palmar grasp Immature grasp in which the palm is used, rather than the fingers, to manipulate an object. Persistence of this immature pattern can be indicative of fine-motor impairment in young children.

Patent ductus arteriosus (PDA) A physical malformation of the heart commonly seen in children with Down syndrome.

Penetrance The degree to which a genetic factor exhibits itself in a given individual; some genetic anomalies are passed from one generation to another with varying degrees of observable effects (varying degrees of penetrance of the trait in question).

Perinatal Period of time extending from week 18 of gestation to 1 week after delivery.

Phenobarbital A medication commonly prescribed for control of seizures; if used in pregnancy, can have deleterious effects on the developing fetus.

Phenylketonuria (PKU) A disorder of metabolism that allows accumulation of excessive phenylalanine in brain tissues, which can lead to mental retardation. Most states require PKU testing of all infants. If present, treatment requires strict control of diet.

Phototherapy Treatment for jaundice using bright lights informally referred to as bililights.

Physicians' Current Procedural Terminology (CPT) A publication of the American Medical Association describing and classifying clinical procedures. The reference is widely used by medical records librarians and third-party payers, such as insurance companies and Medicaid. *CPT* codes can be used in conjunction with *ICD* codes (*see* International Classification of Diseases [ICD]).

Placenta abruptio Detachment of the placenta before birth; a potential cause of spontaneous abortion (miscarriage), hypoxia, or asphyxia in the infant.

Pneumothorax Collection of air and gas in the chest cavity, which can result from too much pressure of an oxygen delivery system.

Post-term delivery Delivery of an infant after the thirty-ninth week of gestation. Post-term babies are at risk for a variety of problems, including language disorders.

Pragmatics A set of sociolinguistic rules related to language usage within the communicative context (*See* Rossetti LM: *The Rossetti Infant-Toddler Language Scale: Examiner's Manual,* East Moline, Ill, 1990, LinguiSystems, pp 8–9.) Early infant-caregiver interactions are the foundation for the learning of pragmatic rules used by the culture to which the family belongs.

Prematurity Delivery of an infant before the thirty-ninth week of gestation. Extreme prematurity, especially if combined with bronchopulmonary dysplasia and grade III or grade IV intraventricular hemorrhage, places the infant at risk for developmental problems, including language disorders.

Preterm The preferred term among medical practitioners for delivery of an infant before the thirty-eighth week of gestation; commonly used by the general public synonymously with *prematurity.*

Prevalence The total rate or proportion of cases in a population at or during a specific period of time.

Prevention Any activity conducted for the purpose of avoiding the occurrence of a disease or disorder (primary prevention), eliminating or curing it if present (secondary prevention), or reducing its negative effects through treatment if amelioration of the condition itself is not possible (tertiary prevention).

Primitive reflexes Motoric responses that develop before birth and persist in infancy. Primitive reflexes are expected to resolve in predictable sequences in favor of voluntary motor control by the end of the first year of life. Persistence of primitive reflexes is a significant diagnostic indicator of developmental problems. Because motor development is intricately interwoven with communicative development, persistent primitive reflexes place infants at risk for communicative delays and disorders.

Prognosis A statement of the probability for full or partial habilitation or rehabilitation based on the professional's assessment in light of all information at hand.

Prone Lying on the stomach or abdomen.

Ptosis A muscular problem in which the eyelid droops; sometimes seen in combination with other craniofacial anomalies associated with developmental delays and disabilities; ptosis also can be a family trait of no particular diagnostic significance.

Public Law 205-17 The 1997 amendments to IDEA reauthorizing and providing funds for special education; provisions for infant-toddler and family services are contained in Part C of this legislation.

Public Law 102-119 The 1991 reauthorization of the Education of the Handicapped Act, including Part H, renaming it as *Individuals with Disabilities Education Act (IDEA).*

Public Law 99-457 The 1986 amendment to PL 94-142 that authorized services to children from 3 to 5 years of age (sec. 619, Part B) gave states the option of providing services to handicapped and at-risk infants, toddlers, and their families (Part B).

Public Law 94-142 The *Education for the Handicapped Act (see also* Individuals with Disabilities Act [IDEA]*).*

Qualified provider A term used for service providers on the multidisciplinary assessment team required under Part C regulations. Each state is allowed to identify the training and credentials required of those who are deemed to be qualified providers, but such designation must be in keeping with the "highest entry-level standards" in the state for each discipline. Practitioners in each state should become familiar with their state's definitional requirements.

Respiratory distress syndrome (RDS) A set of symptoms resulting from oxygen deprivation in the perinatal period; often associated with bronchopulmonary dysplasia.

Retinopathy of prematurity (ROP) A condition caused by excessive or prolonged use of supplementary oxygen in premature babies during the perinatal period, which adversely affects the infant's retina; associated with reduced visual acuity.

Retrognathia Small, underdeveloped mandible that is posterior to the normal position in relation to the maxilla; a trait associated with some syndromes or sequences (e.g., Pierre Robin sequence). Retrognathia can involve significant implications for growth of the head and facial structures and for dental development; it also can be a family trait of no particular developmental significance. It is sometimes confused with a dental underbite, which commonly is present in the condition.

Rubella German measles virus. When rubella is contracted in pregnancy, it causes severe birth defects, including sensory anomalies, heart problems, mental retardation, and deafness.

Screening A process (formal or informal) by which individuals requiring further evaluation or assessment are identified from a general population.

Section 619 A "shorthand" reference to a section of the federal statute that ensures early and continuing care and education for developmentally disabled children at no cost to their families; funding for such services is provided to states under block grants.

Seizure An involuntary lapse of awareness or bodily control resulting from abnormal neural impulses; when used to describe neuromotor aberrations observed in infants and toddlers, seizures can be categorized as idiopathic (peculiar to a given individual and having no easily identified cause), grand mal (involving temporary loss of consciousness along with uncontrolled neuromotor activity), or petit mal (involving a momentary lapse of awareness during which the child may maintain erect body posture and seem to be daydreaming). Spontaneous resolution of seizure activity can occur, but children with seizures are at risk for developmental delays and disorders. Pharmacological treatment is commonly prescribed for persistent seizure activity and as a preventative measure when a history of seizures is present.

Self-stimulation Any habit of a child engaged in for the purpose of providing sensory stimulation or self-calming. Transitory self-stimulation is normal at certain stages of development; unusual, persistent, or excessive forms of self-stimulation (e.g., rocking, arm flapping, spinning) are symptomatic of particular problems, including mental retardation, autism, emotional disorders, and some physical disorders.

Sensorimotor stage development A developmental stage defined by Piaget that is generally inclusive of behaviors characteristic of children between birth and 2 years of age.

Sensory integration therapy A form of therapy based on neurodevelopmental treatment techniques developed by Karl and Berta Bobath for cerebral palsy. The goal of sensory integration therapy is to promote gross motor development in children with impaired neuromotor function. Strategies used in sensory integration therapy have clinical applications in calming some children and making them more receptive to therapies involving instruction and attentional focus. This form of therapy is considered controversial among some early-intervention practitioners.

Sepsis Presence of infection in the blood.

Serological Relating to the study or measurement of components of serum.

Shunt A surgically inserted tube to divert fluid from one part of the body to another; shunts are often used to relieve pressure on the brain caused by excessive accumulation of cerebrospinal fluid in the cranium.

Skin tags Extra bits of skin (with or without cartilage), often abnormally placed, sometimes seen on the head or neck of a child with developmental anomalies; such tissue often represents abnormal migration of facial structures during the embryonic period and can indicate that other problems also occurred during that stage of development.

Sleep apnea *See* Apnea.

Small for gestational age (SGA) The term designates an infant of any gestational age whose weight and size are below expectations for its developmental level. Leading causes of SGA include poor maternal nutrition, maternal illness, or maternal substance abuse. SGA babies are at risk for developmental delays.

Soft neurological signs (SNS) Any neuromotor symptom or physical symptom (or combination thereof) that suggests the possibility of atypical neurological maturation. One sign, taken alone, sometimes raises concern; several signs taken together always warrant further diagnostic assessment. Some children with learning disabilities exhibit an unusual number of soft neurological signs. Research is presently exploring the implications of such signs regarding predicting the risk for learning disabilities among children who exhibit such characteristics. Examples of SNSs include dysdiadochokinesia, astereogenesis, persistence of primitive reflexes, sensory extinction, and diminished dexterity, as well as unusual patterns of form or growth of the hands, feet, and nails and double hair whorls.

State regulation disorder A condition that, for a variety of reasons, causes some infants to be unable to adjust physiological functions such as sleep-wake cycles, level of alertness, or maintenance of body temperature; this difficulty is common in infants suffering from prenatal drug exposure, but can result from other factors.

Stenosis A narrowing of an anatomical passageway (e.g., stenosis of the larynx, stenosis of the external auditory meatus, stenosis of the esophagus).

Subdural hemorrhage Intracranial hemorrhage usually resulting from trauma.

Supine Lying on the back.

Supplementary Security Income (SSI) Federally funded income support for disabled individuals, including infants and toddlers who meet specific eligibility criteria. Current eligibility criteria are available upon request from the local Social Security office or from the national office of the Social Security Administration. Copies also should be available through state education and health agency offices.

Surfactant A substance used in the perinatal period to treat respiratory problems common to premature infants.

Syndactyly Webbing between the fingers or toes; a condition common to some syndromes that also involve anomalies of the head and neck (because the timing of development of those structures is concurrent in embryological formations) and can be associated with communicative disorders in affected children.

Tachycardia Rapid heart rate.

Technology dependent A term used to describe reliance on special equipment (e.g., monitors, supplementary oxygen) to sustain life or to perform specified functions; also refers to infants and toddlers and older individuals who require special devices to assist them in communicating with others; *see* Augmentative communication and Assistive device.

Telecanthus Increased distance between the medial canthi (inner corners of the eye), the presence of which can be either a familial trait or a characteristic of a congenital anomaly.

Temperament Individual differences of social adaptation, self-regulation, and behavior styles of a child.

Teratogen Any agent or factor that produces physical defects in the developing embryo.

Therapeutic positioning The facilitation of specific functions or activities for a given individual through physical positioning (e.g., seating, propping, lying) that reduces or relieves the body's expenditure of energy in the attempt to maintain balance or posture. Therapeutic positioning is usually designed by a physical or occupational therapist. It is imperative that the speech-language pathologist be aware of the benefits of therapeutic positioning when working with neurologically impaired children.

Therapy The application of specific techniques designed to provide a cure or diminution of symptoms or effects of a disease, condition, or behavior. Sometimes used as a synonym for *intervention* or *management*. For the sake of effective communication, multidisciplinary team members need to discuss and agree on the terminology to be used with regard to primary, secondary, and tertiary prevention procedures.

TORCH syndrome Acronym for infections in newborns attributable to any combination of toxoplasmosis, rubella, cytomegalovirus, and herpes virus; TORCH syndrome places a child at risk for hearing loss and language problems.

Toxemia A condition resulting from the spread of bacterial toxins by the bloodstream. Toxemia of pregnancy results from metabolic disturbances during gestation and can result in preeclampsia, a condition that compromises health of the mother and child during delivery.

Toxin Any substance (e.g., heavy metals [e.g., lead], bacterial toxins, or chemical toxins [e.g., alcohol or drugs]) ingested or absorbed by the body that produces a "poisonous" effect and, if left untreated, can produce permanent adverse consequences.

Toxoplasmosis A protozoan disease that can cause lesions of the central nervous system in infants leading to blindness.

Tracheostomy Surgically created airway that allows a patient to breathe through a hole in the neck. Children with tracheostomies usually cannot approximate their vocal cords for phonation. Permanent damage to the vocal cords can occur if prolonged use of the tracheostomy is required to maintain a patent airway.

Treatment Any means used to cure, eliminate, or alleviate the effects of a disease or condition; sometimes used synonymously with *therapy, management*, and *intervention*. Agreement on the use of these terms is essential to effective communication among professionals, and understanding their meanings should be a priority for discussion by members of multidisciplinary teams.

Trisomy An extra chromosome of any chromosomal pair. A common form of trisomy affecting chromosome 21 is Down syndrome.

Very low birth weight (VLBW) Birth weight of less than 1000 g.

WIC Acronym for Special Supplemental Food Program for Women, Infants, and Children, a federally funded, publicly administered maternal and child health nutrition program designed to enhance the health of women of child-bearing age, infants, and young children.

INDEX

Page numbers followed by *f* indicate figures; *t*, tables; *b*, boxes.

A

AAC. *See* Augmentative and alternative communication (AAC).
AAP. *See* American Academy of Pediatrics (AAP).
Aarskog hypertelorism, 62t
ABA. *See* Applied behavioral analysis (ABA).
ABER testing. *See* Auditory brainstem evoked response (ABER) testing.
Aberrations, chromosomal, 37-38
Ablepharon-macrostomia, 62t
Abortion, definition of, 285
ABR. *See* Auditory brain stem response (ABR).
ABR threshold, 115, 115f
ACA. *See* Adjusted chronological age (ACA).
Achondroplasia, 62t
Acoupedic method, 214t
Acoustic method, 214t
Acoustic reflex testing
    in hearing-impaired infants and toddlers, 109
    immittance battery and, 105
Acquired communication disorders, 49
Acquired diseases, communicative disorders and, 38, 39t-40t
Acquired immunodeficiency syndrome (AIDS), 89
Acrocephalopolysyndactyly, carpenter, 62t
Acrocephalosyndactyly, Pfeiffer, 64t
Acrodysostosis, 62t
Acroosteolysis, 62t
Actinic dermatitis, 62t
Acute, definition of, 285
ADAM fetal mutilation, 62t
Adaptations for stimulation, readiness for communication and, 186
Additive risk factors, definition of, 285
ADI-R. *See* Autism Diagnostic Interview-R (ADI-R).
Adjusted chronological age (ACA), definition of, 285
Administrative references, 267-274
ADOS. *See* Autism Diagnostic Observation Schedule (ADOS).
Adult instruction, communication development and, 190-191
Adult language, simplifying, language intervention and, 195
AEP. *See* Auditory-evoked potential (AEP).
AEPS. *See* Assessment, Evaluation, and Programming System (AEPS).
AER. *See* Auditory evoked potential response (AER).
Affective vocal models, language intervention and, 195

Age
    adjusted chronological, definition of, 285
    gestational. *See* Gestational age.
Agency, lead, 12, 291
Ages and Stages Questionnaire, ed 2, 131t
Agyria, 64t
AIDS. *See* Acquired immunodeficiency syndrome (AIDS).
Albers-Schonberg osteopetrosis, 62t
Albinism, Waardenburg central, 66t
Alerting, developmental sequence of auditory skills during first year of life and, 216t
Alexander Graham Bell Association for the Deaf, 269t
Alleles, recombination of, human genome and, 60
Alliance of Genetic Support Groups, 269t
Alopecia, 63t
Alpha-galactosidase B, 66t
Alport nephropathy and deafness, 62t
Als, Heidelese, 13
Alstrom deafness, 62t
Alternative communication, 192, 285
Alternative sensory devices, hearing loss and, 212-213
American Academy
    of Audiology, 24
    for Cerebral Palsy and Developmental Medicine, 269t
    of Neurology, 123, 225
    of Pediatrics (AAP), 8, 15, 24, 96, 123, 135, 225, 270t
American Association for the Care of Children's Health, 270t
American Brittle Bone Association, 270t
American Cleft Palate Educational Foundation, 270t
American Council for the Blind, 270t
American Foundation for Maternal and Child Health, 270t
American Occupational Therapy Association, 24, 270t
American Physical Therapy Association, 270t
American Psychiatric Association, 121
American sign language (AMESLAN; ASL), 214t
American Society for Deaf Children, 270t
American Speech-Language Association, 24
American Speech-Language-Hearing Association (ASHA), 24, 225, 270t
Americans with Disabilties Act of 1990, definition of, 285
AMESLAN. *See* American sign language (AMESLAN; ASL).

Aminoglycoside antibiotics, 49
Amniocentesis, definition of, 285
Amplification, binaural versus monaural, 210-211
Analysis, applied behavioral. *See* Applied
  behavioral analysis (ABA).
Anemia, sickle cell, 65t
Anencephaly, 54-55, 285
Angelman jerky gait, 62t
Aniridia, 62t
Anomaly(ies)
  chromosomal, definition of, 287
  common heritable, 53-55, 54f, 54t
  congenital, 38
  craniofacial, oral-motor and swallow assessment
    and, 241t-243t
  definition of, 285
  isolated versus syndromic forms of, 56t
  nonsyndromic, 53
  oculofacial, 64t
Anoxia, definition of, 285
Antibiotics, aminoglycoside, 49
Apert acrocephaly, 62t
Apert syndrome, 61
Apnea
  definition of, 285
  preterm infants and, 89-90
  sleep, definition of, 294
Applied behavioral analysis (ABA), 136-137, 179
  definition of, 285
  modified, 136-137
Approximations of syllabic content, language
  intervention and, 194
Apraxia
  developmental, of speech, 144-146
  Internet resources for, 277
  of speech, childhood, 146
Arachnodactyly, 66t
Arena-assessment formats, 150-151
Art gallery visit scenario, communication play
  protocol and, 196t
ASD. *See* Autistic spectrum disorder (ASD).
ASHA. *See* American Speech-Language-Hearing
  Association (ASHA).
ASL. *See* American sign language (AMESLAN;
  ASL).
Asperger syndrome, 121-122, 124t-125t, 277-278
Asphyxia, 49
Aspiration, definition of, 285
ASQ. *See* Autism Screening Questionnaire (ASQ).
Assessing Prelinguistic and Linguistic Behaviors,
  163t
Assessment, 141-171
  autistic spectrum disorder and, 121-140
  behavioral threshold, 101-104
  of child competency and difficulty, 255t
  communication, tools for, 158-162, 163t-164t,
    166t-168t
  communicative diagnoses and, 157-162, 163t-164t
  of communicative disorders, role of single and
    multiple risk factors in, 41-47, 44t-45t,
    46t-47t
  of communicative means and functions, cue
    questions in, 254f
  definition of, 286
  developmental, in neonatal intensive care unit,
    95-96, 95t
  developmental delays and disorders and, 35-37

Assessment *(Continued)*
  direct, autistic spectrum disorder and, 129-130
  Evaluation, and Programming System (AEPS),
    163t
  examination, interpretation, and reporting and,
    141-171
  family, 143-149
  feeding, in neonatal intensive care unit, 93-95
  groups of concern to speech-language pathologist
    and, 153-157
  of hearing-impaired infants and toddlers, 101-119
  identification of atypical communicative
    development and, 141-152
  of Infants and Toddlers in Naturalistic
    Contexts, 163t
  interpretation of, to family, 152-153
  language, 133t
  of Mother-Infant Interaction, 163t
  neonatal, for feeding, 239t-240t
  in neonatal intensive care unit, 93-96
  normal development and, 229-247
  norm-referenced scales, definition of, 292
  ongoing, of communication development, 197
  planning of, 158, 159t-160t
  play, 151-152
  of Preterm Infant Behavior, 95t
  reporting results and, 162-166
  sequence for, 159t-160t
  tools and procedures of, 249-265
  traditional, 150-151
  triage concept in, 142-143
Assistant Secretary for Planning and Evaluation
  of the U.S. Department of Health and Human
  Services, 7
Assistive devices
  augmentative and alternative communication
    and, 193
  definition of, 286
Assistive technology
  communication development and, 191-193
  no need for, communication development and,
    193-197
Association
  of Birth Defect Children, 271t
  CHARGE, definition of, 287
  for Persons with Severe Handicaps, 271t
  for Retarded Citizens, 20
Asymmetrical tonic neck reflex (ATN), definition
  of, 286
Asymmetry strabismus, 65t
At risk, definition of, 286
Ataxia, cerebellar, 62t
ATN. *See* Asymmetrical tonic neck reflex (ATN).
Atresia
  definition of, 286
  of larynx, heritable anomalies and, 54
Attachment, infant, readiness for communication
  and, 188
Attending, developmental sequence of auditory
  skills during first year of life and, 216t
Attention deficit disorder, 47t
Attention deficit–hyperactivity disorder, 277
Attributing meaning, language intervention
  and, 194
Atypical communicative development, 141-152
Atypical language development,
  communication impairments and, 10-11

Audiologist, role of, in neonatal intensive care unit, 14
Audiometry, speech, in hearing-impaired infants and toddlers, 104-105
Auditory brain stem response (ABR), 111-117, 114f, 118
  determination of site of peripheral pathology and, 116f
  evaluation of neural integrity and, 114f
  threshold estimation and, 114-116, 115f
Auditory brainstem evoked response (ABER) testing, definition of, 286
Auditory evoked potential response (AER), definition of, 286
Auditory method, 214t
Auditory Numbers Test, 105
Auditory reception, hearing loss and, 202-203
Auditory skills, developmental sequence of, during first year of life, 216t
Auditory stimulation, readiness for communication and, 187
Auditory training, hearing loss and, 215-216, 216t
Auditory-evoked potential (AEP), 111-117
Auditory-visual reception, hearing loss and, 204-205
Augmentative and alternative communication (AAC), 192
Augmentative communication, definition of, 286
Aural habilitation, hearing loss and, 207-218
Autism, 46t, 286
Autism Diagnostic Interview-R (ADI-R), 131t
Autism Diagnostic Observation Schedule (ADOS), 131t
Autism National Committee, 24
Autism Screening Questionnaire (ASQ), 131t
Autism Society of America, 130, 272t
Autistic continuum disorder, 122
Autistic disorder, 124t
Autistic spectrum disorder (ASD), 121-140
  approaches that have proven helpful with infants and toddlers, 136-137
  assessment of, 123-130, 129-130
  case history in, 127-128
  counseling and, 134-135
  definition of, 286
  diagnosis of, in very young children, 123-130, 131t-133t
  differential diagnosis of, 126-130
  direct testing in diagnosis of, 129-130
  earliest indications of, 129
  experimental and emerging treatment elements and, 137
  follow-up care in, 130-138
  information about causes of, 130-134
  Internet resources for, 277-278
  intervention options for, 135-138
  management options for, 135-138
  observation of child in, 128-129
  parent/family interview in, 128
  pervasive developmental disorders and, 121-123
  procedural protocols for, in very young children, 123-130
  review of reports by other professionals in, 128
  tools and procedures for, 130, 131t-133t
  treatment options for, 135-138
  triad of symptoms clusters for definition of, 122
  unproven therapies and, 137-138

Autistic Spectrum Disorders, 130
Autosomal dominant inheritance, 57f
Autosomal dominant rolandic epilepsy, 57
Autosomal recessive inheritance, 57f
Autosomal trisomies, 53

B

Bands, constricting, 62t
Battery, immittance, 105
Battery check, hearing aid, 212
Bayley Scales, 96
Beaked nose, 65t
Beckwith-Wiedemann exomphalos, 62t
Beckwith-Wiedemann syndrome, 35
Behavior
  categories of, 260t
  communication development and, 189
  idiosyncratic, austistic spectrum disorder and, 122
  interactive, levels of, 259t-260t
  observed, recording, 260t-262t
Behavioral analysis, applied. See Applied behavioral analysis (ABA).
Behavioral status, changes in, monitoring, 189-190
Behavioral threshold assessment, 101-104
  in 2- to 3-year-old children, 104
  in neonates, 101-102
  in older infants, 102-104
Behind-the-ear (BTE) hearing aids, 210
Bifid hallux, 64t
Bilateral femoral dysgenesis–unusual facies, 62t
Bilingual-bicultural approach, 214t
Billing, diagnosis codes for, 284t
Binaural amplification, hearing aids and, 210-211
Binaural hearing, 210-211
Binder maxillonasal dysplasia, 62t
Birth defects, Internet resources for, 278
Birth weight
  extremely low, 43
  low, definition of, 291
  very low, 43, 296
Blepharophimosis, 63t
Bloom dwarfism, 62t
Bone dysplasia, 64t
BPD. See Bronchopulmonary dysplasia (BPD).
Brachycephaly, Smith-Magenis, 65t
Brachydactyly, 62t
Bradycardia, definition of, 286
Brain growth and language from birth to 2 years, 231t
Brain injury
  in infancy, toddlers with history of, 193
  traumatic, 46t
Branchial arch disorder, definition of, 286
Branchiooculofacial syndrome, 62t
Broad thumb and hallux, 65t
Bronchopulmonary dysplasia (BPD), 42-43, 89, 286
BTE hearing aids. See Behind-the-ear (BTE) hearing aids.

C

CAM. See Complementary and Alternative Medicine (CAM).
Camptodactyly, 67t
Capitation, managed care and, 19
Care plan, definition of, 287

Caregivers
  interaction of children with, 147-149
  interactions between infants and, facilitation
      of, 185
Carpenter acrocephalopolysyndactyly, 62t
CARS. *See* Childhood Autism Rating Scale
      (CARS).
Case history, autistic spectrum disorder and,
      127-128
Case management, 12, 287
Case manager, definition of, 287
Case studies in communication impairment in
      infants and toddlers, 1-6
CATCH-22, 63t
CDIs. *See* Childhood Development Inventories
      (CDIs).
CEC. *See* Council for Exceptional Children (CEC),
      Division of Early Childhood (DEC).
Census Bureau, 7
Center for Birth Defects Information Services, 271t
Central nervous system maturation, 232t
Centromeric instability, 64t
Cerebellar ataxia, 62t
Cerebral dysfunction, 65t
Cerebral palsy, 47t
  definition of, 287
  Internet resources for, 279
Cerebrocostomandibular syndrome, 62t
Certain severe emotional disorders, 122
Challenges, cognitive, 31
CHARGE association, 62t, 287
Charge nurse, definition of, 287
CHAT. *See* Checklist for Autism in Toddlers
      (CHAT).
Checklist for Autism in Toddlers (CHAT), 132t
Child competency and difficulty, assessment
      of, 255t
Child Neurology Society, 225
Childhood apraxia of speech, 146
Childhood Autism Rating Scale (CARS), 131t
Childhood Development Inventories (CDIs), 132t
Childhood disintegrative disorder, 121-122,
      125t-126t, 149
Children
  areas of competency and difficulty of, identifica-
      tion of, by parents, 255t-259t
  at-risk, determining, for developmental delays
      and disorders, 32-37
  atypical behaviors of, 149
  communication patterns typical of, 146-147
  communicative abilities of, information
      provided by parents about, 143-144, 145t
  communicative disorders in, 174t
  consultation and, 176-177
  deaf, common speech characteristics of, 208t
  handicapped prelanguage, interaction styles of,
      259t-262t
  interaction of
      with caregivers, 147-149
      with family, 16, 17f
  observation of, autistic spectrum disorder and,
      128-129
  promoting functional abilities of, 33-34
  at risk, 32-37
      assessment of, 35-37
      diagnosis of, 35-37
      evaluation of, 35-37

Children *(Continued)*
  prevention and, 34-35
  screening for, 35-37
  screening, referral, and follow-up of, 175-176
  strategies of speech-language pathologist with,
      175-182
  2-year-old to 3-year-old, behavioral threshold
      assessment in, 104
  typical behaviors of, 149
  very young, autistic spectrum disorder and,
      123-130
Chondrodysplasia punctata, 62t
Chondrodystrophy, 65t
Chorionic villus sampling, definition of, 287
Chorioretinal cerebral dysplasia, 52
Chromosomal aberrations, 37-38
Chromosomal anomaly, definition of, 287
Chromosomal disorder, definition of, 287
Chromosome 8 trisomy, 63t
Chromosome 18 trisomy, 56t
Chromosome 21 trisomy, 53, 62t
Chromosome abnormalities, 53
Chromosome 3p+, 62t
Chromosome 4p+, 62t
Chromosome 4p−, 62t
Chromosome 5p−, 62t
Chromosome 9p+, 62t
Chromosome 9p−, 63t
Chromosome 11p+, 62t
Chromosome 18p−, 62t
Chromosome 1q+, 62t
Chromosome 6q−, 62t
Chromosome 7q+, 62t
Chromosome 10q+, 62t
Chromosome 18q−, 62t
Chromosome X, 63t
Chromosome X−, 63t
Chromosome XXY, 63t
Chromosomes, sex, trisomies of, 53
Chronic, definition of, 287
Chronological age, adjusted, definition of, 285
Clasped thumb, 63t
*Classification of Child and Adolescent Mental
      Diagnoses in Primary Care*, 8
Cleft lip, 66t
Cleft palate, 63t, 279
Clefting, 63t
Clefts of larynx, heritable anomalies and, 54
Clinical service delivery model, 25t
Clumsiness, 66t
Cluttering speech, 63t
CMV. *See* Cytomegalovirus (CMV).
Cochlear implants, 212-213, 279, 281t
Cockayne precocious senility, 63t
Codes, diagnosis, Internet resources for, 284t
Coffin-Siris coarse face, 63t
Cognitive delay, 32, 33
Cognitive development, facilitation of, 186-188
Cognitively challenged individual, 31
Cohen hypotonia, 63t
Comelia de Lange Syndrome Foundation, 271t
Commenting context, Communication Play
      Protocol and, 195
Communication
  adult instruction and, 190-191
  alternative, definition of, 285
  assistive technology and, 191-193

Communication *(Continued)*
  augmentative
    and alternative, 192
    definition of, 286
  delayed. *See* Communicative delays.
  development of
    adult instruction and, 190-191
    approaches when assistive technology is not
        required, 193-197
    arena-assessment format and, 150-151
    assessment of, 157-162, 159t-160t
    assistive technology and, 191-193
    atypical, 141-152
    cognitive development and, 186-188
    communication assessment tools and,
        158-162
    communication patterns typical of child and,
        146-147
    communicative diagnoses and, 157-162
    direct management in, 194-197, 196t
    examination of oral mechanism and related
        physical characteristics and, 144-146
    facilitating, in infancy, 184-190
    family assessment in, 143-149
    individual family services plan and, 165-166
    in infancy, facilitation of, 184-190
    infant/toddler checklist for, 252f-253f
    information provided by parents about
        child's communicative abilities and,
        143-144, 145t
    interactions between infant and caregivers
        and, 185
    interpreting of, to family, 152-153
    judgment-based assessment and, 160-161
    late talkers and, 191
    monitoring changes in physical and
        behavioral status and, 189-190
    multidimensional scoring systems and, 162
    multiple strategies and, 161-162
    ongoing assessment as treatment or
        intervention planning and, 197
    physical development to promote readiness
        for communication, 185-186
    play assessment and, 151-152
    predictors of language development and,
        149-150
    psychoemotional disorders associated
        with, 42b
    qualitative scoring systems and, 162
    questionnaires for parent use in determining,
        145t
    report formats and, 166
    reporting results of assessment of, 162-166
    at risk infants and toddlers and, 153-157
    serial observation and analysis of child's
        interactions with familiar caregivers and
        others and, 147-149
    special care necessitated by child's condition
        and, 188-189
    standardized tests and, 158
    toddlers with history of brain injury in
        infancy and, 193
    traditional assessment and, 150-151
    treatment, management, and intervention
        with toddlers and, 190
    triage concept in assessment of, 142-143
    typical child behaviors and, 149

Communication *(Continued)*
  habilitation and, in hearing-impaired infants
      and toddlers. *See* Habilitation and
      communication development in hearing-
      impaired infants and toddlers.
  impaired, problem-solving approaches for
      infants and toddlers with, 182-184
  individualized care and, 173
  lack of need of assistive technology and, 193-197
  late talkers and, 191
  nonverbal, definition of, 292
  ongoing assessment as treatment or
      intervention planning, 197
  optimizing development of, 173-199
  oral, effect of hearing loss on, 201-207
  patterns of, typical of children, 146-147
  power of, language intervention and, 194
  readiness for, facilitation of physical
      development to promote, 185-186
  service-delivery models of, 182
  specifics of treament and intervention in, 184-197
  strategies of speech-language pathologist with
      pediatric population and, 175-182
  and Symbolic Behaviors Scale (CSBS), 133t,
      163t, 183, 264t-265t
  and Symbolic Developmental Profile, 133t
  toddlers with history of brain injury in infancy
      and, 193
  tools for assessment of, 163t-164t
  total, 213
  treatment, management, and intervention in,
      173-199, 174t
Communication assessment tools, 158-162,
    163t-164t
Communication competence, implications of
    developmental delays and disorders in
    infants and toddlers for, 31-48
Communication counseling, autistic spectrum
    disorder and, 135
Communication disorders in infants and toddlers,
    1-29, 44t-45t
  acquired, 38, 39t-40t
  administrative references, 267-274
  assessment of, 141-171, 249-265
  autistic spectrum disorder, 121-140
  causes of, 31-48, 44t-45t
  communication impairment, 1-29
  congenital anomalies, syndromes, sequences,
      and spectrum disorders and, 38
  direct treatment and management of, 179
  diseases and conditions associated with,
      38-41
  early intervention team in, 69-82
  etiologies associated with, 39t-40t, 224t
  examination, interpretation, and reporting of,
      141-171
  genetic and chromosomal aberrations and,
      37-38
  habilitation and communication development
      in hearing-impaired infants and toddlers,
      201-219
  high-incidence, low-visibility, 19
  identification and assessment of hearing-
      impaired infants and toddlers, 101-119
  Internet resources for professionals and
      families, 275-284
  marketing, 221-227

Communication disorders in infants and
    toddlers (Continued)
  medical aspects of. See Medical aspects of
    communication disorders.
  normal development and infant assessment
    tools, 229-247
  optimizing communication development, 173-199
  regulatory, emotional, and mental health
    problems and, 41, 42b
  and related conditions, 46t-47t
  role of speech-language pathologist in neonatal
    intensive care unit, 83-100
  selected medical aspects of, 49-67
  trauma and, 38-41
  treatment, management, and intervention
    targets in, 174t
Communication disorders specialists
  early intervention and, 16-19
  as multidisciplinary team members, 76-81
Communication enhancement, strategies for, from
    CSBS Model, 264t-265t
Communication impairment, 1-29
  case studies in, 1-6
  early intervention and, 15-20
  families and, 7-9, 15-19, 23-24
  framework of family and professional team in,
    20-22
  historical perspective of early intervention in,
    11-15
  managed care and early intervention in, 19-20
  practical approaches to framing issues in, 9-11
  problem-solving approaches for infants and
    toddlers with, 182-184
  professional competencies and, 24-27
  service-delivery models in early intervention in,
    22-23
Communication intervention strategies,
    preintentional, 18
Communication methodologies, hearing loss and,
    213-215, 214t
Communication Play Protocol (CPP), 195, 196t
Communication skills
  affecting early language development, 9t
  early, tools for assessment of, 250t-251t
Communicative abilities of children, information
    provided by parents about, 143-144, 145t
Communicative assessment and diagnosis, items
    essential to, 166t-168t
Communicative competence
  and education, 12-13
  implications of developmental delays and
    disorders in infants and toddlers for, 31-48
Communicative delays
  direct treatment and management of, 179
  etiologies associated with, 39t-40t
  infants and toddlers with, problem-solving
    approaches for, 182-184
  problem-solving approaches for infants and
    toddlers with, 182-184
Communicative development. See Communication,
    development of.
Communicative Development Inventory for
    Infants, 163t
Communicative diagnoses, assessments and,
    157-162, 163t-164t
Communicative disorders. See Communication
    disorders in infants and toddlers.

Communicative impairment, taxonomy of
    risk-factor groups related to, 155t-156t
Communicative means and functions, cue
    questions in assessment of, 254f
Communicative temptations, 194, 263t-264t
Community settings, speech-language pathologist
    and, 81
Competence
  communicative. See Communicative competence.
  professional, communication disorders and,
    24-27, 25t-26t
Competency
  child's, assessment of, 255t-259t
  of speech-language pathologist, 77-79
Complementary and Alternative Medicine
    (CAM), 137
Complex, definition of, 287
Conditions
  definition of, 287
  sequences and, 33-34
Confirmed diagnosis, 36
Congenital, definition of, 287
Congenital anomalies, 38
Congenital communication disorders, 49
Congenital disorders, 50, 283t
Congenital dysphagia, 58
Congenital hearing loss, 213
Connexin 26 mutations, nonsyndromic hearing
    loss and, 58
Conradi-Hunermann, 62t
Consanguineous, definition of, 287
Consonants
  deaf children and, 208t
  hearing loss and, 202-203
  visible speechreading movements and, 204t
Constricting bands, 62t
Consultation
  children and speech-language pathologist and,
    176-177
  definition of, 287
Continuous positive airway pressure (CPAP),
    90, 287
Costello faciocutaneoskeletal syndrome, 63t
Council for Exceptional Children (CEC), Division
    of Early Childhood (DEC), 24, 129
Counseling
  educational, autistic spectrum disorder and, 134
  family, autistic spectrum disorder and, 134
  financial, autistic spectrum disorder and, 134
  genetic. See Genetic counseling.
  individual psychological, autistic spectrum
    disorder and, 134-135
  language, autistic spectrum disorder and, 135
  meeting parental concerns through, 207-209
  with respect to insurance coverage, autistic
    spectrum disorder and, 134
CPAP. See Continuous positive airway pressure
    (CPAP).
CPI. See Physicians' Current Procedural Terminology
    (CPI).
CPP. See Communication Play Protocol (CPP).
CPT. See Current Procedural Terminology (CPT).
Cranial nerves, 231t
Craniofacial disorders
  Internet resources for, 279
  oral-motor and swallow assessment and,
    241t-243t

Craniosynostosis, Shprintzen-Goldberg, 65t
Cri-du-chat syndrome, 53, 62t
Crossovers, human genome and, 60
Crouzon craniofacial dysostosis, 63t
Cryptophthalmia, 63t
CSBS. *See* Communication and Symbolic Behaviors Scale (CSBS).
CSBS Developmental Profile (CSBS-DP), 145t
CSBS-DP. *See* CSBS Developmental Profile (CSBS-DP).
Cue questions, 145t, 163t, 254f
Cued speech, 214t
Cultural considerations, family and, 73-75
Current Procedural Terminology (CPT), 8
Cyanosis, definition of, 288
Cytomegalovirus (CMV), definition of, 288

D

Damping, earmolds of hearing aids and, 210
DAS. *See* Developmental apraxia of speech (DAS).
DASI. *See* Detection of Autism by Infant Sociability Interview (DASI).
Data sharing purposes, diagnosis codes for, Internet resources for, 284t
Database, epidemiological, families as statistics in, 7-9
De Lange synophrys, 63t
Deaf-blind methods, 214t
Deafness, 65t, 67t
    Alport nephropathy and, 62t
    Alstrom, 62t
    common speech characteristics in, 208t
    nonsyndromic, 59
Deafness Management Quotient, 215
DEC. *See* Division of Early Childhood (DEC) of the Council for Exceptional Children (CEC).
Defect, neural tube, definition of, 292
Deficit, developmental, 33
Definitive diagnosis, 36
Delay
    cognitive, 32, 33
    communicative. *See* Communicative delays.
    definition of, 288
    developmental. *See* Developmental delays.
    language, 32, 63t
    of onset of speech without obvious receptive language impairment, 224t
    pervasive developmental, 32
Delayed receptive language development, 224t
Delivery, post-term, definition of, 293
Dementia, Rett, 65t
Demographics, family, 73-75
Denial, parental, communicative assessment and, 157
Denver Developmental Screening Questionnaire, 145t
Department
    of Education, 7, 8-9
    of Health and Human Services, 7
Dependent, technology, definition of, 295
Depressed face, 64t
Dermatitis, actinic, 62t
Descriptive diagnosis, 36
Detection of Autism by Infant Sociability Interview (DASI), 132t

Development
    atypical communicative, assessment in identification of, 141-152
    of auditory skills during first year of life, 216t
    cognitive, facilitation of, 186-188
    communication. *See* Communication, development of.
    disordered, of speech or language, 224t
    of early intervention, role of education legislation in, 11-12
    normal, and infant assessment tools, 229-247
    plateaus in, communication development and, 189
    pragmatic, in infants and toddlers, 236t-237t
    reversals in, communication development and, 189
    sensorimotor stage, definition of, 294
    of sensory skills, hearing loss and, 215-217
    speech, delayed, 65t
    transactional factors in, communication impairments and, 10
Developmental apraxia of speech (DAS), 144-146, 277
Developmental assessment in neonatal intensive care unit, 95-96, 95t
Developmental assessment teams in neonatal intensive care unit, 92
Developmental deficit, 33
Developmental delays, 18, 31-48, 46t
    causes of, 31-48, 42b
    definition of, 288
    diagnosis and assessment of, 41-47
    pervasive, 32
    receiving referrals and determining which children are at risk, 32-37
    single and multiple risk factors in, 41-47
Developmental difference, 32
Developmental disabilities, 33, 288
Developmental disorders, 32-33
    pervasive. *See* Pervasive developmental disorder (PDD).
Developmental domains affecting early language development, 9t
Developmental language disorder (DVD), 157
Developmental model, 36-37
Developmental service delivery model, 26t
Developmentally delayed individual, 31
Device, assistive. *See* Assistive devices.
Diabetes, 62t, 65t
Diagnosis, 36
    autistic spectrum disorder and, 123-130
    communicative, items essential to, 166t-168t
    of communicative disorders, role of single and multiple risk factors in, 41-47, 44t-45t, 46t-47t
    confirmed, 36
    definition of, 288
    definitive, 36
    descriptive, 36
    developmental delays and disorders and, 35-37
    differential, 36, 126-130
    presumptive, 36
Diagnosis codes, Internet resources for, 284t
Diagnostic and Statistical Manual (DSM), 8, 288
Diagnostic and Statistical Manual-IV (DSM-IV), 121, 124t-126t

Diagnostic Classification of Mental Health and Developmental Disorders of Infancy and Early Childhood, 8
Diagnostic classifications of communication impairments, 8-9
Diagnostic guide, implications for normal and deviant patterns of language development and, 234t-235t
Diastrophic dwarfism, 63t
Difference, developmental, 32
Differential diagnosis, 36, 126-130
Difficulty, child's, assessment of, 255t-259t
DiGeorge syndrome, 63t
Digits, hypoplastic fifth, 63t
Dilantin, definition of, 288
Diphthongs
  deaf children and, 208t
  visible speechreading movements and, 204t
Diplegia, facial, Moebius sequence of, 64t
Direct management, communication development and, 194-197, 196t
Direct testing, autistic spectrum disorder and, 129-130
Disability(ies)
  definition of, 7-8
  developmental, 33, 288
  Internet resources for, 280t-281t
  learning, 46t
  multiple, 46t
Disabled, definition of, 97
Discharge planning teams in neonatal intensive care unit, 92
Discrete quality, mendelian disorders and, 55-56
Discrimination, speech, word recognition and, 105
Disease(s), acquired, communicative disorders and, 38, 39t-40t
Disorder(s)
  attention deficit, 47t
  autistic spectrum. *See* Autistic spectrum disorder (ASD).
  branchial arch, definition of, 286
  childhood disintegrative, 149
  chromosomal, definition of, 287
  communication. *See* Communication disorders in infants and toddlers.
  communicative. *See* Communication disorders in infants and toddlers.
  congenital, 50
  craniofacial, 279
  definition of, 288
  developmental, 31-48
  extrapyramidal, 63t
  frequency of, 60-66, 62t-67t
  genetic, definition of, 289
  maternal, teratogens and, 51t
  mendelian, 55-60, 59f
  pervasive developmental, 121-123
  polygenic, 53, 54f, 54t, 55
  psychoemotional, associated with communicative development, 42b
  speech and voice, 65t
  state regulation, definition of, 295
  teratogenic, 61
Disordered development of speech or language, 224t
Disordered receptive language development, 224t

Distance hearing, developmental sequence of auditory skills during first year of life and, 216t
Distortion product, distortion-product otoacoustic emissions and, 110-111
Distortion-product otoacoustic emissions (DPOAEs), 110-111, 112f
Division of Early Childhood (DEC) of the Council for Exceptional Children (CEC), 24, 129
DNA marker, human genome and, 60
Domains, developmental, affecting early language development, 9t
Dominant craniometaphyseal dysplasia, 63t
Dominant inheritance
  autosomal, 57f
  X-linked, 58f
Down syndrome, 52, 61, 62t
DPOAEs. *See* Distortion-product otoacoustic emissions (DPOAEs).
Drugs. *See* Medications.
DSM. See Diagnostic and Statistical Manual (DSM).
DSM-IV. See Diagnostic and Statistical Manual-IV (DSM-IV).
Dubowitz short asymmetric eye slits, 63t
DVD. *See* Developmental language disorder (DVD).
Dwarfism, 63t
  bloom, 62t
  diastrophic, 63t
Dysautonomia, 63t
Dysfunction, definition of, 288
Dysgenesis–unusual facies, bilateral femoral, 62t
Dyslexia, 57
Dysmorphic, definition of, 288
Dysostosis
  Crouzon craniofacial, 63t
  maxillofacial, 64t
  Nager acrofacial, 64t
  Treacher-Collins mandibulofacial, 66t
Dysphagia, congenital, 58
Dysplasia
  binder maxillonasal, 62t
  bone, 63t
  bronchopulmonary, 42-43, 89, 286
  chorioretinal cerebral, 52
  definition of, 288
  ectodermal, 63t
  frontometaphyseal, 63t
  frontonasal, 63t
  retinal, 63t
  spondyloepiphyseal, 65t
  spondylonetaphyseal, X-linked, 65t
Dyspraxia
  Internet resources for, 277
  orofacial, 57
  speech, 57
Dystrophy
  Hallervorden-Spatz infantile neuroaxonal, 63t
  myotonic, 64t
  osteochondromuscular, 64t

E

Ear care, readiness for communication and, 186
Ear infections, readiness for communication and, 186
Ear-level hearing aids, 210
Early and Periodic Screening, Diagnosis, and Testing (EPSDT), 223, 288

Early communication skills, tools for assessment of, 250t-251t
Early intervention
  communications disorders specialists and, 16-19
  communicative competence and education in, 12-13
  families and, 15-19, 17f, 20-22, 23-24
  health care and, 13-15
  high-incidence, low-visibility disorders and, 19
  historical perspective of, 11-15
  infants and, 15-19, 17f
  managed care and, 19-20
  role of education legislation in, 11-12
  service-delivery models in, 22-23
Early intervention team, 69-82
  communication disorders specialists as members of, 76-81
  eco-map and, 72-73, 73f
  expectations of, 75-76, 77t
  family as focus of, 70-76, 77t
  family configurations, demographics, and cultural considerations and, 73-75
  family systems theory and, 70-72
Early interventionist, definition of, 288
Early language development, elements affecting, 9, 9t
Early language sequences affecting early language development, 9t
Earmolds, hearing aids and, 210
Ears, large, 62t
ECMO. *See* Extra-corporeal mechanical oxygenation (ECMO).
Eco-Map, 72-73, 73f
Ecosystem, readiness for communication and, 188
Ectodermal dysplasia, 63t
Ectrodactyly, 63t
Eczema, 64t
Education
  adult, communication development and, 190-191
  communicative competence and, 12-13
  for the Handicapped Act (EHA), 11, 288-289
  meeting parental concerns through, 207-209
  parent, speech-language pathologist and, 177-178
Education legislation, role of, in development of early intervention, 11-12
Education plan, individual, definition of, 290
Educational counseling, autistic spectrum disorder and, 134
EEC, 63t
Efficacy, definition of, 289
Efficiency, definition of, 289
EHA. *See* Education for the Handicapped Act (EHA).
Ehlers-Danlos hyperelasticity, 63t
Eligibility, definition of, 289
Elongated face, 65t
Embryopathy, rubella, 65t
Emissions, otoacoustic. *See* Otoacoustic emissions (OAEs).
Emotional factors
  affecting early language development, 9t
  intonational patterns and, 187
Emotional problems, communicative disorders and, 41, 42b
Empowering of family, 16
Encephalitis, definition of, 289

Encephalocele, 54-55, 289
Encephalopathy, definition of, 289
Endotracheal tube (ET), definition of, 289
English, oral, 214t
Environment
  communicative disorders and, 174t
  developmental sequence of auditory skills during first year of life and, 216t
  effect of, on early language development, 9t
  readiness for communication and, 187-188
Environmental risk, definition of, 289
Environments, naturalistic, 12
EOAEs. *See* Evoked otoacoustic emissions (EOAEs).
Epidemiological database, families as statistics in, 7-9
Epilepsy
  autosomal dominant rolandic, 57
  definition of, 289
Epilepsy Foundation of America, 271t
EPSDT. *See* Early and Periodic Screening, Diagnosis, and Testing (EPSDT).
Estate planning, autistic spectrum disorder and, 134
ET. *See* Endotracheal tube (ET).
Etiology, definition of, 289
Evaluation
  definition of, 289
  developmental delays and disorders and, 35-37
Evoked otoacoustic emissions (EOAEs), 111, 118
Examination, assessment and, 141-171
Exomphalos, Beckwith-Wiedemann, 62t
Exon, definition of, 289
Expectations of family, 75-76, 77t
Experimental treatment elements, autistic spectrum disorder and, 137
Expressive language ability, 10
Extra-corporeal mechanical oxygenation (ECMO), definition of, 289
Extrapyramidal disorder, 63t
Extremely low birth weight (ELBW), 43
Eye slits, Dubowitz short asymmetric, 63t
Eyes, slanted, 65t

F
Face
  Coffin-Siris coarse, 63t
  depressed, 63t
  elongated, 64t
  Freeman-Sheldon whistling, 63t
  Kniest flat, 64t
  Larsen flat, 64t
  long, 62t
  Robinow fetal, 65t
  Simpson dysmorphia bulldog, 65t
  Stickler flat, 65t
  triangular, 63t
Facial diplegia, Moebius sequence of, 64t
Facilitating communicative development in infancy, 184-190
Facio-auriculo-vertebral sequence, 63t
FAE. *See* Fetal alcohol effects (FAE).
FAF. *See* Fetal alcohol effects (FAF).
Failure to thrive (FTT), definition of, 289
Families
  communication disorders and, 23-24, 174t
  definition of, 23

Families *(Continued)*
early intervention and, 15-19, 17f
empowering of, 16
as focus of early intervention team, 70-76
function of, family systems theory and, 71
interaction of, family systems theory and, 71
interaction of children with, 16, 17f
Internet resources for, 275-284, 280t
language intervention and, 195
life cycle of, family systems theory and, 71
professional team and, communication
disorders and, 20-22
as statistics in epidemiological database, 7-9
structure of, family systems theory and, 70
working with, in neonatal intensive care unit,
96-98
Family assessment, 143-149
Family configurations, 73-75
Family counseling, autistic spectrum disorder
and, 134
Family interview, autistic spectrum disorder
and, 128
Family services plan, individual. *See* Individual
family services plan (IFSP).
Family support teams in neonatal intensive care
unit, 92
Family systems theory, 70-72
FAS. *See* Fetal alcohol syndrome (FAS).
Fat pads, definition of, 289
Federal laws and legal information, Internet, 277
Feeder, Haberman, definition of, 290
Feeding
gavage, definition of, 289
neonatal assessment for, 239t-240t
readiness for communication and, 186
Feeding assessment in neonatal intensive care
unit, 93-95
Feeding disorders, infant, 238t
Feeding teams in neonatal intensive care unit, 92
Feet, small puffy, 63t
Femoral dysgenesis–unusual facies, bilateral, 62t
Fetal alcohol effects (FAE), 36, 289
Fetal alcohol growth deficiency, 63t
Fetal alcohol syndrome (FAS), 36, 289
Fetal valproate syndrome, 56t
Fifth digits, hypoplastic, 63t
Financial counseling, autistic spectrum disorder
and, 134
Fingernails, short, 64t
Floating-Harbor short stature, 63t
Floor time, 136, 197
Flush, malar, 63t
Focal lesions, definition of, 289
Foix-Chavany-Marie suprabulbar paresis, 63t
Follow-up of children by speech-language
pathologist, 175-176
Follow-up teams in neonatal intensive care
unit, 92
Fontanel, definition of, 289
Forearms, short, 65t
Formats
arena-assessment, 150-151
report, assessment and, 166
Fragile, 62t
Fragile tissues, 63t
Fragile X syndrome, 122
Freeman-Sheldon whistling face, 63t

Frequency-specific stimuli, testing of hearing
and, 103
Fricatives, auditory reception and, 202-203
Frontometaphyseal dysplasia, 64t
Frontonasal dysplasia, 64t
FTT. *See* Failure to thrive (FTT).
Full-term, definition of, 289
Functional abilities of infants and toddlers,
promoting, 33-34
Functional goals, definition of, 184
Functional skills, definition of, 289

G

Gait, Angelman jerky, 62t
Gangliosidosis, generalized, 66t
Gangliosidosis GM1, 65t
Gavage feeding, definition of, 289
Gene therapy, autistic spectrum disorder and, 137
Genealogical information, inheritance patterns
and, 59
Genealogy chart, 59, 59f
Generalized gangliosidosis, 66t
Genetic aberrations, 37-38
Genetic and Rare Diseases Information Center, 97
Genetic counseling
autistic spectrum disorder and, 134
heritable disorders and, 59
Genetic disorder, definition of, 289
Geneticist, medical, 60
Genetics, Internet resources for, 280t
Genitalia, hypoplastic, 65t
Genome project, 60
Gentamicin, 49
Gestational age, 89
definition of, 289
small for, definition of, 294-295
Gestures, language intervention and, 195
Gigantism, 62t
Sotos cerebral, 65t
Gilles de la Tourette vocal and motor tics, 64t
Glabella, definition of, 289
Glossoptosis, definition of, 289
Goals
functional, definition of, 184
for learner, communication development
and, 183
for partner, communication development and, 183
Goals 2000, 12
Goldenhar syndrome, 56t
Goodness of fit, security and, 188
Grams, weight conversion and, 230t
Grasp, palmar, definition of, 292
Gravida, definition of, 289
Grieving process, child's hearing loss and, 209-209
Group service delivery model, 25t
Growth
brain, and language from birth to 2 years, 231t
physical, communication development and, 189
Growth retardation, 64t
intrauterine, definition of, 291
G-tube, definition of, 290
Gynecomastia, 64t

H

Haberman feeder, 290
Habilitation
aural, hearing loss and, 207-218

Habilitation (Continued)
  and communication development in hearing-
      impaired infants and toddlers, 201-219
    aural rehabilitation, 207-218
    effect of hearing loss on oral communication
        ability, 201-207, 208t
Hallerman-Streiff microcephaly, 64t
Hallervorden-Spatz infantile neuroaxonal
    dystrophy, 64t
Hall-Riggs mental retardation, 64t
Hallux, broad, 64t
Hand movement, purposeful, loss of, 65t
Handicap, 33
  definition of, 290
  mental, 31
Handicapped children
  prelanguage, interaction styles of, 259t-262t
  preschool programs for, 12
Handling and positioning of infants, readiness for
    communication and, 186
Hands
  small puffy, 63t
  ulnar deviation of, 63t
Hanen program, 191
Haphazard marketing, 222
Hazardous procedures, teratogens and, 52t
Head Start, 181
Health
  and Human Services, 7
  Internet resources for, 280t-281t
  mental, Internet resources for, 282t
Health care, early intervention and, 13-15
Hearing
  binaural, 210-211
  distance, developmental sequence of auditory
      skills during first year of life and, 216t
Hearing aids, 209-212
  battery check of, 212
  behind-the-ear, 210
  ear-level, 210
  in-the-canal, 210
  in-the-ear, 210
  listening check of, 212
  orientation to, 211
  types of, 210
  use and care of, 211-212
  visual inspection of, 212
Hearing impairment, 46t, 224t
Hearing loss
  alternative sensory devices and, 212-213
  application of Part C intervention mandates
      and, 180-182
  auditory reception and, 202-203
  auditory training and, 215-216, 216t
  auditory-visual reception and, 204-205
  aural habilitation, 207-218
  binaural amplification and, 210-211
  cochlear implants and, 212-213
  communication methodologies and, 213-215,
      214t
  congenital, 213
  consonants and, 202-203
  development of sensory skills and, 215-217
  direct treatment of communication delays or
      disorders, 179
  earmolds and, 210
  education and, 177-178

Hearing loss (Continued)
  effect of, on oral communication ability, 201-207
  hearing aids and, 209-212
  Internet resources for, 281t
  meeting parental concerns through counseling
      and education and, 207-209
  mild, speech characteristics and, 207
  moderate, speech characteristics and, 207
  monaural amplification and, 210-211
  national effort to make a difference for infants
      and toddlers with special needs and, 181-182
  nonsyndromic, 58
  nonverbal reception and, 205
  oral-language characteristics and, 205-206
  parent training and, 178
  Part V early intervention and, 181
  postlingual, 202, 213
  prelingual, 202, 213
  prevention of, 179-180
  profound, speech characteristics and,
      206-207, 208t
  sensorineural, 212
  sensory perception and, 201-205
  severe, speech characteristics and, 206-207, 208t
  severe-to-profound hearing loss and,
      206-207, 208t
  speech characteristics and, 206-207
  speech training and, 217-218
  use and care of hearing aids, 211-212
  vibrotactile sensory aids and, 213
  visual reception and, 203-204, 204t
  visual training and, 216-217
  vowels and, 202
Hearing-impaired infants and toddlers, 101-119
  auditory brain stem response and, 111-117
  behavioral threshold assessment in, 101-104
  habilitation and communication development
      in. See Habilitation and communication
      development in hearing-impaired infants
      and toddlers.
  identification and assessment of, 101-119
  immittance testing and, 105-109
  neonatal screening and, 117-118
  otoacoustic emissions and, 109-111, 112f
  speech audiometry and, 104-105
Heart malformation, 67t
Help me play with a toy scenario, communication
    play protocol and, 196t
Hemangiomas, 64t
Hemorrhage
  intraventricular, definition of, 291
  subdural, definition of, 295
Heritable anomalies, common, 53-55, 54f, 54t
High-incidence, low-visibility communication
    disorders, 19
Hinks-Dellcrest Center, 41
History
  case, autistic spectrum disorder and, 127-128
  risk, long form of, 243f-245f
HIV. See Human immunodeficiency virus (HIV).
Homocystinuria ectopia lentis, 64t
Horning, earmolds of hearing aids and, 210
Hospital-based multidisciplinary evaluation,
    246f-247f
Human genome, 60
Human immunodeficiency virus (HIV), definition
    of, 290

Human teratogens. *See* Teratogens.
Hunter syndrome, 66t
Hurler syndrome, 66t
Hydrocephalus, 64t
Hydrocephalus, definition of, 290
Hyperbilirubinemia, definition of, 290
Hyperelasticity, Ehlers-Danlos, 63t
Hyperextension, definition of, 290
Hypertelorism, 64t, 67t
    Aarskog, 62t
Hypertelorism, definition of, 290
Hypertonia, definition of, 290
Hypochondroplasia, 64t
Hypogenitalism, 65t
Hypoglossia-hypodactyly, 64t
Hypogonadism, 63t
Hypoplasia, laryngeal, definition of, 291
Hypoplastic fifth digits, 63t
Hypoplastic genitalia, 65t
Hypospadias, 65t
Hypothyroidism, 64t
    Pendred, 64t
Hypotonia
    Cohen, 63t
    Prader-Willi, 64t
Hypotonia, definition of, 290
Hypotrichosis, 64t
Hypoxia
    definition of, 290
    preterm infants and, 89-90

I

I want that toy on the shelf scenario,
    communication play protocol and, 196t
Iatrogenic, definition of, 290
ICD. See International Classification of Diseases (ICD).
ICDL Clinical Practice Guidelines, 123
IDEA. *See* Individuals with Disabilities Education Act (IDEA)
IDEAS. *See* Integrated Developmental Experiences Assessment (IDEAS).
Idiopathic toe walking, 157, 290
Idiosyncratic behaviors, austistic spectrum disorder and, 122
IEP. *See* Individual education plan (IEP).
IFSP. *See* Individual family services plan (IFSP).
Immittance testing, 105-109
    acoustic reflex testing, 109
    in hearing-impaired infants and toddlers, 105-109
    tympanometry, 106-107, 106f, 108f, 108t
Immune deficiency, 64t
Impairment
    communication. *See* Communication impairment.
    hearing, 46t
    language, 46t
    speech, 8, 46t
    visual, readiness for communication and, 186
Implants, cochlear, 212-213, 279, 281t
Incidence, definition of, 290
Incisors, prominent, 63t
Incompetence, palatopharyngeal, 64t
Individual education plan (IEP), definition of, 290
Individual family services plan (IFSP), 12, 77
    assessment and, 165-166
    consultation and, 176
    definition of, 290

Individual psychological counseling, autistic spectrum disorder and, 134-135
Individualized care, communication development and, 173
Individuals with Disabilities Education Act (IDEA), 8-9, 11, 20, 22-23, 24, 70, 134, 290
Infancy
    brain injury in, toddlers with history of, 193
    communicative development in, facilitation of, 184-190
    facilitating communicative development in, 184-190
Infant and Preschool Program at Hinks-Dellcrest Center, 41
Infant assessment tools, normal development and, 229-247
Infant attachment, readiness for communication and, 188
Infant scale of nonverbal interaction, 259t-262t
Infant stress, signs of, 90-92, 91t
Infant/Child Monitoring Questionnaire of Assessment, Evaluation, and Programming System (AEPS), 145t
Infantile oral reflexes, 233t
Infantile reflexes, primitive and postural, of first year, 233t
Infantilism, sexual, 62t
Infants
    assessment of, in neonatal intensive care unit, 93-96
    autistic spectrum disorder and, 121-140
    behavioral organization cues of, 91t
    causes of developmental delays and disorders in, 31-48
    communication disorders in. *See* Communication disorders in infants and toddlers.
    with delayed or impaired communication, problem-solving approaches for, 182-184
    early intervention and, 15-19, 17f
    feeding, sucking, and swallowing disorders of, 238t
    hearing-impaired. *See* Hearing-impaired infants and toddlers.
    interactions between caregivers and, facilitation of, 185
    medically fragile, speech-language pathologist and, 83-100
    older, behavioral threshold assessment in, 102-104
    pragmatic development in, 236t-237t
    preterm, characteristics of, 89-90
    promoting functional abilities of, 33-34
    screening of, for hearing-impairment, 117-118
    services for, marketing of, 223-225, 224t
    with special needs, national effort to make difference for, 181-182
Infant-Toddler and Family Instrument (ITFI), 145t
Infant/toddler checklist for communication and language development, 252f-253f
Infection control in neonatal intensive care unit, 88-89
Infections
    ear, readiness for communication and, 186
    teratogens and, 51t
Inheritance
    autosomal dominant, 57f
    autosomal recessive, 57f

Inheritance *(Continued)*
    X-linked dominant, 58f
    X-linked recessive, 58f
Insurance, counseling with respect to, autistic
    spectrum disorder and, 134
Integrated Developmental Experiences
    Assessment (IDEAS), 164t
Intensity and pitch in deaf children, 208t
Intensive care unit, neonatal. *See* Neonatal
    intensive care unit (NICU).
Interaction
    nonverbal, infant scale of, 259t-262t
    styles of, of handicapped prelanguage children,
      259t-262t
Interactive behavior, levels of, 259t-260t
Interdisciplinary Council on Developmental and
    Learning Disorders, 123, 225
Intermediate tympanogram, 107
International Association for Infant Mental
    Health, 271t
International Classification
    of Diseases (ICD), 8, 290
    of Functioning, Disability, and Health, 8
    of Impairments, Disabilities, and Handicaps, 8
Internet resources for professionals and families,
    275-284
Interpeak latencies in evaluation of neural
    integrity, 113-114
Interpretation, assessment and, 141-171
Intervention
    autistic spectrum disorder and, 121-140
    communication development and, 173-199, 174t
    definition of, 290-291
    early. *See* Early intervention.
    preintentional communication, 18
    tools and procedures of, 249-265
Intervention team, early. *See* Early intervention
    team.
Interventionist, early, definition of, 288
Interview, family, autistic spectrum disorder
    and, 128
In-the-canal (ITC) hearing aids, 210
In-the-ear (ITE) hearing aids, 210
Intonational patterns, emotional content and, 187
Intrauterine growth retardation (IUGR), definition
    of, 291
Intraventricular hemorrhage (IVH), definition
    of, 291
Intubation, definition of, 291
Inventory, phonemic, 146
Isolated forms of anomalies, 56t
ITC hearing aids. *See* In-the-canal (ITC) hearing
    aids.
ITE hearing aids. *See* In-the-ear (ITE) hearing aids.
ITFI. *See* Infant-Toddler and Family Instrument
    (ITFI).
IUGR. *See* Intrauterine growth retardation (IUGR).
IVH. *See* Intraventricular hemorrhage (IVH).

J

Jaundice, definition of, 291
JBA. *See* Judgment-based assessment (JBA).
Jerky gait, Angelman, 62t
Johanson-Blizzard hypoplastic alae nasi, 64t
Joint Commission on Hospital Accreditation, 83
Joint luxations, 64t
Joints, thick, 64t

Journal of the American Medical Association, 123
Judgment-based assessment (JBA), 160-161

K

Kabuki make-up syndrome, 64t
Kanamycin, 49
Kangaroo care in neonatal intensive care unit, 13
Kernicterus, definition of, 291
Kid-Med centers, 15
King-Kopetzky syndrome, 61, 66
Klinefelter syndrome, 62t
Kniest flat face, 63t
Knowledge of speech-language pathologist, 77-79

L

Labeling, language intervention and, 194
Landau-Kleffner syndrome, 122, 149
Langer-Geidion trichorhinophalangeal
    syndrome, 64t
Language
    adult, simplifying, language intervention
      and, 195
    and brain growth from birth to 2 years, 231t
    development of
      implications for normal and deviant patterns
        of, 234t-235t
      infant/toddler checklist for, 252f-253f
      Internet resources for, 283t
      typical and atypical, communication
        impairments and, 10-11
    disordered development of, 224t
    expressive, 10
    hearing loss and, 205-206, 206t
Language ability, receptive, 10
Language assessment tools, 133t
Language counseling, autistic spectrum disorder
    and, 135
Language delay, 63t
Language delayed individual, 32
Language development
    implications for normal and deviant patterns of,
      234t-235t
    predictors of, 149-150
    typical and atypical, communication
      impairments and, 10-11
Language Development Survey, 145t, 164t
Language impairments, 46t
Lanugo, definition of, 291
Large ears, 63t
Large mouth, 62t
Larsen flat face, 64t
Laryngeal hypoplasia, definition of, 291
Larynx, heritable anomalies and, 54
Late talkers, communication development
    and, 191
Latency, interpeak, in evaluation of neural
    integrity, 113-114
Latency-intensity function (LIF), 116, 116f
LBW. *See* Low birth weight (LBW).
Lead agency, 12, 291
Learner, goal for, communication development
    and, 183
Learning disabilities, specific, 46t
Legal information, Internet, 277
Legislation, education, role of, in development of
    early intervention, 11-12
Leopard lentigines, 64t

Leroy syndrome, 66t
Lesions, focal, definition of, 289
Leukomalacia, definition of, 291
Level I nursing care for newborns, 85
Level II nursery
    involvement of speech-language pathologist
        in, 88
    for newborns, 85-86
Level III nursery
    involvement of speech-language pathologist
        in, 87
    for newborns, 85-86
Level IV nursery
    involvement of speech-language pathologist
        in, 87
    for newborns, 86
Libraries, Internet, 276-277
LIF. *See* Latency-intensity function (LIF).
Life cycle, family, family systems theory and, 71
Limb reduction, 63t
Linguistic mapping, 10
Linkage studies, human genome and, 60
Lipomas, 64t
Lips
    cleft, 66t
    Williams patulous, 66t
Listening check of hearing aid, 212
Localization, developmental sequence of auditory
        skills during first year of life and, 216t
Long face, 63t
Lovaas therapy, 179, 291
Low birth weight (LBW), definition of, 291
Luxations, joint, 64t

M

MacArthur Communicative Development
    Inventory: Infant Form and Toddler
    Form, 145t
Macrocephaly, 64t
    definition of, 291
    Weaver, 66t
Macroglossia, 62t
Malar flush, 64t
Male pseudohermaphroditism, 64t
Managed care, early intervention and, 19-20
Management
    case, 12, 287
    communication development and, 173-199, 174t
    definition of, 291
Manager, case, definition of, 287
Mannosidosis alpha B, 66t
Mannosidosis B, 66t
Manually coded English, 214t
Mapping, linguistic, 10
March of Dimes Birth Defects Foundation, 271t
Marketing, 221-227
    haphazard, 222
    ongoing strategies of, 225-226
    organized, 222
    of services for infants and toddlers in
        community, 223-225, 224t
    of speech-language pathologist's services for
        newborns, 222-223
    targeted, 222
Maroteaux-Lamy syndrome, 66t
Maternal and Child Health Services, 223
Maternal disorders, teratogens and, 51t

Maturation, communication development and, 189
Maxillofacial dysostosis, 64t
McKenzie, Lee, 222
Meconium, definition of, 291
Medicaid, 97, 98, 291
Medical aspects of communication disorders,
        49-67, 50f
    chromosome abnormalities, 52-53
    common heritable anomalies, 53-55, 54f, 54t
    effects of teratogens and, 50-52, 51t-52t
    frequencies of disorders, 61-66, 62t-66t
    human genome, 60
    isolated problems versus parts of syndromes,
        55, 56t
    mendelian disorders, 55-60, 57f, 58f, 59f
Medical conditions, Internet resources for, 281t-282t
Medical geneticist, 59
Medical Home initiative of the American
        Academy of Pediatrics, 15
Medical model, 36-37
Medically fragile infants, speech-language
        pathologist and, 83-100
Medications
    Internet resources for, 280t
    teratogens and, 51t
Mendelian disorders, 55-60, 59f
Meningitis, definition of, 291
Meningocele, definition of, 291
Mental deficiency, 62t
Mental health
    communicative disorders and, 41, 42b
    Internet resources for, 282t
Mental retardation, 31, 63t, 67t
    Hall-Riggs, 63t
    X-linked-6, 64t
Mental retardation–Buenos Aires type, 64t
Mental retardation–Verloes type, 64t
Mentally handicapped individual, 31
Mesomelia-synostoses, 64t
Metasites, Internet, 275-276
Microcephaly, 63t, 67t
    definition of, 292
    Hallerman-Streiff, 63t
Micropreemies, speech-language pathologist
        and, 83-100
Microstomia, 66t
Microtia, definition of, 292
Middle-ear pressure, tympanometry and, 107
Mild hearing loss, speech characteristics and, 207
Mild-moderately affected individual, 31
Mitten syndactyly, 62t
Model
    affective vocal, language intervention and, 195
    developmental, 36-37
    medical, 36-37
Moderate hearing loss, speech characteristics
        and, 207
Modified Checklist for Autism in Toddlers, 132t
Moebius sequence of facial diplegia, 64t
Mohr cleft tongue, 64t
Monaural amplification, hearing aids and, 210-211
Monitors, definition of, 292
Morbidity, definition of, 292
Moro reflex, definition of, 292
Morquio syndrome, 66t
Motor stimulation, readiness for communication
        and, 187

Motor tics, Gilles de la Tourette, 64t
Mouth, large, 62t
Mulibrey nanism, 65t
Multichannel vibrotactile sensory aids, 213
Multidimensional scoring systems, assessment and, 162
Multidisciplinary evaluation, hospital-based, 246f-247f
Multidisciplinary service delivery model, 25t
Multidisciplinary team in neonatal intensive care unit, 92
Multiple disabilities, 46t
Multiple pterygium, 64t
Multiple risk factors in diagnosis and assessment in communicative disorders, 41-47, 44t-45t, 46t-47t
Multiple strategies, assessment and, 161-162
Multiple synostoses, 65t
Music, language intervention and, 195
Mutation rate, autosomal dominant mendelian disorder and, 61
Mutilation, ADAM fetal, 62t
Myasthenia, 65t
Myelination, definition of, 292
Myelomeningocele, 54-55, 292
Myopathy
    myotonic, 64t
    Schwartz-Jampel, 65t
Myopia, 66t
Myotonic dystrophy, 65t
Myotonic myopathy, 65t

N
Nager acrofacial dysostosis, 65t
Naming, language intervention and, 194
Nasals, auditory reception and, 202-203
Nasogastric (NG) tube, definition of, 292
National Association
    for Retarded Citizens, 271t
    for Sickle Cell Disease, Inc., 271t
    for the Visually Handicapped, 271t
National Center
    for Clinical Infant Programs, 74
    for Health Statistics, 7
National Down Syndrome Society, 272t
National Easter Seal Society, 272t
National Health Interview Survey, 7, 8
National Information Center for Handicapped Children and Youth, 272t
National Institute(s)
    of Child Health and Human Development, 272t
    of Health (NIH), 15, 118, 130
National Neurofibromatosis Foundation, 272t
National organization(s), 269t-273t
    for Rare Diseases, 272t
National Retinitis Pigmentosa Foundation, 272t
National Tay-Sachs and Allied Diseases Association, 272t
Naturalistic environments, 12
Naturalistic Observation of Preterm Neonate, 95t
NBRS. See Neurobehavioral risk score (NBRS).
NDT. See Neurodevelopmental treatment (NDT).
Neck, webbed, 64t
Necrosis, definition of, 292
Neomycin, 49
Neonatal assessment for feeding, 239t-240t

Neonatal Behavioral Assessment Scale (NBAS), 95t, 96
Neonatal Individualized Developmental Care and Assessment Program (NIDCAP), 93
Neonatal intensive care unit (NICU)
    definition of, 292
    developmental assessment in, 95-96, 95t
    feeding assessment in, 93-95
    infant assessment in, 93-96
    infection control in, 88-89
    influence of work of Heidelese Als on, 13
    level III, involvement of speech-language pathologist in, 87
    level IV, involvement of speech-language pathologist in, 87
    newborn care in, 85-86
    payment for services in, 98
    role of speech-language pathologist in. See Speech-language pathologist (SLP), role of, in neonatal intensive care unit.
    specialized teams in, 92-98
    working with families in, 96-98
Neonatal screening
    age 29 days through 2 years, 117-118
    birth through age 28 days, 117
    for hearing-impairment, 117-118
Neonates
    behavioral threshold assessment in, 101-102
    definition of, 292
Neonatology, Internet resources for, 282t
Neo-oralism, 214t
Nephropathy, Alport, 62t
Neural abnormalities, central nervous system maturation and, 232t
Neural integrity, evaluation of, in hearing-impaired infants and toddlers, 113-114, 114f
Neural tube, anomalies of, 54-55
Neural tube defects
    definition of, 292
    syndromes associated with, 56t
Neurobehavioral risk score (NBRS), 43
Neurodevelopmental treatment (NDT), definition of, 292
Neurofibromatosis, 65t
Neurological lesions and resulting speech and language disorders, 50f
Neurological signs, soft, 146-147, 295
Neurology, Internet resources for, 282t
Neuropathy, Refsum hereditary motor and sensory, 64t
Neurophysiological factors affecting early language development, 9t
Neuropsychologic consequences, central nervous system maturation and, 232t
Nevi, pigmented, 64t
New York State Office of Mental Retardation and Developmental Disabilities, 151
Newborn care options
    level I nursery care, 85
    level II nursery care, 85-86, 88
    level III nursery care, 85-86, 87
    level IV nursery, 86, 87
    neonatal intensive care unit versus other settings for, 85-86
    rooming-in care, 85
Newborns, speech-language pathologist's services for, marketing of, 222-223

NG tube. *See* Nasogastric (NG) tube.
NICU. *See* Neonatal intensive care unit (NICU).
NIDCAP. *See* Neonatal Individualized Developmental Care and Assessment Program (NIDCAP).
NIH. *See* National Institutes of Health (NIH).
Noncategorical preschool programs, 12
Nonspeech sounds, language intervention and, 195
Nonsyndromic anomalies, 53
Nonsyndromic hearing loss, 58, 59
Nonverbal communication, definition of, 292
Nonverbal interaction, infant scale of, 259t-262t
Nonverbal reception, hearing loss and, 205
Noonan pulmonic stenosis, 65t
Normal development and infant assessment tools, 229-247
Norm-referenced scales assessment, definition of, 292
Norrie pseudoglioma of retina, 65t
Northwestern University–Children's Perception of Speech, 105
Nucleotide polymorphism, single, human genome and, 60
Nurse, charge, definition of, 287
Nursery
    level I, for newborns, 85
    level II. *See* Level II nursery.
    level III. *See* Level III nursery.
    level IV. *See* Level IV nursery.
    well-baby, 85
Nursing, Internet resources for, 283t

O

OAEs. *See* Otoacoustic emissions (OAEs).
Obesity, 62t, 63t, 64t
Observation
    of child, autistic spectrum disorder and, 128-129
    serial, of child's interactions with caregivers, 147-149
Observed behavior, recording, 260t-262t
Occiput, definition of, 292
Oculofacial anomalies, 65t
OFD I. *See* Oral-facial-digital (OFD I).
OFD II, 64t
Older infants, behavioral threshold assessment in, 102-104
Oligogenes, human genome and, 60
Ongoing assessment of communication development, 197
Opitz G/BBB syndrome, 58
Opitz hypertelorism, 65t
Oral communication ability, effect of hearing loss on, 201-207
Oral English, 214t
Oral mechanism, examination of, and related physical characteristics, 144-146
Oral method, 214t
Oral reflexes, infantile, 233t
Oral teratoma, 63t
Oral-aural method, 214t
Oral-facial-digital (OFD I), 65t
Oralism, 213
Oral-language characteristics, hearing loss and, 205-206, 206t
Oral-motor assessment, craniofacial anomalies and, 241t-243t
Organized marketing, 222

Orofacial dyspraxia, 57
Osteochondromuscular dystrophy, 65t
Osteogenesis imperfecta, 65t
Osteogenesis imperfecta, definition of, 292
Osteogenesis Imperfecta Foundation, Inc., 272t
Osteopetrosis, Albers-Schonberg, 62t
Osteoporosis, 64t
Otoacoustic emissions, 109-111
    distortion-product, 110-111, 112f
    transient-evoked, 110, 111f
Otoacoustic emissions (OAEs), 111
    distortion-product, 110-111, 112f
    in hearing-impaired infants and toddlers, 109-111, 112f
    transient-evoked, 110, 111f
Otopalatodigital syndrome, 65t
Ototoxin, definition of, 292
Ounces, weight conversion and, 230t

P

Palatopharyngeal incompetence, 65t
Palmar grasp, definition of, 292
Palsy, cerebral, 47t, 287
Parallel talk, language intervention and, 194
Parent education, speech-language pathologist and, 177-178
Parent interview, autistic spectrum disorder and, 128
Parent support groups, grieving process and, child's hearing loss and, 209-209
Parent support teams in neonatal intensive care unit, 92
Parent training, speech-language pathologist and, 178
Parental concerns, meeting, through counseling and education, 207-209
Parental denial, communicative assessment and, 157
Parent-professional partnerships, collaborative activities for, 77t
Parents
    assessment for, of child competency and difficulty, 255t
    identification of child's areas of competency and difficulty by, 255t-259t
    information provided by, about child's communicative abilities, 143-144, 145t
    Internet resources for, 280t
    of Premature and High Risk Infants International, Inc., 273t
Parents' Evaluations of Developmental Status, 143-144
Paresis, Foix-Chavany-Marie suprabulbar, 63t
Part C agencies, 268t-269t
Part C Early Intervention Model, 69
Part C intervention mandates, 180-182
Part H, 11, 12
Part V early intervention, 181
Partner, goal for, communication development and, 183
Patent ductus arteriosus (PDA), definition of, 292
Pathologist, speech-language. *See* Speech-language pathologist (SLP).
Pathology, peripheral, determination of site of, in hearing-impaired infants and toddlers, 116-117, 116f

Payment for services in neonatal intensive care unit, 98
PCPs. *See* Primary care providers (PCPs).
PDA. *See* Patent ductus arteriosus (PDA).
PDD. *See* Pervasive developmental disorder (PDD).
PDD-NOS. *See* Pervasive developmental disorder not otherwise specified (PDD-NOS).
PDDST. *See* Pervasive Developmental Disorders Screening Test (PDDST).
Pediatric population. *See* Children.
Pediatric Speech Intelligibility test, 105
"Pediatrician's Role in the Diagnosis and Management of Autistic Spectrum Disorder in Children," 123
Pendred hypothyroidism, 65t
Penetrance, definition of, 292
Perception, sensory, hearing loss and, 201-205
Pericardial constriction, 65t
Perinatal, definition of, 292
Peripheral pathology, determination of site of, in hearing-impaired infants and toddlers, 116-117, 116f
Pervasive developmental delay, 32
Pervasive developmental disorder (PDD), 121-123, 146
    DSM-IV criteria for, 124t-126t
    earliest indications for, 129
    Internet resources for, 277-278
    not otherwise specified (PDD-NOS), 121-123, 124t, 277-278
Pervasive developmental disorder–autism–Asperger syndrome, 55
Pervasive Developmental Disorders Screening Test (PDDST), 132t
Pervasive Developmental Disorders Screening Test II, 132t
Pfeiffer acrocephalosyndactyly, 65t
Pharmacology. *See* Medications.
Phenobarbital, definition of, 292
Phenotypes, genetic and chromosomal aberrations and, 37
Phenylketonuria (PKU), definition of, 292
Phonemic inventory, 146
Photomyoclonus, 65t
Phototherapy, definition of, 293
Physical development, facilitation of, to promote readiness for communication, 185-186
Physical factors affecting early language development, 9t
Physical growth, communication development and, 189
Physical status, changes in, monitoring, 189-190
Physicians' Current Procedural Terminology (CPI), definition of, 293
Pigmented nevi, 65t
Pitch and intensity in deaf children, 208t
PKU. *See* Phenylketonuria (PKU).
Placenta abruptio, definition of, 293
Plastyspondyly, 64t
Plateaus in development, communication development and, 189
Play
    communication, protocol for, 196t
    language intervention and, 195
    vocal, language intervention and, 194
Play assessment, 151-152

PMT. *See* Prelinguistic Milieu Teaching (PMT).
Pneumothorax, definition of, 293
Policy statements of professional organizations, 273t-274t
Polygenic disorders, 53, 54f, 54t, 55
Polymorphism
    of mendelian disorders, 61
    single nucleotide, human genome and, 60
Popliteal pterygium, 65t
Position and policy statements of professional organizations, 273t-274t
Positioning
    augmentative and alternative communication and, 192
    of infants, readiness for communication and, 186
    language intervention and, 194
    therapeutic, definition of, 295
Postlingual hearing loss, 202, 213
Post-term delivery, definition of, 293
Postural infantile reflexes of first year, 233t
Pounds, weight conversion and, 230t
Power of communication, language intervention and, 194
Practice Parameter: Screening and Diagnosis of Autism, 24, 123
Prader-Willi hypotonia, 65t
Prader-Willi Syndrome Association, 273t
Pragmatic development in infants and toddlers, 236t-237t
Pragmatics
    definition of, 293
    hearing-impaired children and, 206, 206t
Precocious senility, cockayne, 62t
Preemies, speech-language pathologist and, 83-100
Preintentional communication intervention strategies, 18
Prelanguage children, handicapped, interaction styles of, 259t-262t
Prelingual hearing loss, 202, 213
Prelinguistic Milieu Teaching (PMT), 197
Prematurity, definition of, 293
Preschool Language Scale, 164t
Preschool programs for handicapped, 12
Pressure-equalization tubes, communicative development and, 175
Presumptive diagnosis, 36
Preterm, definition of, 293
Preterm infants, characteristics of, 89-90
Prevalence, definition of, 293
Prevention
    definition of, 293
    developmental delays and disorders and, 34-35
    primary, 35
    role of speech-language pathologist in, 179-180
    secondary, 35
    tertiary, 35
Primary care providers (PCPs), managed care and, 19
Primary prevention, 35
Primary tones, distortion-product otoacoustic emissions and, 110-111
Primigravida, definition of, 289
Primitive infantile reflexes of first year, 233t
Primitive reflexes
    definition of, 293
    and postural infantile reflexes of first year, 233t
Primitive reflexes, definition of, 293

Probe effect, acoustic reflex testing and, 109
Probe tone, immittance battery and, 105
Procedural protocols, autistic spectrum disorder and, 123-130
Professional competencies, communication disorders and, 24-27, 25t-26t
Professional denial, communicative assessment and, 157
Professional organizations, position and policy statements of, 273t-274t
Professional team, family and, communication disorders and, 20-22
Professional-parent partnerships, collaborative activities for, 77t
Professionals
    Internet resources for, 275-284
    review of reports by, autistic spectrum disorder and, 128
Profound hearing loss, speech characteristics and, 206-207, 208t
Progeroid short stature, 65t
Prominent incisors, 63t
Prominent nose, 66t
Prone, definition of, 293
Provider, qualified. See Qualified provider.
Pseudohermaphroditism, male, 64t
Pseudo-Hurler syndrome, 66t
Psychoemotional disorders associated with communicative development, 42b
Psychological counseling, individual, autistic spectrum disorder and, 134-135
Psychologists, grieving process and, child's hearing loss and, 209-209
Pterygium, popliteal, 65t
Ptosis, definition of, 293
Public Law 94-142, 11, 293
Public Law 99-457, 11, 293
Public Law 102-119, 11, 20, 293
Public Law 205-17, 293
Public Law 205-17, Part C, 20
Puffy hands and feet, 64t
Pulmonic stenosis, 64t
Pure tones, distortion-product otoacoustic emissions and, 110-111
Pycnodysostosis, 65t

Q

Qualified provider
    definition of, 293-294
    judgment-based assessment and, 160-161
Qualitative scoring systems, assessment and, 162
Questions, cue, 145t, 163t, 254f

R

RDS. See Respiratory distress syndrome (RDS).
Reception
    auditory, hearing loss and, 202-203
    auditory-visual, hearing loss and, 204-205
    nonverbal, hearing loss and, 205
    visual, hearing loss and, 203-204, 204t
Receptive language ability, 10
Receptive language development, delayed, 224t
Receptive-Expressive Emergent Language Scale-2 (REEL-2), 145t
Recessive inheritance
    autosomal, 57f
    X-linked, 58f

Recombination of alleles, human genome and, 60
Recording of observed behaviors, 260t-262t
REEL-2. See Receptive-Expressive Emergent Language Scale-2 (REEL-2).
Referral
    of children by speech-language pathologist, 175-176
    receiving, and determining which children are at risk, developmental delays and disorders and, 32-37
Reflex(es)
    acoustic, testing of. See Acoustic reflex testing.
    asymmetrical tonic neck, definition of, 286
    infantile oral, 233t
    Moro, definition of, 292
    primitive. See Primitive reflexes.
Reflexive auditory skills, development of, during first year of life, 216t
Refsum hereditary motor and sensory neuropathy, 65t
Regulatory problems, communicative disorders and, 41, 42b
Rehabilitation Act of 1973, 8-9
Report formats, assessment and, 166
Reports
    assessment and, 141-171
    review of, by other professionals, autistic spectrum disorder and, 128
Requesting context, Communication Play Protocol and, 195
Residual vision, readiness for communication and, 186
Respiratory considerations, readiness for communication and, 186
Respiratory distress syndrome (RDS), definition of, 294
Responsive Prelinguistic Milieu Teaching (RPMT), 197
Results, reporting, assessment and, 162-166
Retardation
    growth, 63t
    Internet resources for, 283t
    intrauterine growth, definition of, 291
    mental, 31, 62t, 66t
    Hall-Riggs, 63t
Retina, Norrie pseudoglioma of, 64t
Retinal dysplasia, 64t
Retinal yellow dots, 65t
Retinitis pigmentosa, 62t
Retinopathy of prematurity (ROP), definition of, 294
Retrognathia, definition of, 294
Rett dementia, 65t
Rett's disorder, 121-122, 125t
Reversals in development, communication development and, 189
Review of reports by other professionals, autistic spectrum disorder and, 128
Rhythm, language intervention and, 195
Risk factors
    additive, definition of, 285
    environmental, definition of, 289
Risk history, long form of, 243f-245f
Risk score, neurobehavioral, 43
Risk-factor groups, taxonomy of, communicative impairment and, 155t-156t

Robinow fetal face, 65t
Rochester method, 214t
Rolandic epilepsy, autosomal rolandic, 57
Rooming-in care for newborns, 85
ROP. *See* Retinopathy of prematurity (ROP).
Rossetti Infant-Toddler Language Development
  Scale, 164t
Rossetti Infant-Toddler Language Scale, A Measure
  of Communication and Interaction, 133t
Rossetti Infant-Toddler Language Scale: Parent
  Form, 145t
RPMT. *See* Responsive Prelinguistic Milieu
  Teaching (RPMT).
Rubella, definition of, 294
Rubella embryopathy, 65t
Rubenstein-Taybi broad thumbs, 65t
Russel-Silver pseudohydrocephalus, 65t

S
Saethre-Chotzen maxillary hypoplasia, 66t
Sanfilippo syndrome, 66t
Scheie syndrome, 66t
Schindler syndrome, 66t
Schwartz-Jampel myopathy, 66t
Scoring systems, multidimensional, assessment
  and, 162
SCQ. *See* Social Communication Questionnaire
  (SCQ).
Screening
  of children by speech-language pathologist,
    175-176
  definition of, 294
  developmental delays and disorders and, 35-37
  neonatal, for hearing-impairment, 117-118
  universal, of newborns, 117
Screening Tool for Autism in Two-Year-Olds
  (STAT), 133t
Scrotum, shawl, 62t
Search engines, Internet, 275-276
Seckel short stature, 66t
Secondary prevention, 35
Section 619, 294
Security, readiness for communication and, 188
Segmental skills
  in deaf children, 208t
  speech training and, 217
Seizure, definition of, 294
Self-mutilation, 64t
Self-stimulation, definition of, 294
Self-talk, language intervention and, 194
Semantic/Pragmatic Communication Report
  Form, 145t
Semantics, hearing-impaired children and, 206,
  206t
Semivowels, auditory reception and, 202-203
Senility, Cockayne precocious, 62t
Sensorimotor stage development, definition of,
  294
Sensorineural hearing loss, 212
Sensory aids, vibrotactile, 212
Sensory Aids Foundation, 273t
Sensory devices, alternative, hearing loss and,
  212-213
Sensory integration therapy, definition of, 294
Sensory perception, hearing loss and, 201-205
Sensory skills, development of, hearing loss and,
  215-217

Sepsis, definition of, 294
Sequence(s), 38
  early language, affecting early language
    development, 9t
  facio-auriculo-vertebral, 63t
Serial observation of child's interactions with
  familiar caregivers and others, 147-149
Serological, definition of, 294
Service-delivery models
  communication development and, 182
  comparative features of, 25t-26t
  in early intervention, 22-23
Severe hearing loss, speech characteristics and,
  206-207, 208t
Severe-profoundly affected individual, 31
Sex chromosomes, trisomies of, 53
Sexual infantilism, 63t
SGA. *See* Small for gestational age (SGA).
Shawl scrotum, 62t
SHORT. *See* Short stature, hyperextensibility, hernia
  (SHORT).
Short fingernails, 64t
Short forearms, 65t
Short stature, 62t, 63t, 65t, 66t
  Floating-Harbor, 63t
  hyperextensibility, hernia (SHORT), 65t
  progeroid, 64t
  Seckel, 65t
Shprintzen, 67t
Shprintzen-Goldberg craniosynostosis, 66t
Shunt, definition of, 294
Sickle cell anemia, 66t
Sign systems, 214t
Signaling method, augmentative and alternative
  communication and, 192
Signs
  language intervention and, 195
  soft neurological, 146-147, 295
Simosa elongated craniofacial syndrome, 66t
Simpson dysmorphia bulldog face, 66t
Single nucleotide polymorphism (SNP), human
  genome and, 60
Single risk factors, role of, in diagnosis and
  assessment, in communicative disorders, 41-
  47, 44t-45t, 46t-47t
Single-channel vibrotactile sensory aids, 213
Skills
  communication. *See* Communication skills.
  functional, definition of, 289
  segmental, speech training and, 217
  sensory, development of, hearing loss and,
    215-217
  of speech-language pathologist, 77-79
  suprasegmental, speech training and, 217
Skin tags, definition of, 294
Skin-to-skin care in neonatal intensive care unit,
  13
Slanted eyes, 65t
Sleep apnea, definition of, 294
SLP. *See* Speech-language pathologist (SLP).
Small for gestational age (SGA), definition of,
  294-295
Small nose, 64t, 67t
Small puffy hands and feet, 64t
Smith-Lemli-Opitz syndrome, 35
Smith-Magenis brachycephaly, 66t
Smith-Magenis syndrome, 35, 122

SNP. *See* Single nucleotide polymorphism (SNP).
SNS. *See* Soft neurological sign (SNS).
Social Communication Questionnaire (SCQ), 131t
Social Security Administration, 97
Social workers, grieving process and, child's hearing loss and, 209-209
Society for Developmental Pediatrics, 24
Soft neurological sign (SNS), 146-147, 295
Sotos cerebral gigantism, 66t
Soundfield testing, testing of hearing and, 103-104
Sounds, nonspeech, language intervention and, 195
Special care necessitated by child's condition, supporting, 188-189
Specialized teams in neonatal intensive care unit, 92-98
    composition, styles, and roles for speech-language pathologist on, 92-93
    development assessment and, 95-96, 95t
    feeding assessment and, 93-95
    infant assessment and, 93-96
    payment for services rendered and, 98
    working with families and, 96-98
Specific learning disabilities, 46t
Spectrum disorder, 38
    autistic. *See* Autistic spectrum disorder (ASD).
Speech
    childhood apraxia of, 146
    cluttering, 62t
    common characteristics of, of deaf children, 208t
    cued, 214t
    delayed development of, 65t
    delayed onset of, without obvious receptive language impairment, 224t
    development of, Internet resources for, 283t
    developmental apraxia of, 144-146, 277
    disordered development of, 224t
    and language disorders, neurological lesions and, 50f
    visible, 214t
    and voice disorder, 66t
Speech audiometry, 104-105
    in hearing-impaired infants and toddlers, 104-105
    speech detection threshold and, 104
    speech reception threshold and, 105
    word recognition and, 105
Speech characteristics, hearing loss and, 206-207
Speech detection threshold in hearing-impaired infants and toddlers, 104
Speech discrimination
    developmental sequence of auditory skills during first year of life and, 216t
    word recognition and, 105
Speech dyspraxia, 57
Speech impairment, 8, 46t
Speech intelligibility, speech training and, 217
Speech reception threshold (SRT) in hearing-impaired infants and toddlers, 105
Speech training, hearing loss and, 217-218
Speech-language pathologist (SLP), 69, 80
    assessment of sensory characteristics by, 32
    community settings and, 81
    competencies expected of, 77, 78-79
    groups of concern to, 153-157, 155t-156t
    involvement of, in newborn care, 86-88
    knowledge expected of, 77-79

Speech-language pathologist *(Continued)*
    role of, in neonatal intensive care unit, 13-14, 83-100
        characteristics of preterm infants, 89-90
        infection control, 88-89
        medically fragile infants and, 83-100
        micropreemies and, 83-100
        in newborn care, 86-88
        newborn care options in, 85-86
        preemies and, 83-100
        signs of infant stress, 90-92, 91t
        specialized teams and, 92-98
    services of, for newborns, marketing of, 222-223
    skills expected of, 77, 78-79
    strategies of, with pediatric population, 175-182
Speechreading movements, visible, under ideal viewing conditions, 204t
Spina bifida, 54-55
Spina Bifida Association of America, 273t
Spoken Language Predictor Index, 215
Spondyloepiphyseal dysplasia, 66t
Spondylometaphyseal dysplasia, X-linked, 66t
SRT. *See* Speech reception threshold (SRT).
SSI. *See* Supplementary Security Income (SSI).
Standardized tests, communication assessment and, 158
STAT. *See* Screening Tool for Autism in Two-Year-Olds (STAT).
State regulation disorder, definition of, 295
Static admittance, tympanometry and, 107
Statistics, families as, in epidemiological database, 7-9
Stature
    Floating-Harbor short, 63t
    short. *See* Short stature.
Stenosis
    definition of, 295
    of larynx, 53
    Noonan pulmonic, 64t
    pulmonic, 64t
Stickler flat face, 66t
Stimulation, adaptations for, readiness for communication and, 186-187
Stimulus effect, acoustic reflex testing and, 109
Stops, auditory reception and, 202-203
Storage-glutamyl-5-phosphate, 66t
Storage-lysosomal, 65t
Storage-lysosomal IVB, 66t
Storage-lysosomal IVB adult, 66t
Storage-Sialic acid, 67t
Strabismus, asymmetry, 66t
Strategies, communication development and, 184
Streptomycin, 49
Stress
    excessive auditory stimulation of preterm infants and, 91
    families and, 16
    infant, signs of, 90-92, 91t
Subdural hemorrhage, definition of, 295
Sucking disorders, infant, 238t
Supine, definition of, 295
Supplemental Food Program for Women, Infants, and Children (WIC), 15, 296
Supplementary Security Income (SSI), 7, 295
Suprasegmental skills
    in deaf children, 208t
    speech training and, 217

Surfactant, definition of, 295
Surfactant therapy, preterm infants and, 89
Surgery, communicative development and, 175
Survey of Income and Program Participation, 8
Swallowing, assessment of, craniofacial anomalies and, 241t-243t
Swallowing disorders, infant, 238t
Syllabic content, approximations of, language intervention and, 194
Symptoms, spectrum disorders and, 33-34
Syndactyly, 66t
    definition of, 295
    mitten, 62t
Syndactyly I, 67t
Syndrome(s), 38
    associated with neural tube defects, 56t
    branchiooculofacial, 62t
    cerebrocostomandibular, 62t
    communicative component of, 62t-66t
    Costello faciocutaneoskeletal, 63t
    cri-du-chat, 62t
    DiGeorge, 63t
    Down, 62t
    fetal valproate, 56t
    Hunter, 65t
    Hurler, 65t
    Internet resources for, 283t
    Kabuki make-up, 63t
    Klinefelter, 62t
    Langer-Geidion trichorhinophalangeal, 64t
    Leroy, 65t
    Maroteaux-Lamy, 65t
    Morquio, 65t
    Opitz G/BBB, 58
    otopalatodigital, 64t
    parts of, versus isolated medical problems, 55, 56t
    pseudo-Hurler, 65t
    Sanfilippo, 65t
    Scheie, 65t
    Schindler, 65t
    Simosa elongated craniofacial, 65t
    TORCH, definition of, 295
    Turner, 62t
Syndromic forms of anomalies, 56t
Synergistic activities affecting early language development, 9t
Synophrys, De Lange, 63t
Synostoses, multiple, 64t
Syntax, hearing-impaired children and, 206, 206t

T

Tachycardia, definition of, 295
Tactile stimulation, readiness for communication and, 187
Tags, skin, definition of, 294
Talk, parallel, language intervention and, 194
Targeted marketing, 222
Taxonomy of risk-factor groups, communicative impairment and, 155t-156t
TC. See Total communication (TC).
Technology, assistive. See Assistive technology.
Technology dependent, definition of, 295
Telecanthus, definition of, 295
Temperament, definition of, 295
Temporal characteristics in deaf children, 208t
Temptations, communicative, language intervention and, 194

TEOAEs. See Transient-evoked otoacoustic emissions (TEOAEs).
Teratogenic disorders, 61
Teratogens, 51t-52t
    definition of, 295
    effects of, 51t-52t, 80-52
Teratoma, oral, 62t
Tertiary prevention, 35
Testing
    acoustic reflex. See Acoustic reflex testing.
    auditory brainstem evoked response, definition of, 286
    direct, autistic spectrum disorder and, 129-130
    immitance, in hearing-impaired infants and toddlers, 105-109
    soundfield, testing of hearing and, 103-104
    standardized, communication assessment and, 158
Tethered tongue, 66t
Theory, family systems, 70-72
Therapeutic positioning, definition of, 295
Therapy
    definition of, 295
    sensory integration, definition of, 294
    unproven, autistic spectrum disorder and, 137-138
Thick joints, 64t
Threshold estimation in hearing-impaired infants and toddlers, 114-116, 115f
Thumb
    broad, 64t
    clasped, 62t
    Rubenstein-Taybi broad, 65t
Tics, Gilles de la Tourette vocal and motor, 63t
Tissues, fragile, 63t
Tobramycin, 49
Toddlers
    autistic spectrum disorder and, 121-140
    causes of developmental delays and disorders in, 31-48
    communication development in, 190
    communication disorders in. See Communication disorders in infants and toddlers.
    communicative interactions with, 196t
    with delayed or impaired communication, problem-solving approaches for, 182-184
    habilitation and communication development in. See Habilitation and communication development in hearing-impaired infants and toddlers.
    hearing-impaired. See Hearing-impaired infants and toddlers.
    with history of brain injury in infancy, 193
    pragmatic development in, 236t-237t
    promoting functional abilities of, 33-34
    services for, marketing of, 223-225, 224t
    with special needs, national effort to make difference for, 181-182
Toe walking, 157, 290
Tongue
    Mohr cleft, 64t
    tethered, 65t
Tongue protrusion, 64t
Tonic neck reflex, asymmetrical, definition of, 286
TORCH syndrome, definition of, 295
Total communication (TC), 213, 214t
Toxemia, definition of, 295-296
Toxin, definition of, 296

Toxoplasmosis, definition of, 296
Tracheostomy
    communicative development and, 175
    definition of, 296
Traditional assessment, 150-151
Transactional factors in development,
        communication impairments and, 10
Transdisciplinary Play-Based Assessment, 164t
Transdisciplinary service delivery model, 26t
Transient-evoked otoacoustic emissions
        (TEOAEs), 110, 111f
Transitional tympanogram, 107
Trauma
    brain injury and, 46t
    communicative disorders and, 38-41
    teratogens and, 52t
Treacher-Collins mandibulofacial dysostosis, 67t
Treatment
    communication development and, 173-199, 174t
    definition of, 296
    neurodevelopmental, definition of, 292
Triage concept in assessment, 142-143
Triangular face, 63t
Trisomies
    autosomal, 53
    chromosome 18, 56t
    definition of, 296
    of sex chromosomes, 53
Tube
    endotracheal, definition of, 289
    nasogastric, definition of, 292
    pressure-equalization, communicative
        development and, 175
Tuberous sclerosis complex, 122
Turner syndrome, 53, 62t
    "2001 Revised Scope of Practice in Speech-
        Language Pathology," 8
Tympanogram, transitional, 107
Tympanometric configurations, 107, 108f, 108t
Tympanometry
    in hearing-impaired infants and toddlers,
        106-107, 106f, 108f, 108t
    immittance battery and, 105
Typical language development, communication
    impairments and, 10-11

U

Ulnar deviation of hands, 63t
Unisensory method, 214t
United Cerebral Palsy Association, 273t
Universal screening of newborns, 117
Unproven therapies, autistic spectrum disorder
        and, 137-138
U.S. Department
    of Education, 7, 8-9
    of Health and Human Services, 7
Usher retinitis pigmentosa, 67t

V

Van der Woude lip pit/cleft lip, 67t
Velo-cardio-facial, 67t
Venting, earmolds of hearing aids and, 210
Verbal-oral method, 214t
Very low birth weight (VLBW), 43, 296
Vibrotactile sensory aids, 212
Visemes, visual reception and, 203-204
Visible speech, 214t

Visible speechreading movements under ideal
        viewing conditions, 204t
Vision
    augmentative and alternative communication
        and, 192
    residual, readiness for communication and, 186
Visit to art gallery scenario, communication play
        protocol and, 196t
Visual impairment, readiness for communication
        and, 186
Visual reception, hearing loss and, 203-204, 204t
Visual reinforcement audiometry (VRA), 103
Visual stimulation, readiness for communication
        and, 186-187
Visual training, hearing loss and, 216-217
VLBW. See Very low birth weight (VLBW).
Vocabulary usage, hearing-impaired children and,
        206, 206t
Vocal discrimination, developmental sequence of
        auditory skills during first year of life and, 216t
Vocal models, affective, language intervention
        and, 195
Vocal play, language intervention and, 194
Vocal tics, Gilles de la Tourette, 63t
Vocoders, 213
Voice and speech disorder, 65t
Voice defect, 67t
Voice quality in deaf children, 208t
Vowels
    deaf children and, 208t
    hearing loss and, 202
    visible speechreading movements and, 204t
VRA. See Visual reinforcement audiometry (VRA).

W

Waardenburg central albinism, 67t
Walking, toe, 157, 290
Weaver macrocephaly, 67t
Webbed neck, 65t
Webs of larynx, heritable anomalies and, 53
Weight, birth. See Birth weight.
Weight conversion from pounds and ounces to
        grams, 230t
Well-baby nursery for newborns, 85
What's in the container scenario, communication
        play protocol and, 196t
WIC, 15, 296
Wieacker-Wolff syndrome, 57
Williams patulous lips, 67t
Wilson hepatolenticular degeneration, 67t
Withholding objects, language intervention and, 194
Word Intelligibility by Picture Identification, 105
Word recognition in hearing-impaired infants and
        toddlers, 105
Word-class usage, hearing-impaired children and,
        206, 206t
World Health Organization, preterm infant
        classification of, 89

X

X-linked dominant inheritance, 58f
X-linked recessive inheritance, 58f
X-linked spondylometaphyseal dysplasia, 65t

Z

Zero to Three: National Center for Infants,
        Toddlers and Families, 273t

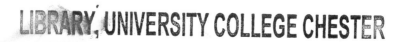